THE DA

VOLUME 2

Dale Harbison Carnegie (November 24, 1888 – November 1, 1955) was an American writer and lecturer and the developer of famous courses in self-improvement, salesmanship, corporate training, public speaking, and interpersonal skills. Born into poverty on a farm in Missouri, he was the author of the bestselling *How to Win Friends and Influence People* (1936), *How to Stop Worrying and Start Living* (1948) and many more self-help books.

THE DALE CARNEGIE OMNIBUS

OMNIBUS

VOLUME 2

RUPA

Published by
Rupa Publications India Pvt. Ltd 2016
7/16, Ansari Road, Daryaganj
New Delhi 110002

Sales centres:
Allahabad Bengaluru Chennai
Hyderabad Jaipur Kathmandu
Kolkata Mumbai

ISBN: 978-81-291-4035-7

First impression 2016

10 9 8 7 6 5 4 3 2 1

Printed at Replika Press Pvt. Ltd, India

CONTENTS

How to Enjoy Your Life and Your Job

PUBLISHER'S NOTE

If you believe in what you are doing, then let nothing hold you up in your work. Much of the best work of the world has been done against seeming impossibilities. The thing is to get the work done. —Dale Carnegie

The simplicity and clarity of Dale Carnegie's thoughts have been guiding readers over the years—in both the personal and professional spheres. Having understood the psychology of a successful personality, he effectively guided his audiences and readers towards active self-improvement, as a cohesive life choice. Succinctly, he tells us how to hone our innate human abilities and put them to effective use. Be it salesmanship or leadership; communication or marketing; or happiness and fulfilment—Carnegie tells us how to make the most of our resources and achieve our fullest potential.

These books, a selection of Carnegie's bestsellers, all must-reads, are now presented in one volume. Be the success you ought to be.

HOW TO STOP WORRYING AND START LIVING

PART 1

1

HOW TO ANALYZE AND
SOLVE WORRY PROBLEMS

Will any magic formula solve *all* worry problems? No, of course not.

Then what *is* the answer? The answer is that we must equip ourselves to deal with different kinds of worries by learning the three basic steps of problem analysis. The three steps are:

- Get the facts.
- Analyze the facts.
- Arrive at a decision—and then act on that decision.

Obvious stuff? Yes, Aristotle taught it—and used it. And you and I must use it too if we are going to solve the problems that are harassing us and turning our days and nights into veritable hells.

Let's take the first rule: *Get the facts.* Why is it so important to get the facts? Because unless we have the facts we can't possibly even attempt to solve our problem intelligently. Without the facts, all we can do is stew around in confusion. My idea? No, that was the idea of the late Herbert E. Hawkes, Dean of Columbia College, Columbia University, for twenty-two years. He had helped two hundred thousand students solve their worry problems; and he told me that *"confusion is the chief cause of worry."* He put it this way—he said: "Half the worry in the world is caused by people trying to make decisions before they have sufficient knowledge on which to base a decision. For example," he said, "if I have a problem which has to be faced at three o'clock next Tuesday, I refuse to even try to make a decision about it until next Tuesday arrives. In the meantime, I concentrate on getting all the facts that bear on the problem. I don't worry," he said. "I don't agonize over my problem. I don't lose any sleep. I simply concentrate on getting the facts. And by the time Tuesday rolls around, if I've got all the facts, the problem usually solves itself!"

I asked Dean Hawkes if this meant he had licked worry entirely. "Yes," he said, "I think I can honestly say that my life is now almost totally devoid of worry. I have found," he went on, "that if a man will devote his time to securing facts in an impartial, objective way, his worries will usually evaporate in the light of knowledge."

Let me repeat that: "If a man will devote his time to securing facts in an impartial, objective way, his worries will usually evaporate in the light of knowledge."

But what do most of us do? If we bother with facts at all—and Thomas Edison said in all seriousness, "There is no expedient to which a man will not resort to avoid the labor of thinking"—if we bother with facts at all, we hunt like bird dogs after the facts that bolster up what we *already* think—and ignore all the others! We want only the facts that justify our acts—the facts that fit in conveniently with our wishful thinking and justify our preconceived prejudices!

Is it any wonder, then, that we find it so hard to get at

the answers to our problems? Wouldn't we have the same trouble trying to solve a second-grade arithmetic problem, if we went ahead on the assumption that two plus two equals five? Yet there are a lot of people in this world who make life a hell for themselves and others by insisting that two plus two equals five—or maybe five hundred!

What can we do about it? We have to keep our emotions out of our thinking; and, as Dean Hawkes put it, we must secure the facts in "an impartial, objective" manner and returned to New York for another try. This time I got a break. One day, while waiting for an interview in a recording-studio office, I played my guitar and sang a song to the girl receptionist: "Jean-nine, I Dream of Lilac Time." While I was singing that song, the man who wrote it—Nat Schildkraut—drifted into the office. Naturally, he was pleased to hear anyone singing his song. So he gave me a note of introduction and sent me down to the Victor Recording Company. I made a record. I was no good—too stiff and self-conscious. So I took the advice of the Victor Recording man; I went back to Tulsa, worked for the railway by day, and at night I sang cowboy songs on a sustaining radio program. I liked that arrangement. It meant that I was keeping my line of supplies open—so I had no worries.

I sang for nine months on radio station KVOO in Tulsa. During that time, Jimmy Long and I wrote a song entitled "That Silver-Haired Daddy of Mine." It caught on. Arthur Sattherly, head of the American Recording Company, asked me to make a recording. It clicked. I made a number of other recordings for fifty dollars each, and finally got a job singing cowboy songs over radio station WLS in Chicago. Salary: forty dollars a week. After singing there for four years, my salary was raised to ninety dollars a week, and I picked up another three hundred dollars doing personal appearances every night in theaters.

Then in 1934, I got a break that opened up enormous possibilities. The League of Decency was formed to clean up the movies. So, Hollywood producers decided to put on cowboy pictures; but they wanted a new kind of cowboy—one who could sing. The man who owned the American Recording Company was also part owner of Republic Pictures. "If you want a singing cowboy," he said to his associates, "I have got one making records for us." That is how I broke into the movies. I started making singing-cowboy pictures for one hundred dollars a week. I had serious doubts about whether I would succeed in pictures, but I didn't worry. I knew I could always go back to my old job.

My success in pictures exceeded my wildest expectations. I now get a salary of one hundred thousand a year plus one half of all the profits on my pictures. However, I realize that this arrangement won't go on forever. But I am not worried. I know that no matter

That is not an easy task when we are worried. When we are worried, our emotions are riding high. But here are two ideas that I have found helpful when trying to step aside from my problems, in order to see the facts in a clear, objective manner.

When trying to get the facts, I pretend that I am collecting this information not for myself, but for some other person. This helps me to take a cold, impartial view of the evidence. This helps me eliminate my emotions.

While trying to collect the facts about the problem that is worrying me, I sometimes pretend that I am a lawyer preparing to argue the other side of the issue. In other words, I try to get all the facts against myself—all the facts that are damaging to my wishes, all the facts I don't like to face.

Then I write down both my side of the case and the other side of the case—and I generally find that the truth lies somewhere in between these two extremities.

Here is the point I am trying to make. Neither you nor I nor Einstein nor the Supreme Court of the United States is brilliant enough to reach an intelligent decision on any problem without first getting the facts. Thomas Edison knew that. At the time of his death, he had two thousand five hundred notebooks filled with facts about the problems he was facing.

So Rule 1 for solving our problems is: *Get the facts.* Let's do what Dean Hawkes did—let's not even attempt to solve our problems without first collecting all the facts in an impartial manner.

However, getting all the facts in the world won't do us any good until we analyze them and interpret them.

I have found from costly experience that it is much easier to analyze the facts after writing them down. In fact, merely writing the facts on a piece of paper and stating our problem clearly goes a long way toward helping us reach a sensible decision. As Charles Kettering puts it: "A problem well stated is a problem half solved."

Let me show you all this as it works out in practice. Since the Chinese say one picture is worth ten thousand words, suppose I show you a picture of how one man put exactly what we are talking about into concrete action.

Let's take the case of Galen Litchfield—a man I have known for several years; one of the most successful American businessmen in the Far East. Mr. Litchfield was in China in 1942, when the Japanese invaded Shanghai. And here is his story as he told it to me while a guest in my home: "Shortly after the Japs took Pearl Harbor," Galen Litchfield began, "they came swarming into Shanghai. I was the manager of the Asia Life Insurance Company in Shanghai. They sent us an 'army liquidator'— he was really an admiral—and gave me orders to assist this man in liquidating our assets. I didn't have any choice in the matter. I could co-operate—or else. And the 'or else' was certain death.

"I went through the motions of doing what I was told, because I had no alternative. But there was one block of securities, worth $750,000, which I left off the list I gave to the admiral. I left that block of securities off the list because they belonged to our Hong Kong organization and had nothing to do with the Shanghai assets. All the same, I feared I might be in hot water if the Japs found out what I had done. And they soon found out.

"I wasn't in the office when the discovery was made, but my head accountant was there. He told me that the Jap admiral flew into a rage, and stamped and swore, and called me a thief and a traitor! I had defied the Japanese army! I knew what that meant. I would be thrown into the Bridgehouse!

"The Bridgehouse! The torture chamber of the Japanese Gestapo! I had had personal friends who had killed themselves rather than be taken to that prison. I had had other friends who had died in that place after ten days of questioning and torture. Now I was slated for the Bridgehouse myself!

"What did I do? I heard the news on Sunday afternoon. I suppose I should have been terrified. And I would have been terrified if I hadn't had a definite technique for solving my problems. For years, whenever I was worried I had always gone to my typewriter and written down two questions—and the answers to these questions:

"*1. What am I worrying about?*

"*2. What can I do about it?*

"I used to try to answer those questions without writing them down. But I stopped that years ago. I found that writing down both the questions and the answers clarifies my thinking. So, that Sunday afternoon, I went directly to my room at the Shanghai YMCA, and got out my typewriter. I wrote:

"1. What am I worrying about?

"I am afraid I will be thrown into the Bridgehouse tomorrow morning.

"Then I typed out the second question:

"2. What can I do about it?

"I spent hours thinking out and writing down the four courses of action I could take—and what the probable consequence of each action would be.

"I can try to explain to the Japanese admiral. But he

'no speak English.' If I try to explain to him through an interpreter, I may stir him up again. That might mean death, for he is cruel, would rather dump me in the Bridgehouse than bother talking about it.

"I can try to escape. Impossible. They keep track of me all the time. I have to check in and out of my room at the YMCA. If I try to escape, I'll probably be captured and shot.

"I can stay here in my room and not go near the office again. If I do, the Japanese admiral will be suspicious, will probably send soldiers to get me and throw me into the Bridgehouse without giving me a chance to say a word.

"I can go down to the office as usual on Monday morning. If I do, there is a chance that the Japanese admiral may be so busy that he will not think of what I did. Even if he does think of it, he may have cooled off and may not bother me. If this happens, I am all right. Even if he does bother me, I'll still have a chance to try to explain to him. So, going down to the office as usual on Monday morning, and acting as if nothing had gone wrong, gives me two chances to escape the Bridgehouse.

"As soon as I thought it all out and decided to accept the fourth plan—to go down to the office as usual on Monday morning—I felt immensely relieved.

"When I entered the office the next morning, the Japanese admiral sat there with a cigarette dangling from his mouth. He glared at me as he always did; and said nothing. Six weeks later—thank God—he went back to Tokyo and my worries were ended.

"As I have already said, I probably saved my life by sitting down that Sunday afternoon and writing out all the various steps I could take and then writing down the probable consequence of each step and calmly coming to a decision. If I hadn't done that, I might have floundered and hesitated and done the wrong thing on the spur of the moment. If I hadn't thought out my problem and come to a decision, I would have been frantic with worry all Sunday afternoon. I wouldn't have slept that night. I would have gone down to the office Monday morning with a harassed and worried look; and that alone might have aroused the suspicion of the Japanese admiral and spurred him to act.

"Experience has proved to me, time after time, the enormous value of arriving at a decision. It is the failure to arrive at a fixed purpose, the inability to stop going round and round in maddening circles, that drives men to nervous breakdowns and living hells. I find that fifty per cent of my worries vanishes once I arrive at a clear, definite decision; and another forty per cent usually vanishes once I start to carry out that decision.

"So I banish about ninety per cent of my worries by taking these four steps:

"1. Writing down precisely what I am worrying about.

"2. Writing down what I can do about it.

"3. Deciding what to do.

"4. Starting immediately to carry out that decision."

Galen Litchfield is now the Far Eastern Director for Starr, Park and Freeman, Inc., 111 John Street, New York, representing large insurance and financial interests.

In fact, as I said before, Galen Litchfield today is one of the most important American businessmen in Asia; and he confessed to me that he owes a large part of his success to this method of analyzing worry and meeting it head-on.

Why is his method so superb? Because it is efficient, concrete, and goes directly to the heart of the problem. On top of all that, it is climaxed by the third and indispensable rule: *Do something about it.* Unless we carry out our action, all our fact-finding and analysis is whistling upwind—it's a sheer waste of energy.

William James said this: "When once a decision is reached and execution is the order of the day, dismiss absolutely all responsibility and care about the outcome." (In this case, William James undoubtedly used the word "care" as a synonym for "anxiety.") He meant—once you have made a careful decision based on facts, *go* into action. Don't stop to reconsider. Don't begin to hesitate, worry and retrace your steps. Don't lose yourself in self-doubting which begets other doubts. Don't keep looking back over your shoulder.

Why don't you employ Galen Litchfield's technique to one of your worries right now?

Here is question No. 1—*What am I worrying about?*

Question No. 2—*What can I do about It?*

Question No. 3—*Here is what I am going to do about it.*

Question No. 4—*When am I going to start doing it?*

"It's not stress that kills us, it is our reaction to it."

—Hans Selye

"Worry is the stomach's worst poison."

—Alfred Nobel

2

HOW TO ELIMINATE FIFTY PER CENT OF YOUR BUSINESS WORRIES

If you are a businessman, you are probably saying to yourself right now: "The title of this chapter is ridiculous. I have been running my business for nineteen years; and I certainly know the answers if anybody does. The idea of anybody trying to tell me how I can eliminate fifty per cent of my business worries—it's absurd!"

Fair enough—I would have felt exactly the same way myself a few years ago if I had seen this title on a chapter. It promises a lot—and promises are cheap.

Let's be very frank about it: *maybe I won't* be able to help you eliminate fifty per cent of your business worries. In the last analysis, no one can do that, except yourself. But what I *can* do is to show you how other people have done it—and leave the rest up to you!

Since worry is that serious, wouldn't you be satisfied if I could help you eliminate even ten per cent of your worries? …Yes? …Good! Well, I am going to show you how one business executive eliminated not fifty per cent of his worries, but seventy-five per cent of all the time he formerly spent in conferences, trying to solve business problems.

Furthermore, I am not going to tell you this story about a "Mr. Jones" or a "Mr. X" or "a man I know in Ohio"—vague stories that you can't check up on. It concerns a very real person—Leon Shimkin, a partner and general manager of one of the foremost publishing houses in these United States: Simon and Schuster, Rockefeller Center, New York 20, New York.

Here is Leon Shimkin's experience in his own words:

"For fifteen years, I spent almost half of every business day holding conferences, discussing problems. Should we do this or that—do nothing at all? We would get tense; twist in our chairs; walk the floor; argue and go around in circles. When night came, I would be utterly exhausted. I fully expected to go on doing this sort of thing for the rest of my life. I had been doing it for fifteen years, and it never occurred to me that there was a better way of doing it. If anyone had told me that I could eliminate three fourths of all the time I spent in those worried conferences, and three fourths of my nervous strain—I would have thought he was a wild-eyed, slap-happy, armchair optimist. Yet I devised a plan that did just that. I have been using this plan for eight years. It has performed wonders for my efficiency, my health, and my happiness.

"It sounds like magic—but like all magic tricks, it is extremely simple when you see how it is done.

"Here is the secret: First, I immediately stopped the procedure I had been using in my conferences for fifteen years—a procedure that began with my troubled associates reciting all the details of what had gone wrong, and ending up by asking: 'What shall we do?' Second, I made a new rule—a rule that everyone who wishes to present a problem to me must first prepare and submit a memorandum answering these four questions:

"Question 1 : What is the problem?

("In the old days we used to spend an hour or two in a worried conference without anyone's knowing specifically and concretely what the real problem was. We used to work ourselves into a lather discussing our troubles without ever troubling to write out specifically what our problem was.)

"Question 2: What is the cause of the problem?

("As I look back over my career, I am appalled at the wasted hours I have spent in worried conferences without ever trying to find out clearly the conditions which lay at the root of the problem.)

"Question 3: What are all possible solutions of the problem?

("In the old days, one man in the conference would suggest one solution. Someone else would argue with him. Tempers would flare. We would often get clear off the subject, and at the end of the conference no one would have written down all the various things we could do to attack the problem.)

"Question 4: What solution do you suggest?

("I used to go into a conference with a man who had spent hours worrying about a situation and going around in circles without ever once thinking through all possible solutions and then writing down: 'This is the solution I recommend.')

"My associates rarely come to me now with their problems. Why? Because they have discovered that in order to answer those four questions they have to get all the facts and think their problems through. And after they have done that they find, in three fourths of the cases, they don't have to consult me at all, because the proper solution has popped out like a piece of bread popping out from an electric toaster. Even in those cases where consultation is necessary, the discussion takes about one third the time formerly required, because it proceeds along an orderly, logical path to a reasoned conclusion.

"Much less time is now consumed in the house of Simon and Schuster in *worrying* and *talking* about what is wrong; and a lot more *action* is obtained toward making those things right."

My friend Frank Bettger, one of the top insurance men in America, tells me he not only reduced his business worries, but nearly doubled his income, by a similar method.

"Years ago," says Frank Bettger, "when I first started to sell insurance, I was filled with a boundless enthusiasm and love for my work. Then something happened. I became so discouraged that I despised my work and thought of giving it up. I think I would have quit—if I hadn't got the idea, one Saturday morning, of sitting down and trying to get at the root of my worries.

"1. I asked myself first, '*Just what is the problem?*' The problem was *that I was not getting high enough returns for the staggering amount of calls I was making.* I seemed to do pretty well at selling a prospect, until the moment came for closing a sale. Then the customer would say, 'Well, I'll think it over, Mr. Bettger. Come and see me again.' It was the time I wasted on these follow-up calls that was causing my depression.

"2. I asked myself, *'What are the possible solutions?'* But to get the answer to that one, I had to study the facts. I got out my record book for the last twelve months and studied the figures.

"I *made an astounding discovery!* Right there in black and white, I discovered that seventy per cent of my sales had been closed on the very first interview! Twenty-three per cent of my sales had been closed on the second interview! And only *seven per cent of* my *sales* had been closed on those third, fourth, fifth, etc., interviews, which were running me ragged and taking up time. In other words, I was wasting fully one half of my working day on a part of my business which was responsible for only seven per cent of my sales!

"3. *'What is the answer?'* The answer was obvious. I immediately cut out all visits beyond the second interview, and spent the extra time building up new prospects. The results were unbelievable. In a very short time, I had raised the cash value of every visit I made from $2.80 to $4.27 a call!"

As I said, Frank Bettger is now one of the best-known life-insurance salesmen in the country. He is with Fidelity Mutual of Philadelphia, and writes a million dollars' worth of policies a year. But he was on the point of giving up. He was on the point of admitting failure—until *analyzing* the problem gave him a boost on the road to success.

Can you apply these questions to *your* business problems? To repeat my challenge—they *can* reduce your worries by fifty per cent. Here they are again:

- What is the problem?
- What is the CAUSE of the problem?
- What are all possible solutions to the problem?
- What solution do you suggest?

"Nothing is permanent in this wicked world—not even our troubles."

—Charlie Chaplin

"Forget the past—the future will give you plenty to worry about."

—George Allen, Sr.

3

"SEVENTY PER CENT OF ALL OUR WORRIES ..."

If I knew how to solve everybody's financial worries, I wouldn't be writing this book, I would be sitting in the White House—right beside the President. But here is one thing I can do: I can quote some authorities on this subject and make some highly practical suggestions, and point out where you can obtain books and pamphlets that will give you additional guidance.

Seventy per cent of all our worries are about money. Most people believe that they would have no more financial worries if they could increase their income by only ten per cent. That is true in many cases, but in a surprisingly large number of cases it is *not* true. For example, while writing this chapter, I interviewed an expert on budgets: Mrs. Elsie Stapleton—a woman who spent years as financial adviser to the customers of Wanamaker's Department Store in New York and of Gimbel's. She has spent additional years as an individual consultant, trying to help people who were frantic with worry about money. She has helped people in all kinds of income brackets, all the way from a porter who earned less than a thousand dollars a year to an executive earning one hundred thousand a year. And this is what she told me: "More money is *not* the answer to most people's financial worries. In fact, I have often seen it happen that an increase in income accomplished nothing but an increase in spending—and an increase in headaches. What causes most people to worry," she said, "is not that they haven't enough money, but that *they don't know how to spend the money they have!*" …You snorted at that last sentence, didn't you? Well, before you snort again, please remember that Mrs. Stapleton did *not* say that was true of *all* people. She said, *"most people."* She didn't mean you. She meant your sisters and your cousins, whom you reckon by the dozens.

A lot of readers are going to say, "I wish this guy Carnegie had my bills to meet, *my* obligations to keep up—on my weekly salary. If he did, I'll bet he would change his tune." Well, I have had my financial troubles: I have worked ten hours a day at hard physical labor in the cornfields and hay barns of Missouri—worked until my one supreme wish was to be free from the aching pains of utter physical exhaustion. I was paid for that grueling work not a dollar an hour, nor fifty cents, nor even ten cents. I was paid five cents an hour for a ten-hour day.

I know what it means to live for twenty years in a house without a bathroom or running water. I know what it means to sleep in bedrooms where the temperature is fifteen degrees below zero. I know what it means to walk miles to save a nickel carfare and have holes in the bottom of my shoes and patches on the seat of my pants.

I know what it means to order the cheapest dish on a restaurant menu, and to sleep with my trousers under the mattress because I couldn't afford to have them pressed by a tailor.

Yet, even during those times, I usually managed to save a few dimes and quarters out of my income because I was *afraid* not to. As a result of this experience, I realized that if you and I long to avoid debt and financial worries, then we have to do what a business firm does: we have to have a plan for spending our money and spend according to that plan. But most of us don't do that.

Here's something to consider—*where your money is concerned, you're in business for yourself!* And it is literally "your business" what you do with your money.

But what are the principles of managing our money? How do we begin to make a budget and a plan? Here are eleven rules.

Rule No. 1: **Get the facts down on paper!**

When Arnold Bennett started out in London fifty years ago to be a novelist, he was poor and hard-pressed. So he kept a record of what he did with every sixpence. Did he wonder where his money was going? No. He knew. He liked the idea so much that he continued to keep such a record even after he became rich, world-famous, and had a private yacht.

You and I, too, will have to get notebooks and start keeping records. For the rest of our lives? No, not necessarily. Experts on budgets recommend that we keep an accurate account of every nickel we spend for at least the first month—and, if possible, for three months. This is to give us an accurate record of where our money goes, so we can draw up a budget.

Oh, you *know* where your money goes? Well, maybe so; but if you do, you are one in a thousand! Mrs. Stapleton tells me it is a common occurrence for men and women to spend hours giving her facts and figures, so she can get them down on paper—then, when they see the result on paper, they exclaim, "Is *that* the way my money goes?" They can hardly believe it. Are *you* like that? Could be.

Rule No. 2: **Get a tailor-made budget that really fits your needs!**

Mrs. Stapleton tells me that two families may live side by side in identical houses, in the very same suburb, have the same number of children in the family, and receive the same income—yet their budgeting needs will be radically different. Why? Because people are different. She says a budget has to be a personal, custom-made job.

The idea of a budget is not to wring all the joy out of life. The idea is to give us a sense of material security—which in many cases means emotional security and freedom from worry. "People who live on budgets," Mrs. Stapleton told me, "are happier people."

But how do you go about it? First, as I said, you must list all expenses. Then get advice.

I asked Mrs. Stapleton, "What would you do, if you lived in a small town, or on a farm, and wanted personal advice on drawing up a budget?" She answered, "I would write to the biggest metropolitan paper published in my territory. I would ask that paper where I could get personal guidance in drawing up a budget—and I would travel all day, if I had to, to get that advice."

Rule No. 3: **Learn how to spend wisely.**

By this I mean: learn how to get the best value for your money. All large corporations have professional buyers and purchasing agents who do nothing but get the very best buys for their firms. As steward and manager of your personal estate, why shouldn't you do likewise?

Rule No. 4: **Don't increase your headaches with your income.**

Mrs. Stapleton told me that the budgets she dreads most to be called into consultation on are family incomes of five thousand a year. I asked her why. "Because" she said, "five thousand a year seems to be a goal to most American families. They may go along sensibly and sanely for years—then, when their income rises to five thousand a year, they think they have 'arrived.' They start branching out. Buy a house in the suburbs 'that doesn't cost any more than renting an apartment.' Buy a car, a lot of new furniture, and a lot of new clothes—and the first thing you know, they are running into the red. They are actually less happy than they were before—because they have bitten off too much with their increase in income."

That is only natural. We all want to get more out of life. But in the long run, which is going to bring us more happiness—forcing ourselves to live within a tight budget, or having dunning letters in the mail and creditors pounding on the front door?

Rule No. 5: **Try to build credit, in the event you must borrow.**

Be sure your insurance policies have a savings aspect, if you want to borrow on them, for this means a cash value. Certain types of insurance, called "term insurance," are merely for your protection over a given period of time and do not build up reserves. These policies are obviously of no use to you for borrowing purposes. Therefore, the rule is: Ask questions! Before you sign for a policy, find out if it has a cash value in case you have to raise money.

Now, suppose you don't have insurance you can borrow on, and you don't have any bonds, but you do own a house, or a car, or some other kind of collateral. Where do you go to borrow? By all means, to a bank! Banks have a reputation to maintain in the community; and they will usually deal with you fairly. Frequently, if you are in a financial jam, the bank will go so far as to discuss your problems with you, make a plan, and help you work your way out of your worry and indebtedness. I repeat, if you have collateral, go to a bank!

However, suppose you are one of the thousands who don't have collateral, don't own any property, and have nothing to offer as guarantee except your wages or salary? Then, as you value your life, heed this word of warning! Do not—*do not*—apply to a "loan company" without making sure that it operates under state license. The 32 states which do have this law, however, the licensed loan companies can usually be depended on. Most of them are ethical, honest, and strictly on the level. They are doing a service to those people who are faced with illness or emergency and have to raise money. They charge a higher rate of interest than the banks, but they have to do this, for they take greater risks and have greater expenses in collecting. But, if you live in a state where loan companies are unregulated, before doing business with any loan company, go to your bank, talk to one of its officers, and ask him to recommend a loan company that he *knows* to be fair.

Rule No. 6: **Protect yourself against illness, fire, and emergency expenses.**

Insurance is available, for relatively small sums, on all kinds of accidents, misfortunes, and conceivable emergencies. I am not suggesting that you cover yourself for everything from slipping in the bathtub to catching German measles—but I *do* suggest that you protect yourself against the major misfortunes that you know *could* cost you money and therefore *do* cost you worry. It's cheap at the price.

For example, I know a woman who had to spend ten days in a hospital last year and, when she came out, was presented a bill—*for exactly eight dollars!* The answer? She had hospital insurance.

Rule No. 7: **Do not have your life-insurance proceeds paid to your widow in cash.**

If you are carrying life insurance to provide for your family after you're gone, do not, I beg of you, have your insurance paid in one lump sum.

What happens to "a new widow with new money"? I'll let Mrs. Marion S. Eberly answer that question. She is head of the Women's Division of the Institute of Life Insurance, 60 East 42nd Street, New York City. She speaks before women's clubs all over America on the wisdom of using life-insurance proceeds to purchase a life income for the widow instead of giving her the proceeds in cash. She tells of one widow who received twenty thousand dollars in cash and lent it to her son to start in the auto-accessory business. The business failed, and she is destitute now. She tells of another widow who was persuaded by a slick real-estate salesman to put most of her life-insurance money in vacant lots that were "sure to double in value within a year." Three years later, she sold the lots for one tenth of what she paid for them. She tells of another widow who had to apply to the Child Welfare Association for the support of her children—within twelve months after she had been left fifteen thousand dollars in life insurance. A hundred thousand similar tragedies could be told.

"The average lifetime of twenty-five thousand dollars left in the hands of a woman is less than seven years." That statement was made by Sylvia S. Porter, financial editor of the *New York Post*, in the *Ladies Home Journal*.

Years ago, *The Saturday Evening Post* said in an editorial: "The ease with which the average widow without business training, and with no banker to advise her, can be wheedled into putting her husband's life-insurance money into wildcat stocks by the first slick salesman who approaches her—is proverbial. Any lawyer or banker can cite a dozen cases in which the entire savings of a thrifty man's lifetime, amassed by years of sacrifice and self-denial, were swept away simply because a widow or an orphan trusted one of the slick crooks who rob women for a livelihood."

If you want to protect your widow and your children, why not take a tip from J. P. Morgan—one of the wisest financiers who ever lived. He left money in his will to sixteen principal legatees. Twelve were women. Did he leave these women cash? No. He left trust funds that insured these women a monthly income for life.

Rule No. 8: **Teach your children a responsible attitude toward money.**

I shall never forget an idea I once read in *Your Life* magazine. The author, Stella Weston Tuttle, described how she was teaching her little girl a sense of responsibility about money. She got an extra checkbook from the bank and gave it to her nine-year-old daughter. When the daughter was given her weekly allowance, she "deposited" the money with her mother, who served as a bank for the child's funds. Then, throughout the week, whenever she wanted a nickel or a dime, she "drew a check" for that amount and kept track of her balance. The little girl not only found that fun, but began to learn real responsibility in handling her money.

An excellent method!

Rule No. 9: **If you are a housewife, maybe you can make a little extra money off your kitchen stove.**

If after you budget your expenses wisely you still find that you don't have enough to make ends meet, you can then do one of two things: you can either scold, fret, worry, and complain, or you can plan to make a little additional money on the side. How? Well, all you have to do to make money is to fill an urgent need that isn't being adequately filled now. That is what Mrs. Nellie Speer, 37-09 83rd Street, Jackson Heights, New York, did. In 1932, she found herself living alone in a three-room apartment. Her husband had died, and both of her children were married. One day, while having some ice cream at a drugstore soda fountain, she noticed that the fountain was also selling bakery pies that looked sad and dreary. She asked the proprietor if he would buy some real home- made pies from her. He ordered two. "Although I was a good cook," Mrs. Speer said, as she told me the story, "I had always had servants when we lived in Georgia, and I had never baked more than a dozen pies in my life. After getting that order for two pies, I asked a neighbor woman how to cook an apple pie. The soda-fountain customers were delighted with my first two home-baked pies—one apple, one lemon. The drugstore ordered five the next day. Then orders gradually came in from other fountains and luncheonettes. Within two years, I was baking five thousand pies a year—I was doing all the work myself in my own tiny kitchen, and I was making a thousand dollars a year clear, without a penny's expense except the ingredients that went into the pies."

The demand for Mrs. Speer's home-baked pastry became so great that she had to move out of her kitchen into a shop and hire two girls to bake for her: pies, cakes, bread, and rolls. During the war, people stood in line for an hour at a time to buy her home-baked foods.

"I have never been happier in my life," Mrs. Speer said. "I work in the shop twelve to fourteen hours a day, but I don't get tired because it isn't work to me. It is an adventure in living. I am doing my part to make people a little happier. I am too busy to be lonesome or worried. My work has filled a gap in my life left vacant by the passing of my mother and husband and my home."

When I asked Mrs. Speer if she felt that other women

who were good cooks could make money in their spare time in a similar way, in towns of ten thousand and up, she replied, "Yes—of course they can!"

Mrs. Ora Snyder will tell you the same thing. She lives in a town of thirty thousand—Maywood, Illinois. Yet she started in business with the kitchen stove and ten cents' worth of ingredients. Her husband fell ill. She had to earn money. But how? No experience. No skill. No capital. Just a housewife. She took the white of an egg and sugar and made some candy on the back of the kitchen stove; then she took her pan of candy and stood near the school and sold it to the children for a penny a piece as they went home. "Bring more pennies tomorrow," she said. "I'll be here every day with my homemade candy." During the first week, she not only made a profit of $4.15, but had also put a new zest into living. She was making both herself and the children happy. No time now for worry.

This quiet little housewife from Maywood, Illinois, was so ambitious that she decided to branch out—to have an agent sell her kitchen-made candy in roaring, thundering Chicago. She timidly approached an Italian selling peanuts on the street. He shrugged his shoulders. His customers wanted peanuts, not candy. She gave him a sample. He liked it, began selling her candy, and made $2.15 profit for Mrs. Snyder on the first day. Four years later, she opened her first store in Chicago. It was only eight feet wide. She made her candy at night and sold it in the daytime. This erstwhile timid housewife, who started her candy factory on her kitchen stove, now has seventeen stores—fifteen of them in the busy Loop district of Chicago.

Here is the point I am trying to make. Nellie Speer, in Jackson Heights, New York, and Mrs. Ora Snyder, in Maywood, Illinois, instead of worrying about finances, did something positive. They started in an extremely small way to make money off the kitchen stove—no overhead, no rent, no advertising, no salaries. Under these conditions, it is almost impossible for a woman to be defeated by financial worries.

Look around you. You will find many needs that are not filled. For example, if you train yourself to be a good cook, you can probably make money by starting cooking classes for young girls right in your own kitchen. You can get your students by ringing door-bells.

Books have been written about how to make money in your spare time; inquire at your public library. There are many opportunities for both men and women. But one word of warning: unless you have a natural gift for selling, don't attempt door-to-door selling. Most people hate it and fail at it.

Rule No. 10: **Don't gamble—ever.**

I am always astounded by the people who hope to make money by betting on the ponies or playing slot machines, I know a man who makes his living by owning a string of these "one-armed bandits," and he has nothing but contempt for the foolish people who are so naïve as to imagine that they can beat a machine that is already rigged against them.

I also know one of the best-known bookmakers in

America. He was a student in my adult-education classes. He told me that with all his knowledge of horse racing, he couldn't make money betting on the ponies. Yet the facts are that foolish people bet six billion dollars a year on the races—six times as much as our total national debt back in 1910. This bookmaker also told me that if he had an enemy that he despised, he could think of no better way of ruining him than by getting him to bet on the races. When I asked him what would happen to the man who played the races according to the tipster sheets, he replied: "You could lose the United States Mint by betting that way."

Rule No. 11: **If we can't possibly improve our financial situation, let's be good to ourselves and stop resenting what can't be changed**.

If we can't possibly improve our financial situation, maybe we can improve our mental attitude toward it. Let's remember that other people have their financial worries, too. We may be worried because we can't keep up with the Joneses; but the Joneses are probably worried because they can't keep up with the Ritzes; and the Ritzes are worried because they can't keep up with the Vanderbilts.

Some of the most famous men in American history have had their financial troubles. Both Lincoln and Washington had to borrow money to make the trip to be inaugurated as President.

If we can't have all we want, let's not poison our days with worry and resentment. Let's be good to ourselves. Let's be philosophical. And philosophy, according to Epictetus, boils down to this: "The essence of philosophy is that a man should so live that his happiness shall depend as little as possible on external things." Here is what Seneca said about it: "If you have what seems to you to be insufficient, then you will be miserable even if you possess the world."

And let's remember that even if we owned the world with a hog-tight fence around it, we could eat only three meals a day and sleep in one bed at a time—even a ditch digger can do that; and he will probably eat with more gusto and sleep more peacefully than Rockefeller.

To lessen financial worries, let's try to follow these eleven rules:

- Get the facts down on paper!
- Get a tailor-made budget that really fits your needs!
- Learn how to spend wisely.
- Don't increase your headaches with your income.
- Try to build credit, in the event you must borrow.
- Protect yourself against illness, fire, and emergency expenses.
- Do not have your life-insurance proceeds paid to your widow in cash.
- Teach your children a responsible attitude toward money.
- If you are a housewife, maybe you can make a little extra money off your kitchen stove.
- Don't gamble—ever.

If we can't possibly improve our financial situation, let's be good to ourselves and stop resenting what can't be changed.

"Worry is a cycle of inefficient thoughts whirling around a center of fear."

—Corrie Ten Boom

"Our fatigue is often caused not by work, but by worry, frustration and resentment."

—Dale Carnegie

PART 2

4

LIVE IN "DAY-TIGHT COMPARTMENTS"

In the spring of 1871, a young man picked up a book and read twenty-one words that had a profound effect on his future. A medical student at the Montreal General Hospital, he was worried about passing the final examination, worried about what to do, where to go, how to build up a practice, how to make a living.

The twenty-one words that this young medical student read in 1871 helped him to become the most famous physician of his generation. He organized the world-famous Johns Hopkins School of Medicine. He became Regius Professor of Medicine at Oxford—the highest honor that can be bestowed upon any medical man in the British Empire. He was knighted by the King of England. When he died, two huge volumes containing 1,466 pages were required to tell the story of his life.

His name was Sir William Osler. Here are the twenty-one words that he read in the spring of 1871—twenty-one words from Thomas Carlyle that helped him lead a life free from worry: *"Our main business is not to see what lies dimly at a distance, but to do what lies clearly at hand."*

Forty-two years later, on a soft spring night when the tulips were blooming on the campus, this man, Sir William Osler, addressed the students of Yale University. He told those Yale students that a man like himself who had been a professor in four universities and had written a popular book was supposed to have "brains of a special quality." He declared that that was untrue. He said that his intimate friends knew that his brains were "of the most mediocre character."

What, then, was the secret of his success? He stated that it was owing to what he called living in "day-tight compartments." What did he mean by that? A few months before he spoke at Yale, Sir William Osler had crossed the Atlantic on a great ocean liner where the captain, standing on the bridge, could press a button and—presto!—there was a clanging of machinery and various parts of the ship were immediately shut off from one another—shut off into watertight compartments. "Now each one of you," Dr. Osler said to those Yale students, "is a much more marvelous organization than the great liner, and bound on a longer voyage. What I urge is that you so learn to control the machinery as to live with 'day-tight compartments' as the most certain way to ensure safety on the voyage. Get on the bridge, and see that at least the great bulkheads are in working order. Touch a button and hear, at every level of your life, the iron doors shutting out the Past—the dead yesterdays. Touch another and shut off, with a metal curtain, the Future—the unborn tomorrows. Then you are safe—safe for today! …Shut off the past! Let the dead past bury its dead…. Shut out the yesterdays which have lighted fools the way to dusty death…. The load of tomorrow, added to that of yesterday, carried today, makes the strongest falter. Shut off the future as tightly as the past…. The future is today…. There is no tomorrow. The day of man's salvation is now.

Waste of energy, mental distress, nervous worries dog the steps of a man who is anxious about the future…. Shut close, then, the great fore and aft bulkheads, and prepare to cultivate the habit of a life of 'day-tight compartments.'"

Did Dr. Osler mean to say that we should not make any effort to prepare for tomorrow? No. Not at all. But he did go on in that address to say that the best possible way to prepare for tomorrow is to concentrate with all your intelligence, all your enthusiasm, on doing today's work superbly today. That is the only possible way you can prepare for the future.

Sir William Osler urged the students at Yale to begin the day with Christ's prayer: "Give us this day our daily bread."

Remember that that prayer asks only for *today's* bread. It doesn't complain about the stale bread we had to eat yesterday; and it doesn't say: "Oh, God, it has been pretty dry out in the wheat belt lately and we may have another drought—and then how will I get bread to eat next fall— or suppose I lose my job—oh, God, how could I get bread then?"

No, this prayer teaches us to ask for today's bread only. Today's bread is the only kind of bread you can possibly eat.

Years ago, a penniless philosopher was wandering through a stony country where the people had a hard time making a living. One day, a crowd gathered about him on a hill, and he gave what is probably the most-quoted speech ever delivered anywhere at any time. This speech contains twenty-six words that have gone ringing down across the centuries: "Take therefore no thought for the morrow; for the morrow shall take thought for the things of itself. Sufficient unto the day is the evil thereof."

Many men have rejected those words of Jesus: "Take no thought for the morrow." They have rejected those words as a counsel of perfection, as a bit of Oriental mysticism. "I *must* take thought for the morrow," they say. "I *must* take out insurance to protect my family. I *must* lay aside money for my old age. I *must* plan and prepare to get ahead."

Right! Of course you must. The truth is that those words of Jesus, translated over three hundred years ago, don't mean today what they meant during the reign of King James. Three hundred years ago the word *thought* frequently meant anxiety. Modern versions of the Bible quote Jesus more accurately as saying: "Have no anxiety for the tomorrow."

By all means take thought for the tomorrow, yes, careful thought and planning and preparation. But have no anxiety.

During the war, our military leaders planned for the morrow, but they could not afford to have any anxiety. "I have supplied the best men with the best equipment we have," said Admiral Ernest J. King, who directed the United States Navy, "and have given them what seems to be the wisest mission. That is all I can do."

"If a ship has been sunk," Admiral King went on, "I can't bring it up. If it is going to be sunk, I can't stop it. I can use my time much better working on tomorrow's problem than by fretting about yesterday's. Besides, if I let those things get me, I wouldn't last long."

Whether in war or peace, the chief difference between good thinking and bad thinking is this: good thinking deals with causes and effects and leads to logical, constructive planning; bad thinking frequently leads to tension and nervous breakdowns.

I recently had the privilege of interviewing Arthur Hays Sulzberger, publisher of one of the most famous newspapers in the world, *The New York Times*. Mr. Sulzberger told me that when the Second World War flamed across Europe, he was so stunned, so worried about the future, that he found it almost impossible to sleep. He would frequently get out of bed in the middle of the night, take some canvas and tubes of paint, look in the mirror, and try to paint a portrait of himself. He didn't know anything about painting, but he painted anyway, to get his mind off his worries. Mr. Sulzberger told me that he was never able to banish his worries and find peace until he had adopted as his motto five words from a church hymn: *One step enough for me.*

Lead, kindly Light...
Keep thou my feet: I do not ask to see
The distant scene; one step enough for me.

One of the most appalling comments on our present way of life is that half of all the beds in our hospitals are reserved for patients with nervous and mental troubles, patients who have collapsed under the crushing burden of accumulated yesterdays and fearful tomorrows. Yet a vast majority of those people would be walking the streets today, leading happy, useful lives, if they had only heeded the words of Jesus: *"Have no anxiety about the morrow"*; or the words of Sir William Osler: *"Live in day-tight compartments."*

You and I are standing this very second at the meeting place of two eternities: the vast past that has endured forever, and the future that is plunging on to the last syllable of recorded time. We can't possibly live in either of those eternities—no, not even for one split second. But, by trying to do so, we can wreck both our bodies and our minds. So let's be content to live the only time we can possibly live: from now until bedtime. "Anyone can carry his burden, however hard, until nightfall," wrote Robert Louis Stevenson. "Anyone can do his work, however hard, for one day. Anyone can live sweetly, patiently, lovingly, purely, till the sun goes down. And this is all that life really means."

Yes, that is all that life requires of us; but Mrs. E.K. Shields, 815 Court Street, Saginaw, Michigan, was driven to despair—even to the brink of suicide—before she learned to live just till bedtime. "In 1937, I lost my husband," Mrs. Shields said as she told me her story. "I was very depressed—and almost penniless. I wrote to my former employer, Mr. Leon Roach, of the Roach-Fowler Company of Kansas City, and got my old job back. I had formerly made my living selling World Books to rural and town school boards. I had sold my car two years previously when my husband became ill; but I managed to scrape together enough money to put a down payment on a used car and started out to sell books again.

"I had thought that getting back on the road would help relieve my depression; but driving alone and eating alone was almost more than I could take. Some of the territory was not very productive, and I found it hard to make those car payments, small as they were.

"In the spring of 1938, I was working out of Versailles, Missouri. The schools were poor, the roads bad; I was so lonely and discouraged that at one time I even considered suicide. It seemed that success was impossible. I had nothing to live for. I dreaded getting up each morning and facing life. I was afraid of everything: afraid I could not meet the car payments; afraid I could not pay my room rent; afraid I would not have enough to eat. I was afraid my health was failing and I had no money for a doctor. All that kept me from suicide were the thoughts that my sister would be deeply grieved, and that I did not have enough money to pay my funeral expenses.

"Then one day I read an article that lifted me out of my despondence and gave me the courage to go on living. I shall never cease to be grateful for one inspiring sentence in that article. It said: 'Every day is a new life to a wise man.' I typed that sentence out and pasted it on the windshield of my car, where I saw it every minute I was driving. I found it wasn't so hard to live only one day at a time. I learned to forget the yesterdays and to not-think of the tomorrows. Each morning I said to myself, 'Today is a new life.'

"I have succeeded in overcoming my fear of loneliness, my fear of want. I am happy and fairly successful now and have a lot of enthusiasm and love for life. I know now that I shall never again be afraid, regardless of what life hands me. I know now that I don't have to fear the future. I know now that I can live one day at a time—and that 'Every day is a new life to a wise man.'"

Who do you suppose wrote this verse:

Happy the man, and happy he alone,
He, who can call to-day his own:
He who, secure within, can say:
"To-morrow, do thy worst, for I have liv'd to-day."

Those words sound modern, don't they? Yet they were written thirty years before Christ was born, by the Roman poet Horace.

One of the most tragic things I know about human nature is that all of us tend to put off living. We are all dreaming of some magical rose garden over the horizon—instead of enjoying the roses that are blooming outside our windows today.

Why are we such fools—such tragic fools?

"How strange it is, our little procession of life!" wrote Stephen Leacock. "The child says, 'When I am a big boy.' But what is that? The big boy says, 'When I grow up.' And then, grown up, he says, 'When I get married.' But to be married, what is that after all? The thought changes to 'When I'm able to retire.' And then, when retirement comes, he looks back over the landscape traversed; a cold wind seems to sweep over it; somehow he has missed it all, and it is gone. Life, we learn too late, is in the living, in the tissue of every day and hour."

The late Edward S. Evans of Detroit almost killed

himself with worry before he learned that life "is in the living, in the tissue of every day and hour." Brought up in poverty, Edward Evans made his first money by selling newspapers, then worked as a grocer's clerk. Later, with seven people dependent upon him for bread and butter, he got a job as an assistant librarian. Small as the pay was, he was afraid to quit. Eight years passed before he could summon up the courage to start out on his own. But once he started, he built up an original investment of fifty-five borrowed dollars into a business of his own that made him twenty thousand dollars a year. Then came a frost, a killing frost. He endorsed a big note for a friend—and the friend went bankrupt. Quickly on top of that disaster came another: the bank in which he had all his money collapsed. He not only lost every cent he had, but was plunged into debt for sixteen thousand dollars. His nerves couldn't take it. "I couldn't sleep or eat," he told me. "I became strangely ill. *Worry and nothing but worry*," he said, *"brought on this illness.* One day as I was walking down the street, I fainted and fell on the sidewalk. I was no longer able to walk. I was put to bed and my body broke out in boils. These boils turned inward until just lying in bed was agony. I grew weaker every day. Finally my doctor told me that I had only two more weeks to live. I was shocked. I drew up my will, and then lay back in bed to await my end. No use now to struggle or worry. I gave up, relaxed, and went to sleep. I hadn't slept two hours in succession for weeks; but now with my earthly problems drawing to an end, I slept like a baby. My exhausting weariness began to disappear. My appetite returned. I gained weight.

"A few weeks later, I was able to walk with crutches. Six weeks later, I was able to go back to work. I had been making twenty thousand dollars a year; but I was glad now to get a job for thirty dollars a week. I got a job selling blocks to put behind the wheels of automobiles when they are shipped by freight. I had learned my lesson now. No more worry for me—no more regret about what had happened in the past—no more dread of the future. I concentrated all my time, energy, and enthusiasm into selling those blocks." Edward S. Evans shot up fast now. In a few years, he was president of the company—the Evans Products Company. It has been listed on the New York Stock Exchange for years. If you ever fly over Greenland you may land on Evans Field—a flying field named in his honor. Yet Edward S. Evans never would have achieved these victories if he hadn't learned to live in day-tight compartments.

John Ruskin had on his desk a simple piece of stone on which was carved one word: TODAY. And while I haven't a piece of stone on my desk, I do have a poem pasted on my mirror where I can see it when I shave every morning—a poem that Sir William Osler always kept on his desk—a poem written by the famous Indian dramatist, Kalidasa:

SALUTATION TO THE DAWN

Look to this day!
For it is life, the very life of life.
In its brief course
Lie all the verities and realities of your existence:

The bliss of growth The glory of action The splendor of achievement,

For yesterday is but a dream And tomorrow is only a vision,

But today well lived makes every yesterday a dream of happiness

And every tomorrow a vision of hope.

Look well, therefore, to this day!

Such is the salutation to the dawn.

So, the first thing you should know about worry is this: if you want to keep it out of your life, do what Sir William Osler did:

- Shut the iron doors on the past and the future. Live in day-tight compartments.
- Why not ask yourself these questions, and write down the answers?
- Do I tend to put off living in the present in order to worry about the future, or to yearn for some "magical rose garden over the horizon"?
- Do I sometimes embitter the present by regretting things that happened in the past—that are over and done with?
- Do I get up in the morning determined to "Seize the day"—to get the utmost out of these twenty-four hours?
- Can I get more out of life by "living in day-tight compartments"?
- When shall I start to do this? Next week? ... Tomorrow? ... *Today?*

"Every day brings a choice: to practice stress or to practice peace."
—Joan Borysenko

"Life is too short to worry about anything. You had better enjoy it because the next day promises nothing."
—Eric Davis

5

A MAGIC FORMULA

Would you like a quick, sure-fire recipe for handling worry situations—a technique you can start using right away, before you go any further in reading this book?

Then let me tell you about the method worked out by Willis H. Carrier, the brilliant engineer who launched the air-conditioning industry, and who is now head of the world-famous Carrier Corporation, in Syracuse, New York. It is one of the best techniques I ever heard of for solving worry problems, and I got it from Mr. Carrier personally when we were having lunch together one day at the Engineers' Club in New York.

"When I was a young man," Mr. Carrier said, "I worked for the Buffalo Forge Company in Buffalo, New York. I was handed the assignment of installing a gas-cleaning device in a plant of the Pittsburgh Plate Glass Company at Crystal City, Missouri—a plant costing millions of dollars. The purpose of this installation was to remove the impurities from the gas so it could be burned without injuring the engines. This method of cleaning gas was new. It had been tried only once before—and under different conditions. In my work at Crystal City, Missouri, unforeseen difficulties arose. It worked after a fashion—but not well enough to meet the guarantee we had made.

"I was stunned by my failure. It was almost as if

someone had struck me a blow on the head. My stomach, my insides, began to twist and turn. For a while I was so worried I couldn't sleep.

"Finally, common sense reminded me that worry wasn't getting me anywhere; so I figured out a way to handle my problem without worrying. It worked superbly. I have been using this same anti-worry technique for more than thirty years. It is simple. Anyone can use it. It consists of three steps:

"Step I. *I analyzed the situation fearlessly and honestly and figured out what was the worst that could possibly happen as a result of this failure.* No one was going to jail me or shoot me. That was certain. True, there was a chance that I would lose my position; and there was also a chance that my employers would have to remove the machinery and lose the twenty thousand dollars we had invested.

"Step II. *After figuring out what was the worst that could possibly happen, I reconciled myself to accepting it, if necessary.* I said to myself: This failure will be a blow to my record, and it might possibly mean the loss of my job; but if it does, I can always get another position. Conditions could be much worse; and as far as my employers are concerned—well, they realize that we are experimenting with a new method of cleaning gas, and if this experience costs them twenty thousand dollars, they can stand it. They can charge it up to research, for it is an experiment.

"After discovering the worst that could possibly happen and reconciling myself to accepting it, if necessary, an extremely important thing happened: I immediately relaxed and felt a sense of peace that I hadn't experienced in days.

"Step III. *From that time on, I calmly devoted my time and energy to trying to improve upon the worst which I had already accepted mentally.*

"I now tried to figure out ways and means by which I might reduce the loss of twenty thousand dollars that we faced. I made several tests and finally figured out that if we spent another five thousand for additional equipment, our problem would be solved. We did this, and instead of the firm losing twenty thousand, we made fifteen thousand.

"I probably would never have been able to do this if I had kept on worrying, because one of the worst features about worrying is that it destroys our ability to concentrate. When we worry, our minds jump here and there and everywhere, and we lose all power of decision. However, when we force ourselves to face the worst and accept it mentally, we then eliminate all these vague imaginings and put ourselves in a position in which we are able to concentrate on our problem.

"This incident that I have related occurred many years ago. It worked so superbly that I have been using it ever since; and, as a result, my life has been almost completely free from worry."

Now, why is Willis H. Carrier's magic formula so valuable and so practical, psychologically speaking? Because it yanks us down out of the great gray clouds in which we fumble around when we are blinded by worry. It plants our feet good and solid on the earth. We know where we stand. And if we haven't solid ground under us, how in creation can we ever hope to think anything through?

The same idea was expressed by Lin Yutang in his widely read book, *The Importance of Living.* "True peace of mind," said this Chinese philosopher, "comes from accepting the worst. Psychologically, I think, it means a release of energy."

That's it, exactly! Psychologically, it means a new release of energy! When we have accepted the worst, we have nothing more to lose. And that automatically means—we have *everything* to gain! "After facing the worst," Willis H. Carrier reported, "I immediately relaxed and felt a sense of peace that I hadn't experienced in days. From that time on, I was able to *think.*"

Makes sense, doesn't it? Yet millions of people have wrecked their lives in angry turmoil, because they refused to accept the worst; refused to try to improve upon it; refused to salvage what they could from the wreck. Instead of trying to reconstruct their fortunes, they engaged in a bitter and "violent contest with experience"—and ended up victims of that brooding fixation known as melancholia.

Would you like to see how someone else adopted Willis H. Carrier's magic formula and applied it to his own problem? Well, here is one example, from a New York oil dealer who was a student in my classes.

"I was being blackmailed!" this student began. "I didn't believe it was possible—I didn't believe it could happen outside of the movies—but I was actually being blackmailed! What happened was this: the oil company of which I was the head had a number of delivery trucks and a number of drivers. At that time, OPA regulations were strictly in force, and we were rationed on the amount of oil we could deliver to any one of our customers. I didn't know it, but it seems that certain of our drivers had been delivering oil short to our regular customers, and then reselling the surplus to customers of their own.

"The first inkling I had of these illegitimate transactions was when a man who claimed to be a government inspector came to see me one day and demanded hush money. He had got documentary proof of what our drivers had been doing, and he threatened to turn this proof over to the District Attorney's office if I didn't cough up.

"I knew, of course, that I had nothing to worry about—personally, at least. But I also knew that the law says a firm is responsible for the actions of its employees. What's more, I knew that if the case came to court, and it was aired in the newspapers, the bad publicity would ruin my business. And I was proud of my business—it had been founded by my father twenty-four years before.

"I was so worried I was sick! I didn't eat or sleep for three days and nights. I kept going around in crazy circles. Should I pay the money—five thousand dollars—or should I tell this man to go ahead and do his damnedest? Either way I tried to make up my mind, it ended in nightmare.

"Then, on Sunday night, I happened to pick up the booklet on *How to Stop Worrying* which I had been given in my Carnegie class in public speaking. I started to read it, and came across the story of Willis H. Carrier. 'Face the worst,' it said. So I asked myself, 'What is the worst that can happen if I refuse to pay up, and these blackmailers turn their records over to the District Attorney?'

"The answer to that was: 'The ruin of my business—that's the worst that can happen. I can't go to jail. All that can happen is that I shall be ruined by the publicity.'

"I then said to myself, 'All right, the business *is* ruined. I accept that mentally. What happens next?'

"Well, with my business ruined, I would probably have to look for a job. That wasn't bad. I knew a lot about oil—there were several firms that might be glad to employ me…. I began to feel better. The blue funk I had been in for three days and nights began to lift a little. My emotions calmed down…. And to my astonishment, I was able to *think*.

"I was clearheaded enough now to face Step III—*improve on the worst*. As I thought of solutions, an entirely new angle presented itself to me. If I told my attorney the whole situation, he might find a way out which I hadn't thought of. I know it sounds stupid to say that this hadn't even occurred to me before—but of course I hadn't been thinking, I had only been *worrying!* I immediately made up my mind that I would see my attorney first thing in the morning—and then I went to bed and slept like a log!

"How did it end? Well, the next morning my lawyer told me to go and see the District Attorney and tell him the truth. I did precisely that. When I finished I was astonished to hear the D.A. say that this blackmail racket had been going on for months and that the man who claimed to be a 'government agent' was a crook wanted by the police. What a relief to hear all this after I tormented myself for three days and nights wondering whether I should hand over five thousand dollars to this professional swindler!

"This experience taught me a lasting lesson. Now, whenever I face a pressing problem that threatens to worry me, I give it what I call 'the old Willis H. Carrier formula.'"

If you think Willis H. Carrier had troubles—listen: you ain't heard nothin' yet. Here is the story of Earl P. Haney, who lives at 52 Wedgemere Avenue, Winchester, Massachusetts. Here is the story as he told it to me himself on November 17, 1948, in the Hotel Statler in Boston.

"Back in the twenties," he said, "I was so worried that ulcers began eating the lining of my stomach. One night, I had a terrible hemorrhage. I was rushed to a hospital connected with the School of Medicine of Northwestern University in Chicago. My weight dropped from 175 pounds to 90 pounds. I was so ill I was warned not even to lift my hand. Three doctors, including a celebrated ulcer specialist, said my case was 'incurable.' I lived on alkaline powders and a tablespoonful of half milk and half cream every hour. A nurse put a rubber tube down into my stomach every night and morning and pumped out the contents.

"This went on for months…. Finally, I said to myself: 'Look here, Earl Haney, if you have nothing to look forward to except a lingering death, you might as well make the most of the little time you have left. You have always wanted to travel around the world before you die; so if you are ever going to do it, you'll have to do it now.'

"When I told my physicians I was going to travel around the world and pump out my own stomach twice a day, they were shocked. Impossible! They had never heard of such a thing. They warned me that if I started around the world, I would be buried at sea. 'No, I won't,' I replied. 'I have promised my relatives that I will be buried in the family plot at Broken Bow, Nebraska. So I am going to take my casket with me.'

"I arranged for a casket, put it aboard ship, and then made arrangements with the steamship company—in the event of my death—to put my corpse in a freezing compartment and keep it there till the liner returned home. I set out on my trip, imbued with the spirit of old Omar:

> *Ah, make the most of what we yet may spend,*
> *Before we too into the Dust descend;*
> *Dust into Dust, and under Dust, to lie,*
> *Sans Wine, sans Song, sans Singer, and—sans End!*

"The moment I boarded the *S.S. President Adams* in Los Angeles and headed for the Orient, I felt better. I gradually gave up my alkaline powders and my stomach pump. I was soon eating all kinds of foods—even strange native mixtures and concoctions that were guaranteed to kill me. As the weeks went by, I even smoked long, black cigars and drank highballs. I enjoyed myself more than I had in years! We ran into monsoons and typhoons which should have put me in my casket, if only from fright— but I got an enormous kick out of all this adventure.

"I played games aboard the ship, sang songs, made new friends, stayed up half the night. When we reached China and India, I realized that the business cares that I had faced back home were paradise compared to the poverty and hunger in the Orient. I stopped all my senseless worrying and felt fine. When I got back to America, I had gained ninety pounds and I had almost forgotten had ever had a stomach ulcer. I had never felt better in my life. I went back to business and haven't been ill a day since."

Earl P. Haney told me he realizes now that he was unconsciously using the selfsame principles that Willis H. Carrier used to conquer worry.

"First, I asked myself, 'What is the worst that could possibly happen?' The answer was death.

"Second, I prepared myself to accept death. I had to. There was no choice. The doctors said my case was hopeless.

"Third, I tried to improve the situation by getting the utmost enjoyment out of life for the short time I had left. ... If," he continued, "if I had gone on worrying after boarding that ship, I have no doubt that I would have made the return voyage inside my coffin. But I relaxed—and I forgot all my troubles. And this calmness of mind gave me a new birth of energy which actually saved my life."

So, Rule 2 is: If you have a worry problem, apply the magic formula of Willis H. Carrier by doing these three things:

- Ask yourself, "What is the worst that can possibly happen?"

- Prepare to accept it if you have to.
- Then calmly proceed to improve on the worst.

"You're only here for a short visit. Don't hurry, don't worry. And be sure to smell the flowers along the way."
—Walter Hagen

"If only the people who worry about their liabilities would think about the riches they do possess, they would stop worrying."
—Dale Carnegie

6

WHAT WORRY MAY DO TO YOU

Some time ago, a neighbor rang my doorbell one evening
and urged me and my family to be vaccinated against
smallpox. He was only one of thousands of volunteers
who were ringing doorbells all over New York City.
Frightened people stood in lines for hours at a time to be
vaccinated. Vaccination stations were opened not only in
all hospitals, but also in firehouses, police precincts, and
in large industrial plants. More than two thousand
doctors and nurses worked feverishly day and night,
vaccinating crowds. The cause of all this excitement?
Eight people in New York City had smallpox—and two
had died. Two deaths out of a population of almost eight
million.

Now, I have lived in New York for over thirty-seven
years; and no one has ever yet rung my doorbell to warn
me against the emotional sickness of worry—an illness
that, during the last thirty-seven years, has caused ten
thousand times more damage than smallpox.

No doorbell ringer has ever warned me that one person
out of ten now living in these United States will have a
nervous breakdown—induced in the vast majority of
cases by worry and emotional conflicts. So I am writing
this chapter to ring your doorbell and warn you.

The great Nobel prize winner in medicine, Dr. Alexis
Carrel, said, "Businessmen who do not know how to

fight worry die young." And so do housewives and horse doctors and bricklayers.

A few years ago, I spent my vacation motoring through Texas and New Mexico with Dr. O.F. Gober—one of the medical executives of the Santa Fe railway. His exact title was chief physician of the Gulf, Colorado and Santa Fe Hospital Association. We got to talking about the effects of worry, and he said: "Seventy per cent of all patients who come to physicians could cure themselves if' they only got rid of their fears and worries. Don't think for a moment that I mean that their ills are imaginary," he said. "Their ills are as real as a throbbing toothache and sometimes a hundred times more serious. I refer to such illnesses as nervous indigestion, some stomach ulcers, heart disturbances, insomnia, some headaches, and some types of paralysis.

"These illnesses are real. I know what I am talking about," said Dr. Gober, "for I myself suffered from a stomach ulcer for twelve years.

"Fear causes worry. Worry makes you tense and nervous and affects the nerves of your stomach and actually changes the gastric juices of your stomach from normal to abnormal and often leads to stomach ulcers."

Dr. W. C. Alvarez, of the Mayo Clinic, said: "Ulcers frequently flare up or subside according to the hills and valleys of emotional stress."

That statement was backed up by a study of 15,000 patients treated for stomach disorders at the Mayo Clinic. Four out of five had no physical basis whatever for their stomach illnesses. Fear, worry, hate, supreme selfishness, and the inability to adjust themselves to the world of reality—these were largely the causes of their stomach illnesses and stomach ulcers…. Stomach ulcers can kill you. According to *Life* magazine, they now stand tenth in our list of fatal diseases.

I recently had some correspondence with Dr. Harold C. Habein of the Mayo Clinic. He read a paper at the annual meeting of the American Association of Industrial Physicians and Surgeons, saying that he had made a study of 176 business executives whose average age was 44.3 years. *He reported that slightly more than a third of these executives suffered from one of three ailments peculiar to high-tension* living—*heart disease, digestive-tract ulcers, and high blood pressure.* Think of it—a third of our business executives are wrecking their bodies with heart disease, ulcers, and high blood pressure before they even reach forty-five. What price success! And they aren't even buying success! Can any man possibly be a success who is paying for business advancement with stomach ulcers and heart trouble? What shall it profit a man if he gains the whole world—and loses his health? Even if he owned the whole world, he could sleep in only one bed at a time and eat only three meals a day. Even a ditchdigger can do that—and probably sleep more soundly and enjoy his food more than a high-powered executive. Frankly, I would rather be a sharecropper down in Alabama with a banjo on my knee than wreck my health at forty-five by trying to run a railroad or a cigarette company.

And speaking of cigarettes—the best-known cigarette manufacturer in the world recently dropped dead from heart failure while trying to take a little recreation in the Canadian woods. He amassed millions—and fell dead at sixty-one. He probably traded years of his life for what is called "business success".

In my estimation, this cigarette executive with all his millions was not half as successful as my father—a Missouri farmer—who died at eighty-nine without a dollar.

The famous Mayo brothers declared that more than half of our hospital beds are occupied by people with nervous troubles. Yet, when the nerves of these people are studied under a high-powered microscope in a post-mortem examination, their nerves in most cases are apparently as healthy as the nerves of Jack Dempsey. Their "nervous troubles" are caused not by a physical deterioration of the nerves, but by emotions of futility, frustration, anxiety, worry, fear, defeat, despair. Plato said that "the greatest mistake physicians make is that they attempt to cure the body without attempting to cure the mind; yet the mind and body are one and should not be treated separately!"

It took medical science twenty-three hundred years to recognize this great truth. We are just now beginning to develop a new kind of medicine called *psychosomatic* medicine—a medicine that treats both the mind and the body. It is high time we are doing that, for medical science has largely wiped out the terrible *diseases caused by physical* germs—diseases such as smallpox, cholera, yellow fever, and scores of other scourges that swept untold millions into untimely graves. But medical science has been unable to cope with the mental and physical wrecks caused, not by germs, but by emotions of worry, fear, hate, frustration, and despair. Casualties caused by these emotional diseases are mounting and spreading with catastrophic rapidity.

Doctors figure that one American in every twenty now alive will spend a part of his life in an institution for the mentally ill. One out of every six of our young men called up by the draft in the Second World War was rejected as mentally diseased or defective.

What causes insanity? No one knows all the answers. But it is highly probable that in many cases fear and worry are contributing factors. The anxious and harassed individual who is unable to cope with the harsh world of reality breaks off all contact with his environment and retreats into a private dream world of his own making, and this solves his worry problems.

Worry can make even the most stolid person ill. General Grant discovered that during the closing days of the Civil War. The story goes like this: Grant had been besieging Richmond for nine months. General Lee's troops, ragged and hungry, were beaten. Entire regiments were deserting at a time. Others were holding prayer meetings in their tents—shouting, weeping, and seeing visions. The end was close. Lee's men set fire to the cotton and tobacco ware-houses in Richmond, burned the arsenal, and fled from the city at night while towering flames roared up into darkness. Grant was in hot pursuit, banging away at the Confederates from both sides and the rear, while Sheridan's cavalry was heading them off in front, tearing up railway lines and capturing supply trains.

Grant, half blind with a violent sick headache, fell behind his army and stopped at a farmhouse. "I spent the night," he records in his *Memoirs,* "in bathing my feet in hot water and mustard, and putting mustard plasters on my wrists and the back part of my neck, hoping to be cured by morning."

The next morning, he was cured instantaneously. And the thing that cured him was not a mustard plaster, but a horseman galloping down the road with a letter from Lee, saying he wanted to surrender.

"When the officer [bearing the message] reached me," Grant wrote, "I was still suffering with the sick headache, but the instant I saw the contents of the note, I was cured."

Obviously it was Grant's worries, tensions, and emotions that made him ill. He was cured instantly the moment his emotions took on the hue of confidence, achievement, and victory.

Seventy years later, Henry Morgenthau, Jr., Secretary of the Treasury in Franklin D. Roosevelt's cabinet, discovered that worry could make him so ill that he was dizzy. He records in his diary that he was terribly worried when the President, in order to raise the price of wheat, bought 4,400,000 bushels in one day. He says in his diary: "I felt literally dizzy while the thing was going on. I went home and went to bed for two hours after lunch."

If I want to see what worry does to people, I don't have to go to a library or a physician. I can look out of the window of my home where I am writing this book; and I can see, within one block, one house where worry caused a nervous breakdown—and another house where a man worried himself into diabetes. When the stock market went down, the sugar in his blood and urine went up.

When Montaigne, the illustrious French philosopher, was elected Mayor of his home town—Bordeaux—he said to his fellow citizens: "I am willing to take your affairs into my hands but not into my liver and lungs."

This neighbor of mine took the affairs of the stock market into his blood stream—and almost killed himself.

If I want to be reminded of what worry does to people, I don't need to look at my neighbors' houses. I can look at this very room where I am writing now and be reminded that a former owner of this house worried himself into an untimely grave.

Worry can put you into a wheel chair with rheumatism and arthritis. Dr. Russell L. Cecil, of the Cornell University Medical School, is a world-recognized authority on arthritis; and he has listed four of the commonest conditions that bring on arthritis:

1. Marital shipwreck.
2. Financial disaster and grief.
3. Loneliness and worry.
4. Long-cherished resentments.

Naturally, these four emotional situations are far from being the only causes of arthritis. There are many different kinds of arthritis—due to various causes. But, to repeat, the *commonest conditions* that bring on arthritis are the four listed by Dr. Russell L. Cecil. For example, a friend of mine was so hard hit during the depression that the gas company shut off the gas and the bank foreclosed the mortgage on the house. His wife suddenly had a painful attack of arthritis—and, in spite of medicine and diets, the arthritis continued until their financial situation improved.

Worry can even cause tooth decay. Dr. William I.L. McGonigle said in an address before the American Dental Association that "unpleasant emotions such as those caused by worry, fear, nagging ...may upset the body's calcium balance and cause tooth decay." Dr. McGonigle told of a patient of his who had always had a perfect set of teeth until he began to worry over his wife's sudden illness. During the three weeks she was in the hospital, he developed nine cavities—cavities brought on by worry.

Have you ever seen a person with an acutely overactive thyroid?

I have, and I can tell you they tremble; they shake; they look like someone half scared to death—and that's about what it amounts to. The thyroid gland, the gland that regulates the body, has been thrown out of kilter. It speeds up the heart—the whole body is roaring away at full blast like a furnace with all of its drafts wide open. And if this isn't checked, by operation or treatment, the victim may die, may "burn himself out."

A short time ago I went to Philadelphia with a friend of mine who has this disease. We consulted Dr. Israel Bram, 1633 Spruce Street—a famous specialist who has been treating this type of ailment for thirty-eight years. Here is the advice he had hanging on the wall of his waiting room—painted on a large wooden sign. I copied it down on the back of an envelope while I was waiting:

Relaxation and Recreation

The most relaxing recreating forces are a healthy religion, sleep, music, and laughter.

Have faith in God—learn to sleep well—

Love good music—see the funny side of life—

And health and happiness will be yours.

The first question he asked this friend of mine was: "What emotional disturbance brought on this condition?" He warned my friend that, if he didn't stop worrying, he could get other complications: heart trouble, stomach ulcers, or diabetes. "All of these diseases," said that eminent doctor, "are cousins, first cousins." Sure, they're first cousins—they're all worry diseases!

When I interviewed Merle Oberon, she told me that she refused to worry because she knew that worry would destroy her chief asset on the motion-picture screen: her good looks.

"When I first tried to break into the movies," she told me, "I was worried and scared. I had just come from India, and I didn't know anyone in London, where I was trying to get a job. I saw a few producers, but none of them hired me; and the little money I had began to give out. For two weeks I lived on nothing but crackers and water. I was not only worried now. I was hungry. I said to myself, 'Maybe you're a fool. Maybe you will *never* break into the movies. After all, you have no experience, you've never acted at all—what have you to offer but a rather pretty face?'

"I went to the mirror. And when I looked in that mirror, I saw what worry was doing to my looks! I saw the lines it was forming.

I saw the anxious expression. So I said to myself, 'You've got to stop this at once! You can't afford to worry. The only thing you have to offer at all is your looks, and worry will ruin them!'"

Few things can age and sour a woman and destroy her looks as quickly as worry. Worry curdles the expression. It makes us clench our jaws and lines our faces with wrinkles. It forms a permanent scowl. It may turn the hair gray, and, in some cases, even make it fall out. It can ruin the complexion—it can bring on all kinds of skin rashes, eruptions, and pimples.

Heart disease is the number-one killer in America today. During the Second World War, almost a third of a million men were killed in combat; but during that same period, heart disease killed two million civilians—and one million of those casualties were caused by the kind of heart disease that is brought on by worry and high-tension living. Yes, heart disease is one of the chief reasons why Dr. Alexis Carrel said: "Businessmen who do not know how to fight worry die young."

The African Americans down South and the Chinese rarely have the kind of heart disease brought on by worry, because they take things calmly. Twenty times as many doctors as farm workers die from heart failure. The doctors lead tense lives—and pay the penalty.

"The Lord may forgive us our sins," said William James, "but the nervous system never does."

Here is a startling and almost incredible fact: more Americans commit suicide each year than die from the five most common communicable diseases.

Why? The answer is largely: Worry.

When the cruel Chinese war lords wanted to torture their prisoners, they would tie their prisoners hand and foot and put them under a bag of water that constantly dripped…dripped…dripped…day and night. These drops of water constantly falling on the head finally became like the sound of hammer blows—and drove men insane. This same method of torture was used during the Spanish Inquisition and in German concentration camps under Hitler.

Worry is like the constant drip, drip, drip of water; and the constant drip, drip, drip of worry often drives men to insanity and suicide.

When I was a country lad in Missouri, I was half scared to death by listening to Billy Sunday describe the hell-fires of the next world. But he never even mentioned the hell-fires of physical agony that worriers may have to face here and now. For example, if you are a chronic worrier, you may be stricken someday with one of the most excruciating pains ever endured by man: angina pectoris.

Boy, if that ever hits you, you will scream with agony. Your screams will make the sounds in Dante's *Inferno* sound like *Babes in Toyland*. You will say to yourself then, "Oh, God, oh, God, if I can ever get over this, I will never worry about anything—ever." (If you think I am exaggerating, ask your family physician.)

Do you love life? Do you want to live long and enjoy good health? Here is how you can do it. I am quoting Dr. Alexis Carrel again: He said, "*Those who keep the peace of their inner selves in the midst of the tumult of the modern city are immune from nervous diseases."*

Can you keep the peace of your inner self in the midst of the tumult of a modern city? If you are a normal person, the answer is "Yes. Emphatically, yes." Most of us are stronger than we realize. We have inner resources that we have probably never tapped. As Thoreau said in his immortal book, *Walden:* "I know of no more encouraging fact than the unquestionable ability of man to elevate his life by a conscious endeavor…. If one advances confidently in the direction of his dreams, and endeavors to live the life he has imagined, he will meet with a success unexpected in common hours."

Surely, many of the readers of this book have as much will power and as many inner resources as Olga K. Jarvey has. Her address is Box 892, Coeur d'Alene, Idaho. She discovered that under the most tragic circumstances she could banish worry. I firmly believe that you and I can also—if we apply the old, old truths discussed in this volume. Here is Olga K. Jarvey's story as she wrote it for me: "Eight and a half years ago, I was condemned to die—a slow, agonizing death—of cancer. The best medical brains of the country, the Mayo brothers, confirmed the sentence. I was at a dead-end street, the ultimate gaped at me! I was young. I did not want to die! In my desperation, I phoned to my doctor at Kellogg and cried out to him the despair in my heart. Rather impatiently he upbraided me, 'What's the matter, Olga, haven't you any fight in you? Sure, you will die if you keep on crying. Yes, the worst has overtaken you. O.K.—

face the facts! Quit worrying! And then do something about it!' Right then and there I took an oath, an oath so solemn that the nails sank deep into my flesh and cold chills ran down my spine: '*I am not going to worry! I am not going to cry! And if there is anything to mind over matter, I am going to win! I am going to LIVE!*'

"The usual amount of X ray in such advanced cases, where they cannot apply radium, is $10 minutes a day for 30 days. They gave me X ray for 1472 minutes a day for 49 days; and although my bones stuck out of my emaciated body like rocks on a barren hillside, and although my feet were like lead, I *did not worry!* Not once did I cry! I *smiled!* Yes, I actually *forced* myself to smile.

"I am not so idiotic as to imagine that merely smiling can cure cancer. But I do believe that a cheerful mental attitude helps the body fight disease. At any rate, I experienced one of the miracle cures of cancer. I have never been healthier than in the last few years, thanks to those challenging, fighting words: 'Face the facts: Quit worrying; then do something about it!'"

I am going to close this chapter by repeating its title: the words of Dr. Alexis Carrel: "*Businessmen who do not know how to fight worry die young.*"

The fanatical followers of the prophet Mohammed often had verses from the Koran tattooed on their breasts. I would like to have the title of this chapter tattooed on the breast of every reader of this book: "Businessmen who do not know how to fight worry die young."

Was Dr. Carrel speaking of *you?*

Could be.

"Some of us think holding on makes us strong; but sometimes it is letting go."

—Herman Hesse

"Worry is interest paid on trouble before it comes due."

—William Ralph Inge

PART 3

7

HOW TO CROWD WORRY
OUT OF YOUR MIND

I shall never forget the night, a few years ago, when Marion J. Douglas was a student in one of my classes. (I have not used his real name. He requested me, for personal reasons, not to reveal his identity.) But here is his real story as he told it before one of our adult-education classes. He told us how tragedy had struck at his home, not once, but twice. The first time he had lost his five-year-old daughter, a child he adored. He and his wife thought they couldn't endure that first loss; but, as he said, "Ten months later God gave us another little girl—and she died in five days."

This double bereavement was almost too much to bear. "I couldn't take it," this father told us. "I couldn't sleep, I couldn't eat, I couldn't rest or relax. My nerves were utterly shaken and my confidence gone." At last he went to doctors; one recommended sleeping pills and another recommended a trip. He tried both, but neither remedy helped. He said, "My body felt as if it were encased in a vise, and the jaws of the vise were being drawn tighter and tighter." The tension of grief—if you have ever been paralyzed by sorrow, you know what he meant.

"But thank God, I had one child left—a four-year-old son. He gave me the solution to my problem. One afternoon as I sat around feeling sorry for myself, he asked: 'Daddy, will you build a boat for me?' I was in no mood to build a boat; in fact, I was in no mood to do anything. But my son is a persistent little fellow! I had to give in.

"Building that toy boat took about three hours. By the time it was finished, I realized that those three hours spent building that boat were the first hours of mental relaxation and peace that I had had in months!

"That discovery jarred me out of my lethargy and caused me to do a bit of thinking—the first real thinking I had done in months. I realized that it is difficult to worry while you are busy doing something that requires planning and thinking. In my case, building the boat had knocked worry out of the ring. So I resolved to keep busy.

"The following night, I went from room to room in the house, compiling a list of jobs that ought to be done. Scores of items needed to be repaired: bookcases, stair steps, storm windows, window shades, knobs, locks, leaky faucets. Astonishing as it seems, in the course of two weeks I had made a list of 242 items that needed attention.

"During the last two years I have completed most of them. Besides, I have filled my life with stimulating activities. Two nights per week I attend adult-education classes in New York. I have gone in for civic activities in my home town and I am now chairman of the school board. I attend scores of meetings. I help collect money for the Red Cross and other activities. I am so busy now that I have no time for worry."

No time for worry! That is exactly what Winston

Churchill said when he was working eighteen hours a day at the height of the war. When he was asked if he worried about his tremendous responsibilities, he said, "I'm too busy. I have no time for worry."

Charles Kettering was in that same fix when he started out to invent a self-starter for automobiles. Mr. Kettering was, until his recent retirement, vice-president of General Motors in charge of the world-famous General Motors Research Corporation. But in those days, he was so poor that he had to use the hayloft of a barn as a laboratory. To buy groceries, he had to use fifteen hundred dollars that his wife had made by giving piano lessons; later, had to borrow five hundred dollars on his life insurance. I asked his wife if she wasn't worried at a time like that. "Yes," she replied, "I was so worried I couldn't sleep; but Mr. Kettering wasn't. He was too absorbed in his work to worry."

The great scientist, Pasteur, spoke of "the peace that is found in libraries and laboratories." Why is peace found there? Because the men in libraries and laboratories are usually too absorbed in their tasks to worry about themselves. Research men rarely have nervous breakdowns. They haven't time for such luxuries.

Why does such a simple thing as keeping busy help to drive out anxiety? Because of a law—one of the most fundamental laws ever revealed by psychology. And that law is: that it is utterly impossible for any human mind, no matter how brilliant, to think of more than *one thing* at any given time. You don't quite believe it? Very well, then, let's try an experiment.

Suppose you lean back right now, close your eyes, and try, at the same instant, to think of the Statue of Liberty and of what you plan to do tomorrow morning. (Go ahead, try it.)

You found out, didn't you, that you could focus on either thought *in turn,* but never on both simultaneously? Well, the same thing is true in the field of emotions. We cannot be pepped up and enthusiastic about doing something exciting and feel dragged down by worry at the very same time. One kind of emotion drives out the other. And it was that simple discovery that enabled Army psychiatrists to perform such miracles during the war.

When men came out of battle so shaken by the experience that they were called "psychoneurotic," Army doctors prescribed "Keep 'em busy" as a cure.

Every waking minute of these nerve-shocked men was filled with activity—usually outdoor activity, such as fishing, hunting, playing ball, golf, taking pictures, making gardens, and dancing. They were given no time for brooding over their terrible experiences.

"Occupational therapy" is the term now used by psychiatry when work is prescribed as though it were a medicine. It is not new. The old Greek physicians were advocating it five hundred years before Christ was born!

The Quakers were using it in Philadelphia in Ben Franklin's time. A man who visited a Quaker sanitarium in 1774 was shocked to see that the patients who were mentally ill were busy spinning flax. He thought these poor unfortunates were being exploited—until the Quakers explained that they found that their patients actually improved when they did a little work. It was soothing to the nerves.

Any psychiatrist will tell you that work—keeping busy—is one of the best anesthetics ever known for sick nerves. Henry W. Longfellow found that out for himself when he lost his young wife. His wife had been melting some sealing wax at a candle one day, when her clothes caught on fire. Longfellow heard her cries and tried to reach her in time; but she died from the burns. For a while, Longfellow was so tortured by the memory of that dreadful experience that he nearly went insane; but, fortunately for him, his three small children needed his attention. In spite of his own grief, Longfellow undertook to be father and mother to his children. He took them for walks, told them stories, played games with them, and immortalized their companionship in his poem The *Children's Hour.* He also translated Dante; and all these duties combined kept him so busy that he forgot himself entirely, and regained his peace of mind. As Tennyson declared when he lost his most intimate friend, Arthur Hallam, "I must lose myself in action, lest I wither in despair."

Most of us have little trouble "losing ourselves in action" while we have our noses to the grindstone and are doing our day's work. But the hours after work—they are the dangerous ones. Just when we're free to enjoy our own leisure, and ought to be happiest—that's when the blue devils of worry attack us. That's when we begin to wonder whether we're getting anywhere in life; whether we're in a rut; whether the boss "meant anything" by that remark he made today; or whether we're getting bald.

When we are not busy, our minds tend to become a near-vacuum. Every student of physics knows that "nature abhors a vacuum." The nearest thing to a vacuum that you and I will probably ever see is the inside of an incandescent electric-light bulb. Break that bulb—and nature forces air in to fill the theoretically empty space.

Nature also rushes in to fill the vacant mind. With what? Usually with emotions. Why? Because emotions of worry, fear, hate, jealousy, and envy are driven by primeval vigor and the dynamic energy of the jungle. Such emotions are so violent that they tend to drive out of our minds all peaceful, happy thoughts and emotions.

James L. Mursell, professor of education, Teachers College, Columbia, puts it very well when he says: "Worry is most apt to ride you ragged not when you are in action, but when the day's work is done. Your imagination can run riot then and bring up all sorts of ridiculous possibilities and magnify each little blunder. At such a time," he continues, "your mind is like a motor operating without its load. It races and threatens to burn out its bearings or even to tear itself to bits. The remedy for worry is to get completely occupied doing something constructive."

But you don't have to be a college professor to realize this truth and put it into practice. During the war, I met a housewife from Chicago who told me how she discovered for herself that "the remedy for worry is to get completely occupied doing something constructive." I met this woman and her husband in the dining car while

I was traveling from New York to my farm in Missouri. (Sorry I didn't get their names—I never like to give examples without using names and street addresses—details that give authenticity to a story.)

This couple told me that their son had joined the armed forces the day after Pearl Harbor. The woman told me that she had almost wrecked her health worrying over that only son. Where was he? Was he safe? Or in action? Would he be wounded? Killed?

When I asked her how she overcame her worry, she replied: "I got busy." She told me that at first she had dismissed her maid and tried to keep busy by doing all her housework herself. But that didn't help much. "The trouble was," she said, "that I could do my housework almost mechanically, without using my mind. So I kept on worrying while making the beds and washing the dishes. I realized I needed some new kind of work that would keep me busy both mentally and physically every hour of the day. So I took a job as a saleswoman in a large department store.

"That did it," she said. "I immediately found myself in a whirl-wind of activity: customers swarming around me, asking for prices, sizes, colors. Never a second to think of anything except my immediate duty; and when night came, I could think of nothing except getting off my aching feet. As soon as I ate dinner, I fell into bed and instantly became unconscious. I had neither the time nor the energy to worry."

She discovered for herself what John Cowper Powys meant when he said, in *The Art of Forgetting the*

Unpleasant: "A certain comfortable security, a certain profound inner peace, a kind of happy numbness, soothes the nerves of the human animal when absorbed in its allotted task."

And what a blessing that it is so! Osa Johnson, the world's most famous woman explorer, recently told me how she found release from worry and grief. You may have read the story of her life. It is called *I Married Adventure.* If any woman ever married adventure, she certainly did. Martin Johnson married her when she was sixteen and lifted her feet off the sidewalks of Chanute, Kansas, and set them down on the wild jungle trails of Borneo. For a quarter of a century, this Kansas couple traveled all over the world, making motion pictures of the vanishing wild life of Asia and Africa. Back in America nine years ago, they were on a lecture tour, showing their famous films. They took a plane out of Denver, bound for the Coast. The plane plunged into a mountain. Martin Johnson was killed instantly. The doctors said Osa would never leave her bed again. But they didn't know Osa Johnson. Three months later, she was in a wheel chair, lecturing before large audiences. In fact, she addressed over a hundred audiences that season—all from a wheel chair. When I asked her why she did it, she replied: "I did it so that I would have no time for sorrow and worry."

Osa Johnson had discovered the same truth that Tennyson had sung about a century earlier: "I must lose myself in action, lest I wither in despair."

Admiral Byrd discovered this same truth when he lived

all alone for five months in a shack that was literally buried in the great glacial icecap that covers the South Pole—an icecap that holds nature's oldest secrets—an icecap covering an unknown continent larger than the United States and Europe combined. Admiral Byrd spent five months there alone. No other living creature of any kind existed within a hundred miles. The cold was so intense that he could hear his breath freeze and crystallize as the wind blew it past his ears. In his book *Alone*, Admiral Byrd tells all about those five months he spent in bewildering and soul-shattering darkness. The days were as black as the nights. He had to keep busy to preserve his sanity.

"At night," he says, "before blowing out the lantern, I formed the habit of blocking out the morrow's work. It was a case of assigning myself an hour, say, to the Escape Tunnel, half an hour to leveling drift, an hour to straightening up the fuel drums, an hour to cutting bookshelves in the walls of the food tunnel, and two hours to renewing a broken bridge in the man-hauling sledge...."

"It was wonderful," he says, "to be able to dole out time in this way. It brought me an extraordinary sense of command over myself...." And he adds, "Without that or an equivalent, the days would have been without purpose; and without purpose they would have ended, as such days always end, in disintegration."

*Note that last again: "Without purpose, the days would have ended, as such days always end, in disintegration."**

---

*From *Alone*, by Richard E. Byrd. Copyright, 1938, by Richard E. Byrd. Courtesy of G. P. Putnam's Sons.

If you and I are worried, let's remember that we can use good old-fashioned work as a medicine. That was said by no less an authority than the late Dr. Richard C. Cabot, formerly professor of clinical medicine at Harvard. In his book *What Men Live By*, Dr. Cabot says, "As a physician, I have had the happiness of seeing work cure many persons who have suffered from trembling palsy of the soul which results from overmastering doubts, hesitations, vacillation and fear.... Courage given us by our work is like the self-reliance which Emerson has made forever glorious.

If you and I don't keep busy—if we sit around and brood—we will hatch out a whole flock of what Charles Darwin used to call the "wibber gibbers. And the "wibber gibbers" are nothing but old-fashioned gremlins that will run us hollow and destroy our power of action and our power of will.

I know a businessman in New York who fought the "wibber gibbers" by getting so busy that he had no time to fret and stew. His name is Tremper Longman, and his office is at 40 Wall Street. He was a student in one of my adult-education classes; and his talk on conquering worry was so interesting, so impressive, that I asked him to have a late supper with me after class; and we sat in a restaurant until long past midnight, discussing his experiences. Here is the story he told me: "Eighteen years ago, I was so worried I had insomnia. I was tense, irritated, and jittery. I felt I was headed for a nervous breakdown.

"I had reason to be worried. I was treasurer of the Crown Fruit and Extract Company, 418 West Broadway,

New York. We had half a million dollars invested in strawberries packed in gallon tins. For twenty years, we had been selling these gallon tins of straw-berries to manufacturers of ice cream. Suddenly our sales stopped because the big ice-cream makers, such as National Dairy and Borden's, were rapidly increasing their production and were saving money and time by buying strawberries packed in barrels.

"Not only were we left with half a million dollars in berries we couldn't sell, but we were also under contract to buy a million dollars more of strawberries in the next twelve months! We had already borrowed $350,000 from the banks. We couldn't possibly pay off or renew these loans. No wonder I was worried!

"I rushed out to Watsonville, California, where our factory was located, and tried to persuade our president that conditions had changed, that we were facing ruin. He refused to believe it. He blamed our New York office for all the trouble—poor salesmanship.

"After days of pleading, I finally persuaded him to stop packing more strawberries and to sell our new supply on the fresh berry market in San Francisco. That almost solved our problems. I should have been able to stop worrying then; but I couldn't. Worry is a habit; and I had that habit.

"When I returned to New York, I began worrying about everything; the cherries we were buying in Italy, the pineapples we were buying in Hawaii, and so on. I was tense, jittery, couldn't sleep; and, as I have already said, I was heading for a nervous breakdown.

"In despair, I adopted a way of life that cured my insomnia and stopped my worries. I got busy. I got so busy with problems demanding all my faculties that I had no time to worry. I had been working seven hours a day. I now began working fifteen and sixteen hours a day. I got down to the office every morning at eight o'clock and stayed there every night until almost midnight. I took on new duties, new responsibilities. When I got home at midnight, I was so exhausted when I fell in bed that I became unconscious in a few seconds.

"I kept up this program for about three months. I had broken the habit of worry by that time, so I returned to a normal working day of seven or eight hours. This event occurred eighteen years ago. I have never been troubled with insomnia or worry since then."

George Bernard Shaw was right. He summed it all up when he said: *"The secret of being miserable is to have the leisure to bother about whether you are happy or not."* So don't bother to think about it! Spit on your hands and get busy. Your blood will start circulating; your mind will start ticking—and pretty soon this whole positive upsurge of life in your body will drive worry from your mind. Get busy. *Keep* busy. It's the cheapest kind of medicine there is on this earth—and one of the best.

To break the worry habit, here is Rule 1:

KEEP BUSY. THE WORRIED PERSON MUST LOSE HIMSELF IN ACTION, LEST HE WITHER IN DESPAIR.

"You can only lose what you cling to."

—Buddha

"Don't worry about being a star, worry about doing good work, and all that will come to you."

—Ice Cube

8

DON'T LET THE BEETLES GET YOU DOWN

Here is a dramatic story that I'll probably remember as long as I live. It was told to me by Robert Moore, of 14 Highland Avenue, Maplewood, New Jersey.

"I learned the biggest lesson of my life in March, 1945," he said. "I learned it under 276 feet of water off the coast of Indo-China. I was one of eighty-eight men aboard the submarine *Baya* S.S. 318. We had discovered by radar that a small Japanese convoy was coming our way. As daybreak approached, we submerged to attack. I saw through the periscope a Jap destroyer escort, a tanker, and a mine layer. We fired three torpedoes at the destroyer escort, but missed. Something went haywire in the mechanics of each torpedo. The destroyer, not knowing that she had been attacked, continued on. We were getting ready to attack the last ship, the mine layer, when suddenly she turned and came directly at us. (A Jap plane had spotted us under sixty feet of water and had radioed our position to the Jap mine layer.) We went down to 150 feet, to avoid detection, and rigged for a depth charge. We put extra bolts on the hatches; and, in order to make our sub absolutely silent, we turned off the fans, the cooling system, and all electrical gear.

"Three minutes later, all hell broke loose. Six depth charges exploded all around us and pushed us down to the ocean floor—a depth of 276 feet. We were terrified.

90

To be attacked in less than a thousand feet of water is dangerous—less than five hundred feet is almost always fatal. And we were being attacked in a trifle more than half of five hundred feet of water—just about knee-deep, as far as safety was concerned. For fifteen hours, that Jap mine layer kept dropping depth charges. If a depth charge explodes within seventeen feet of a sub, the concussion will blow a hole in it. Scores of these depth charges exploded within fifty feet of us. We were ordered 'to secure'—to lie quietly in our bunks and remain calm.

'I was so terrified I could hardly breathe. 'This is death,' I kept saying to myself over and over. 'This is death! ... This is death!' With the fans and cooling system turned off, the air inside the sub was over a hundred degrees; but I was so chilled with fear that I put on a sweater and a fur-lined jacket; and still I trembled with cold. My teeth chattered. I broke out in a cold, clammy sweat. The attack continued for fifteen hours. Then ceased suddenly. Apparently the Jap mine layer had exhausted its supply of depth charges, and steamed away. Those fifteen hours of attack seemed like fifteen million years. All my life passed before me in review. I remembered all the bad things I had done, all the little absurd things I had worried about. I had been a bank clerk before I joined the Navy. I had worried about the long hours, the poor pay, the poor prospects of advancement. I had worried because I couldn't own my own home, couldn't buy a new car, couldn't buy my wife nice clothes. How I had hated my old boss, who was always nagging and scolding! I remembered how I would come home at night sore and grouchy and quarrel with my wife over trifles. I had worried about a scar on my forehead—a nasty cut from an auto accident.

"How big all those worries seemed years ago! But how absurd they seemed when depth charges were threatening to blow me to kingdom come. I promised myself then and there that if I ever saw the sun and the stars again, I would never, never worry again. Never! Never!! Never!!! I learned more about the art of living in those fifteen terrible hours in that submarine than I had learned by studying books for four years in Syracuse University."

We often face the major disasters of life bravely—and then let the trifles, the "pains in the neck," get us down. For example, Samuel Pepys tells in his Diary about seeing Sir Harry Vane's head chopped off in London. As Sir Harry mounted the platform, he was not pleading for his life, but was pleading with the executioner not to hit the painful boil on his neck!

That was another thing that Admiral Byrd discovered down in the terrible cold and darkness of the polar nights—that his men fussed more about the "pains in the neck" than about the big things. They bore, without complaining, the dangers, the hardships, and the cold that was often eighty degrees below zero. "But," says Admiral Byrd, "I know of bunkmates who quit speaking because each suspected the other of inching his gear into the other's allotted space; and I knew of one who could not eat unless he could find a place in the mess hall out of sight of the Fletcherist who solemnly chewed his food twenty-eight times before swallowing.

"In a polar camp," says Admiral Byrd, "little things like that have the power to drive even disciplined men to the edge of insanity."

And you might have added, Admiral Byrd, that "little things" in marriage drive people to the edge of insanity and cause "half the heartaches in the world."

At least, that is what the authorities say. For example, Judge Joseph Sabath of Chicago, after acting as arbiter in more than forty thousand unhappy marriages, declared: "Trivialities are at the bottom of most marital unhappiness"; and Frank S. Hogan, District Attorney of New York County, says, "Fully half the cases in our criminal courts originate in little things. Barroom bravado, domestic wrangling, an insulting remark, a disparaging word, a rude action—those are the little things that lead to assault and murder. Very few of us are cruelly and greatly wronged. It is the small blows to our self-esteem, the indignities, the little jolts to our vanity, which cause half the heartaches in the world."

When Eleanor Roosevelt was first married, she "worried for days" because her new cook had served a poor meal. "But if that happened now," Mrs. Roosevelt says, "I would shrug my shoulders and forget it." Good. That is acting like an adult emotionally. Even Catherine the Great, an absolute autocrat, used to laugh the thing off when the cook spoiled a meal.

Mrs. Carnegie and I had dinner at a friend's house in Chicago. While carving the meat, he did something wrong. I didn't notice it; and I wouldn't have cared even if I had noticed it. But his wife saw it and jumped down his throat right in front of us. "John," she cried, "watch what you are doing! Can't you ever learn to serve properly!"

Then she said to us: "He is always making mistakes. He just doesn't try." Maybe he didn't try to carve; but I certainly give him credit for trying to live with her for twenty years. Frankly, I would rather have eaten a couple of hot dogs with mustard—in an atmosphere of peace—than to have dined on Peking duck and shark fins while listening to her scolding.

Shortly after that experience, Mrs. Carnegie and I had some friends at our home for dinner. Just before they arrived, Mrs. Carnegie found that three of the napkins didn't match the table-cloth.

"I rushed to the cook," she told me later, "and found that the other three napkins had gone to the laundry. The guests were at the door. There was no time to change. I felt like bursting into tears! All I could think was, 'Why did this stupid mistake have to spoil my whole evening?' Then I thought—well—why let it? I went in to dinner, determined to have a good time. And I did. I would much rather our friends think I was a sloppy housekeeper," she told me, "than a nervous, bad-tempered one. And anyhow, as far as I could make out, no one noticed the napkins!"

A well-known legal maxim says: *De minimis non curat lex*—"the law does not concern itself with trifles." And neither should the worrier—if he wants peace of mind.

Much of the time, all we need to overcome the annoyance of trifles is to affect a shifting of emphasis—set up a new, and pleasurable, point of view in the mind.

My friend Homer Croy, who wrote *They Had to See Paris* and a dozen other books, gives a wonderful example of how this can be done. He used to be driven half crazy, while working on a book, by the rattling of the radiators in his New York apartment. The steam would bang and sizzle—and he would sizzle with irritation as he sat at his desk.

"Then," says Homer Croy, "I went with some friends on a camping expedition. While listening to the limbs crackling in the roaring fire, I thought how much they sounded like the cracking of the radiators. Why should I like one and hate the other? When I went home I said to myself, 'The crackling of the limbs in the fire was a pleasant sound; the sound of the radiators is about the same—I'll go to sleep and not worry about the noise.' *And I did.* For a few days I was conscious of the radiators; but soon I forgot all about them.

"And so it is with many petty worries. We dislike them and get into a stew, all because we exaggerate their importance...."

Disraeli said: "Life is too short to be little." "Those words," said André Maurois in *This Week* magazine, "have helped me through many a painful experience: often we allow ourselves to be upset by small things we should despise and forget.... Here we are on this earth, with only a few more decades to live, and we lose many irreplaceable hours brooding over grievances that, in a year's time, will be forgotten by us and by everybody. No, let us devote our life to worth-while actions and feelings, to great thoughts, real affections and enduring undertakings. For life is too short to be little."

Even so illustrious a figure as Rudyard Kipling forgot at times that "Life is too short to be little." The result? He and his brother-in-law fought the most famous court battle in the history of Vermont—a battle so celebrated that a book has been written about it: *Rudyard Kipling's Vermont Feud*.

The story goes like this: Kipling married a Vermont girl, Caroline Balestier, built a lovely home in Brattleboro, Vermont; settled down and expected to spend the rest of his life there. His brother-in-law, Beatty Balestier, became Kipling's best friend. The two of them worked and played together.

Then Kipling bought some land from Balestier, with the understanding that Balestier would be allowed to cut hay off it each season. One day, Balestier found Kipling laying out a flower garden on this hayfield. His blood boiled. He hit the ceiling. Kipling fired right back. The air over the Green Mountains of Vermont turned blue!

A few days later, when Kipling was out riding his bicycle, his brother-in-law drove a wagon and a team of horses across the road suddenly and forced Kipling to take a spill. And Kipling—the man who wrote, "If you can keep your head when all about you are losing theirs and blaming it on you"—he lost his own head, and swore out a warrant for Balestier's arrest! A sensational trial followed. Reporters from the big cities poured into the town. The news flashed around the world. Nothing was settled. This quarrel caused Kipling and his wife to abandon their American home for the rest of their lives.

All that worry and bitterness over a mere trifle! A load of hay.

Pericles said, twenty-four centuries ago: "Come, gentlemen, we sit too long on trifles." We do, indeed!

Here is one of the most interesting stories that Dr. Harry Emerson Fosdick ever told—a story about the battles won and lost by a giant of the forest:

On the slope of Long's Peak in Colorado lies the ruin of a gigantic tree. Naturalists tell us that it stood for some four hundred years. It was a seedling when Columbus landed at San Salvador, and half grown when the Pilgrims settled at Plymouth. During the course of its long life it was struck by lightning fourteen times, and the innumerable avalanches and storms of four centuries thundered past it. It survived them all. In the end, however, an army of beetles attacked the tree and leveled it to the ground. The insects ate their way through the bark and gradually destroyed the inner strength of the tree by their tiny but incessant attacks. A forest giant which age had not withered, nor lightning blasted, nor storms subdued, fell at last before beetles so small that a man could crush them between his forefinger and his thumb.

Aren't we all like that battling giant of the forest? Don't we manage somehow to survive the rare storms and avalanches and lightning blasts of life, only to let our hearts be eaten out by little beetles of worry—little beetles that could be crushed between a finger and a thumb?

A few years ago, I traveled through the Teton National Park, in Wyoming, with Charles Seifred, highway superintendent for the state of Wyoming, and some of his friends. We were all going to visit the John D. Rockefeller estate in the park. But the car in which I was riding took the wrong turn, got lost, and drove up to the entrance of the estate an hour after the other cars had gone in. Mr. Seifred had the key that unlocked the private gate, so he waited in the hot, mosquito-infested woods for an hour until we arrived. The mosquitoes were enough to drive a saint insane. But they couldn't triumph over Charles Seifred. While waiting for us, he cut a limb off an aspen tree—and made a whistle of it. When we arrived, was he cussing the mosquitoes? No, he was playing his whistle. I have kept that whistle as a memento of a man who knew how to put trifles in their place.

To break the worry habit before it breaks you, here is Rule 2:

LET'S NOT ALLOW OURSELVES TO BE UPSET BY SMALL THINGS WE SHOULD DESPISE AND FORGET. REMEMBER "LIFE IS TOO SHORT TO BE LITTLE."

"When I let go of what I am, I become what I might be. When I let go of what I have, I receive what I need."

—Tao Te Ching

"I never worry about the problem. I worry about the solution."

—Shaquille O'Neal

9

A LAW THAT WILL OUTLAW
MANY OF YOUR WORRIES

As a child, I grew up on a Missouri farm; and one day, while helping my mother pit cherries, I began to cry. My mother said, "Dale, what in the world are you crying about?" I blubbered, "I'm afraid I am going to be buried alive!"

I was full of worries in those days. When thunderstorms came, I worried for fear I would be killed by lightning. When hard times came, I worried for fear we wouldn't have enough to eat. I worried for fear I would go to hell when I died. I was terrified for fear an older boy, Sam White, would cut off my big ears—as he threatened to do. I worried for fear girls would laugh at me if I tipped my hat to them. I worried for fear no girl would ever be willing to marry me. I worried about what I would say to my wife immediately after we were married. I imagined that we would be married in some country church, and then get in a surrey with fringe on the top and ride back to the farm …but how would I be able to keep the conversation going on that ride back to the farm? How? How? I pondered over that earth-shaking problem for many an hour as I walked behind the plow.

As the years went by, I gradually discovered that ninety-nine per cent of the things I worried about never happened.

For example, as I have already said, I was once terrified of lightning; but I now know that the chances of my being killed by lightning in any one year are, according to the National Safety Council, only one in three hundred and fifty thousand.

My fear of being buried alive was even more absurd: I don't imagine that—even back in the days before embalming was the rule—that one person in ten million was buried alive; yet I once cried for fear of it.

One person out of every eight dies of cancer. If I had wanted something to worry about, I should have worried about cancer—instead of being killed by lightning or being buried alive.

To be sure, I have been talking about the worries of youth and adolescence. But many of our adult worries are almost as absurd. You and I could probably eliminate nine tenths of our worries right now if we would cease our fretting long enough to discover whether, *by the law of averages,* there was any real justification for our worries.

The most famous insurance company on earth—Lloyd's of London—has made countless millions of dollars out of the tendency of everybody to worry about things that rarely happen. Lloyd's of London bets people that the disasters they are worrying about will never occur. However, *they don't call it betting. They call it insurance. But it is really betting based on the law of averages.* This great insurance firm has been going strong for two hundred years; and unless human nature changes, it will still be going strong fifty centuries from now by insuring shoes and ships and sealing wax against disasters that, *by the law of averages,* don't happen nearly so often as people imagine.

If we examine the law of averages, we will often be astounded at the facts we uncover. For example, if I knew that during the next five years I would have to fight in a battle as bloody as the Battle of Gettysburg, I would be terrified. I would take out all the life insurance I could get. I would draw up my will and set all my earthly affairs in order. I would say, "I'll probably never live through that battle, so I had better make the most of the few years I have left." Yet the facts are that, according to the law of averages, it is just as dangerous, just as fatal, to try to live from age fifty to age fifty-five in peacetime as it was to fight in the Battle of Gettysburg. What I am trying to say is this: in times of peace, just as many people die per thousand between the ages of fifty and fifty-five as were killed per thousand among the 163,000 soldiers who fought at Gettysburg.

I wrote several chapters of this book at James Simpson's Num-Ti-Gah Lodge, on the shore of Bow Lake in the Canadian Rockies. While stopping there one summer, I met Mr. and Mrs. Herbert H. Salinger, of 2298 Pacific Avenue, San Francisco. Mrs. Salinger, a poised, serene woman, gave me the impression that she had never worried. One evening in front of the roaring fireplace, I asked her if she had ever been troubled by worry. "Troubled by it?" she said.

"My life was almost *ruined* by it. Before I learned to conquer worry, I lived through eleven years of self-made hell. I was irritable and hot-tempered. I lived under terrific tension. I would take the bus every week from my home in San Mateo to shop in San Francisco. But even while shopping, I worried myself into a dither: maybe I had left the electric iron connected on the ironing board. Maybe the house had caught fire. Maybe the maid had run off and left the children. Maybe they had been out on their bicycles and been killed by a car. In the midst of my shopping, I would often worry myself into a cold perspiration and rush out and take the bus home to see if everything was all right. No wonder my first marriage ended in disaster.

"My second husband is a lawyer—a quiet, analytical man who never worries about anything. When I became tense and anxious, he would say to me, 'Relax. Let's think this out…. What are you really worrying about? Let's examine the law of averages and see whether or not it is likely to happen.'

"For example, I remember the time we were driving from Albuquerque, New Mexico, to the Carlsbad Caverns—driving on a dirt road—when we were caught in a terrible rainstorm.

"The car was slithering and sliding. We couldn't control it. I was positive we would slide off into one of the ditches that flanked the road; but my husband kept repeating to me: 'I am driving very slowly. Nothing serious is likely to happen. Even if the car does slide into the ditch, by the law of averages, we won't be hurt.' His calmness and confidence quieted me.

"One summer we were on a camping trip in the Touquin Valley of the Canadian Rockies. One night, we were camping seven thousand feet above sea level, when a storm threatened to tear our tents to shreds. The tents were tied with guy ropes to a wooden platform. The outer tent shook and trembled and screamed and shrieked in the wind. I expected every minute to see our tent torn loose and hurled through the sky. I was terrified! But my husband kept saying: 'Look, my dear, we are traveling with Brewsters' guides. Brewsters know what they are doing. They have been pitching tents in these mountains for sixty years. This tent has been here for many seasons. It hasn't blown down yet and, by the law of averages, it won't blow away tonight; and even if it does, we can take shelter in another tent. So relax.... I did; and I slept soundly the balance of the night.

"A few years ago an infantile-paralysis epidemic swept over our part of California. In the old days, I would have been hysterical. But my husband persuaded me to act calmly. We took all the precautions we could: we kept our children away from crowds, away from school and the movies. By consulting the Board of Health, we found out that even during the worst infantile-paralysis epidemic that California had ever known up to that time, only 1835 children had been stricken in the entire state of California. And that the usual number was around two hundred or three hundred. Tragic as those figures are, we nevertheless felt that, according to the law of averages, the chances of any one child being stricken were remote.

"'By the law of averages, it won't happen.' That phrase has destroyed ninety per cent of my worries; and it has made the past twenty years of my life beautiful and peaceful beyond my highest expectations."

General George Crook—probably the greatest Indian fighter in American history—says on page 77 of his *Autobiography* that "nearly all the worries and unhappiness" of the Indians "came from their imagination, and not from reality."

As I look back across the decades, I can see that that is where most of my worries came from also. Jim Grant told me that that had been his experience, too. He owns the James A. Grant Distributing Company, 204 Franklin Street, New York City. He orders from ten to fifteen carloads of Florida oranges and grapefruit at a time. He told me that he used to torture himself with such thoughts as: What if there's a train wreck? What if my fruit is strewn all over the countryside? What if a bridge collapses as my cars are going across it? Of course, the fruit was insured; but he feared that if he didn't deliver his fruit on time, he might risk the loss of his market. He worried so much that he feared he had stomach ulcers and went to a doctor. The doctor told him there was nothing wrong with him except jumpy nerves. "I saw the light then," he said, "and began to ask myself questions. I said to myself: 'Look here, Jim Grant, how many fruit cars have you handled over the years?' The answer was: 'About twenty-five thousand.' Then I asked myself: 'How many of those cars were ever wrecked?' The answer was: 'Oh—maybe five.' Then I said to myself: 'Only five—out of twenty-five thousand? Do you know what that means? A ratio of five thousand to one! In other words, by the law of averages, based on experience, the chances are five thousand to one against one of your cars ever being wrecked. So what are you worried about?'

"Then I said to myself: 'Well, a bridge may collapse!' Then I asked myself: 'How many cars have you actually lost from a bridge collapsing?' The answer was—'None.' Then I said to myself: 'Aren't you a fool to be worrying yourself into stomach ulcers over a bridge which has never yet collapsed, and over a railroad wreck when the chances are five thousand to one against it!'

"When I looked at it that way," Jim Grant told me, "I felt pretty silly. I decided then and there to let the law of averages do the worrying for me—and I have not been troubled with my 'stomach ulcer' since!"

When Al Smith was Governor of New York, I heard him answer the attacks of his political enemies by saying over and over: "Let's examine the record ... let's examine the record." Then he proceeded to give the facts. The next time you and I are worrying about what may happen, let's take a tip from wise old Al Smith: "let's examine the record and see what basis there is, if any, for our gnawing anxieties." That is precisely what Frederick J. Mahlstedt did when he feared he was lying in his grave. Here is his story as he told it to one of our adult-education classes in New York:

"Early in June, 1944, I was lying in a slit trench near Omaha Beach. I was with the 999th Signal Service Company, and we had just 'dug in' in Normandy. As I looked around at that slit trench—just a rectangular hole in the ground—I said to myself, 'This looks just like a grave.' When I lay down and tried to sleep in it, it felt like a grave. I couldn't help saying to myself, *'Maybe this is my grave.'* When the German bombers began coming over at 11 p.m., and the bombs started falling, I was scared stiff. For the first two or three nights I couldn't sleep at all. By the fourth or fifth night, I was almost a nervous wreck. I knew that if I didn't do something, I would go stark crazy. So I reminded myself that five nights had passed, and I was still alive; and so was every man in our outfit. Only two had even been injured, and they had been hurt, not by German bombs, but by falling flak, from our own antiaircraft guns.

I decided to stop worrying by doing something constructive. So I built a thick wooden roof over my slit trench, to protect myself from flak. I thought of the vast area over which my unit was spread. I told myself that the only way I could be killed in that deep, narrow slit trench was by a direct hit; and I figured out that the chance of a direct hit on me was not one in ten thousand. After a couple of nights of looking at it in this way, I calmed down and slept even through the bomb raids!"

The United States Navy used the statistics of the law of averages to buck up the morale of their men. One ex-sailor told me that when he and his shipmates were assigned to high-octane tankers, they were worried stiff. They all believed that if a tanker loaded with high-octane gasoline was hit by a torpedo, it exploded and blew everybody to kingdom come.

But the U.S. Navy knew otherwise; so the Navy issued exact figures, showing that out of one hundred tankers hit by torpedoes, sixty stayed afloat; and of the forty that did sink, only five sank in less than ten minutes. That meant time to get off the ship—it also meant casualties were exceedingly small. Did this help morale? "This knowledge of the law of averages wiped out my jitters," said Clyde W. Maas, of 1969 Walnut Street, St. Paul, Minnesota—the man who told this story. "The whole crew felt better. We knew we had a chance; and that, by the law of averages, we probably wouldn't be killed."

To break the worry habit before it breaks you—here is Rule 3:

"LET'S EXAMINE THE RECORD." LET'S ASK OURSELVES: "WHAT ARE THE CHANCES, ACCORDING TO THE LAW OF AVERAGES, THAT THIS EVENT I AM WORRYING ABOUT WILL EVER OCCUR?"

"The greatest weapon against stress is our ability to choose one thought over another."
—William James

"When you begin to worry, go find something to do."
—Joyce Meyer

10

CO-OPERATE WITH THE INEVITABLE

When I was a little boy, I was playing with some of my friends in the attic of an old, abandoned log house in northwest Missouri. As I climbed down out of the attic, I rested my feet on a window sill for a moment—and then jumped. I had a ring on my left fore-finger; and as I jumped, the ring caught on a nailhead and tore off my finger.

I screamed. I was terrified. I was positive I was going to die. But after the hand healed, I never worried about it for one split second. What would have been the use? ... I accepted the inevitable.

Now I often go for a month at a time without even thinking about the fact that I have only three fingers and a thumb on my left hand.

A few years ago, I met a man who was running a freight elevator in one of the downtown office buildings in New York. I noticed that his left hand had been cut off at the wrist. I asked him if the loss of that hand bothered him. He said, "Oh, no, I hardly ever think about it. I am not married; and the only time I ever think about it is when I try to thread a needle."

It is astonishing how quickly we can accept almost any situation—if we have to—and adjust ourselves to it and forget about it.

I often think of an inscription on the ruins of a

fifteenth-century cathedral in Amsterdam, Holland. This inscription says in Flemish: "It is so. It cannot be otherwise."

As you and I march across the decades of time, we are going to meet a lot of unpleasant situations that are so. They cannot be otherwise. We have our choice. We can either accept them as inevitable and adjust ourselves to them, or we can ruin our lives with rebellion and maybe end up with a nervous breakdown.

Here is a bit of sage advice from one of my favorite philosophers, William James. "*Be willing to* have *it* so," he said. "*Acceptance of what has happened is the first step to overcoming the consequences of any misfortune.*" Elizabeth Connley, of 2840 NE 49th Avenue, Portland, Oregon, had to find that out the hard way. Here is a letter that she wrote me recently: "On the very day that America was celebrating the victory of our armed forces in North Africa," the letter says, "I received a telegram from the War Department: my nephew—the person I loved most—was missing in action. A short time later, another telegram arrived saying he was dead.

"I was prostrate with grief. Up to that time, I had felt that life had been very good to me. I had a job I loved. I had helped to raise this nephew. He represented to me all that was fine and good in young manhood. I had felt that all the bread I had cast upon the waters was coming back to me as cake! ... Then came this telegram. My whole world collapsed. I felt there was nothing left to live for. I neglected my work; neglected my friends. I let everything go. I was bitter and resentful. Why did my loving nephew have to be taken? Why did this good boy—with life all before him—why did he have to be killed? I couldn't accept it. My grief was so over-whelming that I decided to give up my work, and go away and hide myself in my tears and bitterness.

"I was clearing out my desk, getting ready to quit, when I came across a letter that I had forgotten—a letter from this nephew who had been killed, a letter he had written to me when my mother had died a few years ago. 'Of course, we will all miss her,' the letter said, 'and especially you. But I know you'll carry on. Your own personal philosophy will make you do that. I shall never forget the beautiful truths you taught me. Wherever I am, or how far apart we may be, I shall always remember that you taught me to smile, and to take whatever comes, like a man.'

"I read and reread that letter. It seemed as if he were there beside me, speaking to me. He seemed to be saying to me: 'Why don't you do what you taught me to do? Carry on, no matter what happens. Hide your private sorrows under a smile and carry on.'

"So, I went back to my work. I stopped being bitter and re-bellious. I kept saying to myself: 'It is done. I can't change it. But I can and will carry on as he wished me to do. I threw all my mind and strength into my work. I wrote letters to soldiers—to other people's boys. I joined an adult-education class at night—seeking out new interests and making new friends. I can hardly believe the change that has come over me. I have ceased mourning over the past that is forever gone. I am living each day now with joy—just as my nephew would have wanted me to do. I have made peace with life. I have accepted my fate. I am now living a fuller and more complete life than I have ever known."

Elizabeth Connley, out in Portland, Oregon, learned what all of us will have to learn sooner or later: namely, that we must accept and co-operate with the inevitable. "It is so. It cannot be otherwise." That is not an easy lesson to learn. Even kings on their thrones have to keep reminding themselves of it. The late George V had these framed words hanging on the wall of his library in Buckingham Palace: "Teach me neither to cry for the moon nor over spilt milk." The same thought is expressed by Schopenhauer in this way: "A good supply of resignation is of the first importance in providing for the journey of life."

Obviously, circumstances alone do not make us happy or unhappy. It is the way we react to circumstances that determines our feelings. Jesus said that the kingdom of heaven is within you. That is where the kingdom of hell is, too.

We can all endure disaster and tragedy and triumph over them—if we have to. We may not think we can, but we have surprisingly strong inner resources that will see us through if we will only make use of them. We are stronger than we think.

The late Booth Tarkington always said: "I could take anything that life could force upon me except one thing: blindness. I could never endure that."

Then one day, when he was along in his sixties,

Tarkington glanced down at the carpet on the floor. The colors were blurred. He couldn't see the pattern. He went to a specialist. He learned the tragic truth: he was losing his sight. One eye was nearly blind; the other would follow. That which he feared most had come upon him.

And how did Tarkington react to this "worst of all disasters"? Did he feel, "This is it! This is the end of my life"? No, to his amazement, he felt quite gay. He even called upon his humor. Floating "specks" annoyed him; they would swim across his eyes and cut off his vision. Yet when the largest of these specks would swim across his sight, he would say, "Hello! There's Grandfather again! Wonder where he's going on this fine morning!"

How could fate ever conquer a spirit like that? The answer is it couldn't. When total darkness closed in, Tarkington said, "I found I could take the loss of my eyesight, just as a man can take anything else. If I lost *all five* of my senses, I know I could live on inside my mind. For it is in the mind we see, and in the mind we live, whether we know it or not."

In the hope of restoring his eyesight, Tarkington had to go through more than twelve operations within one year. With *local* anesthetic! Did he rail against this? He knew it had to be done. He knew he couldn't escape it, so the only way to lessen his suffering was to take it with grace. He refused a private room at the hospital and went into a ward, where he could be with other people who had troubles, too. He tried to cheer them up. And when he had to submit to repeated operations—fully conscious of what was being done to his eyes—he tried to remember how fortunate he was. "How wonderful!" he said. "How wonderful, that science now has the skill to operate on anything so delicate as the human eye!" The average man would have been a nervous wreck if he had had to endure more than twelve operations and blindness. Yet Tarkington said, "I would not exchange this experience for a happier one." It taught him acceptance. It taught him that nothing life could bring him was beyond his strength to endure. It taught him, as John Milton discovered, that "It is not miserable to be blind, it is only miserable not to be able to endure blindness." Margaret Fuller, the famous New England feminist, once offered as her credo: "I accept the Universe!"

When grouchy old Thomas Carlyle heard that in England, he snorted, "By gad, she'd better!" Yes, and by gad, you and I had better accept the inevitable, too!

If we rail and kick against it and grow bitter, we won't change the inevitable; but we will change ourselves. I know. I have tried it.

I once refused to accept an inevitable situation with which I was confronted. I played the fool and railed against it, and rebelled. I turned my nights into hells of insomnia. I brought upon myself everything I didn't want. Finally, after a year of self-torture, I had to accept what I knew from the outset I couldn't possibly alter.

I should have cried out years ago with old Walt Whitman:

Oh, to confront night, storms, hunger,
Ridicule, accident, rebuffs as the trees and animals do.

I spent twelve years working with cattle; yet I never

saw a Jersey cow running a temperature because the pasture was burning up from a lack of rain or because of sleet and cold or because her boyfriend was paying too much attention to another heifer. The animals confront night, storms, and hunger calmly; so they never have nervous breakdowns or stomach ulcers; and they never go insane.

Am I advocating that we simply bow down to *all* the adversities that come our way? Not by a long shot! That is mere fatalism. As long as there is a chance that we can save a situation, let's fight! But when common sense tells us that we are up against something that is so—and cannot be otherwise—then, in the name of our sanity, let's not "look before and after and pine for what is not." The late Dean Hawkes of Columbia University told me that he had taken a Mother Goose rhyme as one of his mottoes:

For every ailment under the sun,
There is a remedy, or there is none;
If there be one, try to find it;
If there be none, never mind it.

While writing this book, I interviewed a number of the leading businessmen of America; and I was impressed by the fact that they co-operated with the inevitable and led lives singularly free from worry. If they hadn't done that, they would have cracked under the strain. Here are a few examples of what I mean:

J.C. Penney, founder of the nation-wide chain of Penney stores, said to me: "I wouldn't worry if I lost every dollar I have because I don't see what is to be gained by worrying. I do the best job I possibly can; and leave the results in the laps of the gods."

Henry Ford told me much the same thing. "When I can't handle events," he said, "I let them handle themselves."

When I asked K.T. Keller, president of the Chrysler Corporation, how he kept from worrying, he replied: "When I am up against a tough situation, if I can do anything about it, I do it. If I can't, I just forget it. I never worry about the future, because I know no man living can possibly figure out what is going to happen in the future. There are so many forces that will affect that future! Nobody can tell what prompts those forces—or understand them. So why worry about them?" K.T. Keller would be embarrassed if you told him he is a philosopher. He is just a good businessman, yet he has stumbled on the same philosophy that Epictetus taught in Rome nineteen centuries ago. "There is only one way to happiness," Epictetus taught the Romans, "and that is to cease worrying about things which are beyond the power of our will."

Sarah Bernhardt, the "divine Sarah," was an illustrious example of a woman who knew how to co-operate with the inevitable. For half a century, she had been the reigning queen of the theater on four continents—the best-loved actress on earth. Then when she was seventy-one and broke—she had lost all her money—her physician, Professor Pozzi of Paris, told her he would have to amputate her leg. While crossing the Atlantic, she had fallen on deck during a storm, and injured her leg severely.

Phlebitis developed. Her leg shrank. The pain became so intense that the doctor felt her leg had to be amputated. He was almost afraid to tell the stormy, tempestuous "divine Sarah" what had to be done. He fully expected that the terrible news would set off an explosion of hysteria. But he was wrong. Sarah looked at him a moment, and then said quietly, "If it has to be, it has to be." It was fate.

As she was being wheeled away to the operating room, her son stood weeping. She waved to him with a gay gesture and said cheer-fully: "Don't go away. I'll be right back."

On the way to the operating room she recited a scene from one of her plays. Someone asked her if she were doing this to cheer herself up. She said: "No, to cheer up the doctors and nurses. It will be a strain on them."

After recovering from the operation, Sarah Bernhardt went on touring the world and enchanting audiences for another seven years.

"When we stop fighting the inevitable," said Elsie MacCormick in *a Reader's Digest* article, "we release energy which enables us to create a richer life."

No one living has enough emotion and vigor to *fight* the inevitable and, at the same time, enough left over to create a new life. Choose one or the other. You can either bend with the inevitable sleetstorms of life—or you can resist them and break!

I saw that happen on a farm I own in Missouri. I planted a score of trees on that farm. At first, they grew with astonishing rapidity. Then a sleetstorm encrusted each twig and branch with a heavy coating of ice. Instead of bowing gracefully to their burden, these trees proudly resisted and broke and split under the load—and had to be destroyed. They hadn't learned the wisdom of the forests of the North. I have traveled hundreds of miles through the evergreen forests of Canada, yet I have never seen a spruce or a pine broken by sleet or ice. These evergreen forests know how to bend, how to bow down their branches, how to co-operate with the inevitable.

The masters of jujitsu teach their pupils to "bend like the willow; don't resist like the oak."

Why do you think your automobile tires stand up on the road and take so much punishment? At first, the tire manufacturers tried to make a tire that would resist the shocks of the road. It was soon cut to ribbons. Then they made a tire that would absorb the shocks of the road. That tire could "take it." You and I will last longer, and enjoy smoother riding, if we learn to absorb the shocks and jolts along the rocky road of life.

What will happen to you and me if we resist the shocks of life instead of absorbing them? What will happen if we refuse to "bend like the willow" and insist on resisting like the oak? The answer is easy. We will set up a series of inner conflicts. We will be worried, tense, strained, and neurotic.

If we go still further and reject the harsh world of reality and retreat into a dream world of our own making, we will then be insane.

During the war, millions of frightened soldiers had either to accept the inevitable or break under the strain. To illustrate, let's take the case of William H. Casselius,

7126 67th Street, Glendale, New York. Here is a prize-winning talk he gave before one of my adult-education classes in New York:

"Shortly after I joined the Coast Guard, I was assigned to one of the hottest spots on this side of the Atlantic. I was made a supervisor of explosives. Imagine it. Me! A cracker salesman becoming a supervisor of explosives! The very thought of finding yourself standing on top of thousands of tons of TNT is enough to chill the marrow in a cracker salesman's bones. I was given only two days of instruction; and what I learned filled me with even more terror. I'll never forget my first assignment. On a dark, cold, foggy day, I was given my orders on the open pier of Caven Point, Bayonne, New Jersey.

"I was assigned to Hold No. 5 on my ship. I had to work down in that hold with five longshoremen. They had strong backs, but they knew nothing whatever about explosives. And they were loading blockbusters, each one of which contained a ton of TNT—enough explosive to blow that old ship to kingdom come. These blockbusters were being lowered by two cable slings. I kept saying to myself: Suppose one of those cables slipped—or broke! Oh, boy! Was I scared! I trembled. My mouth was dry. My knees sagged. My heart pounded. But I couldn't run away. That would be desertion. I would be disgraced— my parents would be disgraced—and I might be shot for desertion. I couldn't run. I had to stay. I kept looking at the careless way those longshoremen were handling those blockbusters. The ship might blow up any minute. After an hour or more of this spine-chilling terror, I began to use a little common sense. I gave myself a good talking to. I said, 'Look here! So you are blown up. So what! You will never know the difference! It will be an easy way to die. Much better than dying by cancer. Don't be a fool. You can't expect to live forever! You've got to do this job—or be shot. So you might as well like it.'

"I talked to myself like that for hours; and I began to feel at ease. Finally, I overcame my worry and fears by forcing myself to accept an inevitable situation.

"I'll never forget that lesson. Every time I am tempted now to worry about something I can't possibly change, I shrug my shoulders and say, 'Forget it.' I find that it works—even for a cracker salesman." Hooray! Let's give three cheers and one cheer more for the cracker salesman of the *Pinafore*.

Outside the crucifixion of Jesus, the most famous death scene in all history was the death of Socrates. Ten thousand centuries from now, men will still be reading and cherishing Plato's immortal description of it—one of the most moving and beautiful passages in all literature. Certain men of Athens—jealous and envious of old barefooted Socrates—trumped up charges against him and had him tried and condemned to death. When the friendly jailer gave Socrates the poison cup to drink, the jailer said: "*Try to bear lightly what needs must be.*" Socrates did. He faced death with a calmness and resignation that touched the hem of divinity.

"*Try to bear lightly what needs must be.*" Those words were spoken 399 years before Christ was born; but this worrying old world needs those words today more than ever before: *"Try to bear lightly what needs must be."*

During the past eight years, I have been reading practically every book and magazine article I could find that dealt even remotely with banishing worry.... Would you like to know what is the best single bit of advice about worry that I have ever discovered in all that reading? Well, here it is—summed up in twenty-seven words— words that you and I ought to paste on our bathroom mirrors, so that each time we wash our faces we could also wash away all worry from our minds. This priceless prayer was written by Dr. Reinhold Niebuhr, Professor of Applied Christianity, Union Theoogical Seminary, Broadway at 120th Street, New York.

God grant me the serenity
To accept the things I cannot change;
The courage to change the things I can;
And the wisdom to know the difference.

To break the worry habit before it breaks you, Rule 4 is:

CO-OPERATE WITH THE INEVITABLE.

"Stress is the trash of modern life—we all generate it but if you don't dispose of it properly, it will pile up and overtake your life."

—Terri Guillemets

"By forgetting the past and by throwing myself into other interests, I forget to worry."

—Jack Dempsey

11

PUT A "STOP-LOSS" ORDER ON
YOUR WORRIES

Would you like to know how to make money in Wall Street? Well, so would a million other people—and if I knew the answer, this book would sell for ten thousand dollars a copy. However, there's one good idea that some successful operators use. This story was told to me by Charles Roberts, an investment counselor with offices at 17 East 42nd Street, New York.

"I originally came to New York from Texas with twenty thousand dollars which my friends had given me to invest in the stock market," Charles Roberts told me. "I thought," he continued, "that I knew the ropes in the stock market; but I lost every cent. True, I made a lot of profit on some deals; but I ended up by losing everything.

"I did not mind so much losing my own money," Mr. Roberts explained, "but I felt terrible about having lost my friends' money, even though they could well afford it. I dreaded facing them again after our venture had turned out so unfortunately, but, to my astonishment, they not only were good sports about it, but proved to be incurable optimists.

"I knew I had been trading on a hit-or-miss basis and depending largely on luck and other people's opinions. As H. I. Phillips said, I had been 'playing the stock market by ear.'

"I began to think over my mistakes and I was determined that before I went back into the market again, I would try to find out what it was all about. So I sought out and became acquainted with one of the most successful speculators who ever lived: Burton S. Castles. I believed I could learn a great deal from him because he had long enjoyed the reputation of being successful year after year and I knew that such a career was not the result of mere chance or luck.

"He asked me a few questions about how I had traded before and then told me what I believe is the most important principle in trading. He said, 'I put a stop-loss order on every market commitment I make. If I buy a stock at, say, fifty dollars a share, I immediately place a stop-loss order on it at forty-five.' That means that when and if the stock should decline as much as five points below its cost, it would be sold automatically, thereby limiting the loss to five points.

"'If your commitments are intelligently made in the first place,' the old master continued, 'your profits will average ten, twenty-five, or even fifty points. Consequently, by limiting your losses to five points, you can be wrong more than half of the time and still make plenty of money.'

"I adopted that principle immediately and have used it ever since. It has saved my clients and me many thousands of dollars.

"After a while I realized that the stop-loss principle could be used in other ways besides in the stock market. I began to place stop-loss orders on other worries besides financial ones. I began to place a stop-loss order on any and every kind of annoyance and resentment that came to me. It has worked like magic.

"For example, I often have a luncheon date with a friend who is rarely on time. In the old days, he used to keep me stewing around for half my lunch hour before he showed up. Finally, I told him about my stop-loss orders on my worries. I said, 'Bill, my stop-loss order on waiting for you is exactly ten minutes. If you arrive more than ten minutes late, our luncheon engagement will be sold down the river—and I'll be gone.'"

Man how I wish I had had the sense, years ago, to put stop-loss orders on my impatience, on my temper, on my desire for self-justification, on my regrets, and on all my mental and emotional strains. Why didn't I have the horse sense to size up each situation that threatened to destroy my peace of mind and say to myself: "See here, Dale Carnegie, this situation is worth just so much fussing about—and no more"? …Why didn't I?

However, I must give myself credit for a little sense on one occasion, at least. And it was a serious occasion, too—a crisis in my life—when I stood watching my dreams and my plans for the future and the work of years vanish into thin air. It happened like this. In my early thirties, I had decided to spend my life writing novels. I was going to be a second Frank Norris or Jack London or Thomas Hardy. I was so in earnest that I spent two years in Europe—where I could live cheaply with dollars during the period of wild, printing-press money that followed the First World War. I spent two years there, writing my magnum opus. I called it *The Blizzard.* The title was a natural, for the reception it got among publishers was as cold as any blizzard that ever howled across the plains of the Dakotas. When my literary agent told me it was worthless, that I had no gift, no talent, for fiction, my heart almost stopped. I left his office in a daze. I couldn't have been more stunned if he had hit me across the head with a club. I was stupefied. I realized that I was standing at the crossroads of life, and had to make a tremendous decision. What should I do? Which way should I turn? Weeks passed before I came out of the daze. At that time, I had never heard of the phrase "put a stop-loss order on your worries." But as I look back now, I can see that I did just that. I wrote off my two years of sweating over that novel for just what they were worth—a noble experiment—and went forward from there. I re- turned to my work of organizing and teaching adult-education classes, and wrote biographies in my spare time— biographies and non-fiction books such as the one you are reading now.

Am I glad now that I made that decision? Glad? Every time I think about it now I feel like dancing in the street for sheer joy!

I can honestly say that I have never spent a day or an hour since, lamenting the fact that I am not another Thomas Hardy.

One night a century ago, when a screech owl was screeching in the woods along the shores of Walden Pond, Henry Thoreau dipped his goose quill into his homemade ink and wrote in his diary: "The cost of a thing is the amount of what I call life, which is required to be exchanged for it immediately or in the long run."

To put it another way: we are fools when we overpay for a thing in terms of what it takes out of our very existence.

Yet that is precisely what Gilbert and Sullivan did. They knew how to create gay words and gay music, but they knew distressingly little about how to create gaiety in their own lives. They created some of the loveliest light operas that ever delighted the world: *Patience*, *Pinafore*, *The Mikado*. But they couldn't control their tempers. They embittered their years over nothing more than the price of a carpet! Sullivan ordered a new carpet for the theater they had bought. When Gilbert saw the bill, he hit the roof. They battled it out in court, and never spoke to one another again as long as they lived. When Sullivan wrote the music for a new production, he mailed it to Gilbert; and when Gilbert wrote the words, he mailed them back to Sullivan. Once they had to take a curtain call together, but they stood on opposite sides of the stage and bowed in different directions, so they wouldn't see one another. They hadn't the sense to put a stop-loss order on their resentments, as Lincoln did.

Once, during the Civil War, when some of Lincoln's friends were denouncing his bitter enemies, Lincoln said, "You have more of a feeling of personal resentment than I have. Perhaps I have too little of it; but I never thought it paid. A man doesn't have the time to spend half his life in quarrels. If any man ceases to attack me, I never remember the past against him."

I wish an old aunt of mine—Aunt Edith—had had Lincoln's forgiving spirit. She and Uncle Frank lived on a mortgaged farm that was infested with cockleburs and cursed with poor soil and ditches. They had tough going—had to squeeze every nickel. But Aunt Edith loved to buy a few curtains and other small items to brighten up their bare home. She bought these small luxuries on credit at Dan Eversole's drygoods store in Maryville, Missouri. Uncle Frank worried about their debts. He had a farmer's horror of running up bills, so he secretly told Dan Eversole to stop letting his wife buy on credit. When she heard that, she hit the roof—and she was still hitting the roof about it almost fifty years after it had happened. I have heard her tell the story—not once, but many times. The last time I ever saw her, she was in her late seventies. I said to her, "Aunt Edith, Uncle Frank did wrong to humiliate you; but don't you honestly feel that your complaining about it almost half a century after it happened is infinitely worse than what he did?" (I might as well have said it to the moon.)

Aunt Edith paid dearly for the grudge and bitter memories that she nourished. She paid for them with her own peace of mind.

When Benjamin Franklin was seven years old, he made a mistake that he remembered for seventy years. When he was a lad of seven, he fell in love with a whistle. He was so excited about it that he went into the toyshop, piled all his coppers on the counter, and demanded the whistle without even asking its price. "I then came home," he wrote to a friend seventy years later, "and went whistling all over the house, much pleased with my whistle." But when his older brothers and sisters found out that he had paid far more for his whistle than he should have paid, they gave him the horse laugh; and, as he said, "I cried with vexation."

Years later, when Franklin was a world-famous figure, and Ambassador to France, he still remembered that the fact that he had paid too much for his whistle had caused him "more chagrin than the whistle gave him pleasure."

But the lesson it taught Franklin was cheap in the end. "As I grew up," he said, "and came into the world and observed the actions of men, I thought I met with many, very many, who gave *too much for the whistle*. In short, I conceive that a great part of the miseries of mankind are brought upon them by the false estimates they have made of the value of things, and by their *giving too much for their whistles.*"

Gilbert and Sullivan paid too much for their whistle. So did Aunt Edith. So did Dale Carnegie—on many occasions. And so did the immortal Leo Tolstoy, author of two of the world's greatest novels, *War and Peace* and *Anna Karenina.* According to *The Encyclopadia Britannica*, Leo Tolstoy was, during the last twenty years of his life, "probably the most venerated man in the whole world." For twenty years before he died—from 1890 to 1910—an unending stream of admirers made pilgrimages to his home in order to catch a glimpse of his face, to hear the sound of his voice, or even touch the hem of his garment. Every sentence he uttered was taken down in a notebook, almost as if it were a "divine revelation." But when it came to living—to ordinary living—well, Tolstoy had even less sense at seventy than Franklin had at seven! He had no sense at all.

Here's what I mean. Tolstoy married a girl he loved very dearly. In fact, they were so happy together that they used to get on their knees and pray to God to let them continue their lives in such sheer, heavenly ecstasy. But the girl Tolstoy married was jealous by nature.

She used to dress herself up as a peasant and spy on his movements, even out in the woods. They had fearful rows. She became so jealous, even of her own children, that she grabbed a gun and shot a hole in her daughter's photograph. She even rolled on the floor with an opium bottle held to her lips, and threatened to commit suicide, while the children huddled in a corner of the room and screamed with terror.

And what did Tolstoy do? Well, I don't blame the man for smashing up the furniture—he had good provocation. But he did far worse than that. He kept a private diary! Yes, a diary, in which he placed all the blame on his wife! That was his "whistle"! He was determined to make sure that coming generations would exonerate him and put the blame on his wife. And what did his wife do, in answer to this? Why, she tore pages out of his diary and burned them, of course. She started a diary of her own, in which she made *him* the villain. She even wrote a novel, entitled *Whose Fault?*, in which she depicted her husband as a household fiend and herself as a martyr.

All to what end? Why did these two people turn the only home they had into what Tolstoy himself called "a lunatic asylum"? Obviously, there were several reasons. One of those was their burning desire to impress you and me. Yes, we are the posterity whose opinion they were worried about! Do we give a hoot in Hades about which one was to blame? No, we are too concerned with our own problems to waste a minute thinking about the Tolstoys. What a price these two wretched people paid for their whistle! Fifty years of living in a veritable hell—just because neither of them had the sense to say, "Stop!" Because neither of them had enough judgment of values to say, "Let's put a stop-loss order on this thing instantly. We are squandering our lives. Let's say 'Enough' now!"

Yes, I honestly believe that this is one of the greatest secrets to true peace of mind—a decent sense of values. And I believe we could annihilate fifty percent of all our worries at once if we would develop a sort of private gold standard—a gold standard of what things are worth to us in terms of our lives.

So, to break the worry habit before it breaks you, here is Rule 5:

Whenever we are tempted to throw good money after bad in terms of human living, let's stop and ask ourselves these three questions:

How much does this thing I am worrying about really matter to me?

At what point shall I set a "stop-loss" order on this worry—and forget it?

Exactly how much shall I pay for this whistle? Have I already paid more than it is worth?

"Let yourself be open and life will be easier. A spoon of salt in a glass of water makes the water undrinkable. A spoon of salt in a lake is almost unnoticed."

—The Buddha

"As a rule, men worry more about what they can't see than about what they can."

—Julius Caesar

12

DON'T TRY TO SAW SAWDUST

As I write this sentence, I can look out of my window and see some dinosaur tracks in my garden—dinosaur tracks embedded in shale and stone. I purchased those dinosaur tracks from the Peabody Museum of Yale University; and I have a letter from the curator of the Peabody Museum, saying that those tracks were made 180 million years ago. Even a Mongolian idiot wouldn't dream of trying to go back 180 million years to change those tracks. Yet that would not be any more foolish than worrying because we can't go back and change what happened 180 seconds ago—and a lot of us are doing just that. To be sure, we may do something to *modify the effects* of what happened 180 seconds ago; but we can't possibly change the event that occurred then.

There is only one way on God's green footstool that the past can be constructive; and that is by calmly analyzing our past mistakes and profiting by them—and forgetting them.

I know that is true; but have I always had the courage and sense to do it? To answer that question, let me tell you about a fantastic experience I had years ago. I let more than three hundred thousand dollars slip through my fingers without making a penny's profit. It happened like this: I launched a large-scale enterprise in adult education, opened branches in various cities, and spent money lavishly in overhead and advertising. I was so busy with teaching that I had neither the time nor the desire to look after finances. I was too naïve to realize that I needed an astute business manager to watch expenses.

Finally, after about a year, I discovered a sobering and shocking truth. I discovered that in spite of our enormous intake, we had not netted any profit whatever. After discovering that, I should have done two things. First, I should have had the sense to do what George Washington Carver, the Negro scientist, did when he lost forty thousand dollars in a bank crash—the savings of a lifetime. When someone asked him if he knew he was bankrupt, he replied, "Yes, I heard"—and went on with his teaching. He wiped the loss out of his mind so completely that he never mentioned it again.

Here is the second thing I should have done: I should have analyzed my mistakes and learned a lasting lesson.

But frankly, I didn't do either one of these things. Instead, I went into a tailspin of worry. For months I was in a daze. I lost sleep and I lost weight. Instead of learning a lesson from this enormous mistake, I went right ahead and did the same thing again on a smaller scale!

It is embarrassing for me to admit all this stupidity; but I discovered long ago that "it is easier to teach twenty what were good to be done than to be one of the twenty to follow mine own teaching."

How I wish that I had had the privilege of attending the George Washington High School here in New York and studying under Mr. Brandwine—the same teacher who taught Allen Saunders, of 939 Woodycrest Avenue,

Bronx, New York!

Mr. Saunders told me that the teacher of his hygiene class, Mr. Brandwine, taught him one of the most valuable lessons he had ever learned. "I was only in my teens," said Allen Saunders as he told me the story, "but I was a worrier even then. I used to stew and fret about the mistakes I had made. If I turned in an examination paper, I used to lie awake and chew my fingernails for fear I hadn't passed. I was always living over the things I had done, and wishing I'd done them differently; thinking over the things I had said, and wishing I'd said them better.

"Then one morning, our class filed into the science laboratory, and there was the teacher, Mr. Brandwine, with a bottle of milk prominently displayed on the edge of the desk. We all sat down, staring at the milk, and wondering what it had to do with the hygiene course he was teaching. Then, all of a sudden, Mr. Brandwine stood up, swept the bottle of milk with a crash into the sink—and shouted, 'Don't cry over spilt milk!'

"He then made us all come to the sink and look at the wreckage. 'Take a good look,' he told us, 'because I want you to remember this lesson the rest of your lives. That milk is gone—you can see it's down the drain; and all the fussing and hair-pulling in the world won't bring back a drop of it. With a little thought and prevention, that milk might have been saved. But it's too late now—all we can do is write it off, forget it, and go on to the next thing.'

"That one little demonstration," Allen Saunders told me, "stuck with me long after I'd forgotten my solid geometry and Latin. In fact, it taught me more about practical living than anything else in my four years of high school. It taught me to keep from spilling milk if I could; but to forget it completely, once it was spilled and had gone down the drain."

Some readers are going to snort at the idea of making so much over a hackneyed proverb like "Don't cry over spilt milk." I know it is trite, commonplace, and a platitude. I know we have heard it a thousand times. But I also know that these hackneyed proverbs contain the very essence of the distilled wisdom of all ages. They have come out of the fiery experience of the human race and have been handed down through countless generations. If we were to read everything that has ever been written about worry by the great scholars of all time, we would never read anything more basic or more profound than such hackneyed proverbs as "Don't cross your bridges until you come to them" and "Don't cry over spilt milk." If we only applied those two proverbs—instead of snorting at them—we wouldn't need this book at all. In fact, if we applied most of the old proverbs, we would lead almost perfect lives. However, knowledge isn't power until it is applied; and the purpose of this book is not to tell you something new. The purpose of this book is to remind you of what you already know and to kick you in the shins and inspire you to do something about applying it.

I have always admired a man like the late Fred Fuller Shedd, who had a gift for stating an old truth in a new and picturesque way. He was editor of the *Philadelphia*

Bulletin; and, while addressing a college graduating class, he asked, "How many of you have ever sawed wood? Let's see your hands." Most of them had. Then he enquired, "How many of you have ever sawed *sawdust?*" No hands went up.

"Of course, you can't saw sawdust!" Mr. Shedd exclaimed. "It's already sawed! And it's the same with the past. When you start worrying about things that are over and done with, you're merely trying to saw sawdust."

When Connie Mack, the grand old man of baseball, was eighty-one years old, I asked him if he had ever worried over games that were lost.

"Oh, yes, I used to," Connie Mack told me. "But I got over that foolishness long years ago. I found out it didn't get me anywhere at all. You can't grind any grain," he said, "with water that has already gone down the creek."

No, you can't grind any grain—and you can't saw any logs with water that has already gone down the creek. But you can saw wrinkles in your face and ulcers in your stomach.

I had dinner with Jack Dempsey last Thanksgiving; and he told me over the turkey and cranberry sauce about the fight in which he lost the heavyweight championship to Tunney. Naturally, it was a blow to his ego. "In the midst of that fight," he told me, "I suddenly realized I had become an old man.... At the end of the tenth round, I was still on my feet, but that was about all. My face was puffed and cut, and my eyes were nearly closed.... I saw the referee raise Gene Tunney's hand in token of victory.... I was no longer champion of the world. I started back in the rain—back through the crowd to my dressing room. As I passed, some people tried to grab my hand. Others had tears in their eyes.

"A year later, I fought Tunney again. But it was no use. I was through forever. It was hard to keep from worrying about it all, but I said to myself, 'I'm not going to live in the past or cry over spilt milk. I am going to take this blow on the chin and not let it floor me.'"

And that is precisely what Jack Dempsey did. How? By saying to himself over and over, "I won't worry about the past"? No, that would merely have forced him to think of his past worries. He did it by accepting and writing off his defeat and then concentrating on plans for the future. He did it by running the Jack Dempsey Restaurant on Broadway and the Great Northern Hotel on 57th Street. He did it by promoting prize fights and giving boxing exhibitions. He did it by getting so busy on something constructive that he had neither the time nor the temptation to worry about the past. "I have had a better time during the last ten years," Jack Dempsey said, "than I had when I was champion."

Mr. Dempsey told me that he had not read many books; but, without knowing it, he was following Shakespeare's advice: "Wise men ne'er sit and wail their loss, but cheerily seek how to redress their harms."

As I read History and Biography and observe people under trying circumstances, I am constantly astonished and inspired by some people's ability to write off their worries and tragedies and go on living fairly happy lives.

I once paid a visit to Sing Sing, and the thing that

astonished me most was that the prisoners there appeared to be about as happy as the average person on the outside. I commented on it to Lewis E. Lawes—then warden of Sing Sing—and he told me that when criminals first arrive at Sing Sing, they are likely to be resentful and bitter. But after a few months, the majority of the more intelligent ones write off their misfortunes and settle down and accept prison life calmly and make the best of it. Warden Lawes told me about one Sing Sing prisoner—a gardener—who *sang* as he cultivated the vegetables and flowers inside the prison walls.

That Sing Sing prisoner who sang as he cultivated the flowers showed a lot more sense than most of us do. He knew that

The Moving Finger writes; and, having writ,
Moves on: nor all your Piety nor Wit Shall lure it back to cancel half a Line,
Nor all your Tears wash out a Word of it.

So why waste the tears? Of course, we have been guilty of blunders and absurdities! And so what? Who hasn't? Even Napoleon lost one-third of all the important battles he had fought. Perhaps our batting average is no worse than Napoleon's. Who knows?

And, anyhow, all the king's horses and all the king's men can't put the past together again. So let's remember Rule 7:

DON'T TRY TO SAW SAWDUST.

"My need to solve the problem is the problem."
—Anonymous

"Above all else, remember that worrying is totally useless. Worrying will not solve your problem."
—Joyce Meyer

PART 4

13

HOW TO ADD ONE HOUR A DAY TO YOUR WAKING LIFE

Why am I writing a chapter on preventing fatigue in a book on preventing worry? That is simple: fatigue often produces worry, or, at least, it makes you susceptible to worry. Any medical student will tell you that fatigue lowers physical resistance to the common cold and hundreds of other diseases; and any psychiatrist will tell you that fatigue also lowers your resistance to the emotions of fear and worry. So preventing fatigue tends to prevent worry.

Did I say "*tends* to prevent worry"? That is putting it mildly. Dr. Edmund Jacobson goes much further. Dr. Jacobson has written two books on relaxation: *Progressive Relaxation* and *You Must Relax;* and as director of the University of Chicago Laboratory for Clinical Physiology, he has spent years conducting investigations in using relaxation as a method in medical practice. He declares that any nervous or emotional state "fails to exist in the presence of complete relaxation." That is another way of saying: *You cannot continue to worry if you relax.*

So, to prevent fatigue and worry, the first rule is: Rest often. Rest before you get tired.

Why is that so important? Because fatigue accumulates with astonishing rapidity. The United States Army has discovered by repeated tests that even young men—men toughened by years of Army training—can march better, and hold up longer, if they throw down their packs and rest ten minutes out of every hour. So the Army forces them to do just that. Your heart is just as smart as the U. S. Army. Your heart pumps enough blood through your body every day to fill a railway tank car. It exerts enough energy every twenty-four hours to shovel twenty tons of coal onto a platform three feet high. It does this incredible amount of work for fifty, seventy, or maybe ninety years. How can it stand it? Dr. Walter B. Cannon, of the Harvard Medical School, explains it. He says, "Most people have the idea that the heart is working all the time. As a matter of fact, there is a definite rest period after each contraction. *When beating at a moderate rate of seventy pulses per minute, the heart is actually working only nine hours out of the twenty-four. In the aggregate its rest periods total a full fifteen hours per day.*"

During World War II, Winston Churchill, in his late sixties and early seventies, was able to work sixteen hours a day, year after year, directing the war efforts of the British Empire. A phenomenal record. His secret? He worked in bed each morning until eleven o'clock, reading reports, dictating orders, making telephone calls, and holding important conferences. After lunch, he went to bed again and slept for an hour. In the evening, he went to bed once more and slept for two hours before having dinner at eight. He didn't cure fatigue. He didn't have to cure it. He prevented it. Because he rested frequently, he was able to work on, fresh and fit, until long past midnight.

The original John D. Rockefeller made two extraordinary records. He accumulated the greatest fortune the world had ever seen up to that time and he also lived to be ninety-eight. How did he do it? The chief reason, of course, was because he had inherited a tendency to live long. Another reason was his habit of taking a half-hour nap in his office every noon. He would lie down on his office couch—and not even the President of the United States could get John D. on the phone while he was having his snooze!

In his excellent book, *Why Be Tired?* Daniel W. Josselyn observes, "Rest is not a matter of doing absolutely nothing. *Rest is repair*." There is so much repair power in a short period of rest that even a five-minute nap will help to forestall fatigue! Connie Mack, the grand old man of baseball, told me that if he doesn't take an afternoon nap before a game, he is all tuckered out at around the fifth inning. But if he does go to sleep, if for only five minutes, he can last throughout an entire double-header without feeling tired.

When I asked Eleanor Roosevelt how she was able to carry such an exhausting schedule during the twelve years she was in the White House, she said that before meeting a crowd or making a speech, she would often sit in a chair or davenport, close her eyes, and relax for twenty minutes.

I recently interviewed Gene Autry in his dressing room at the Madison Square Garden, where he was the star attraction at the world's championship rodeo. I noticed an army cot in his dressing room. "I lie down there every afternoon," Gene Autry said, "and get an hour's nap between performances. When I am making pictures in Hollywood," he continued, "I often relax in a big easy chair and get two-or three ten-minute naps a day. They buck me up tremendously."

Edison attributed his enormous energy and endurance to his habit of sleeping whenever he wanted to.

I interviewed Henry Ford shortly before his eightieth birthday. I was surprised to see how fresh and fine he looked. I asked him the secret. He said, "I never stand up when I can sit down; and I never sit down when I can lie down."

Horace Mann, "the father of modern education," did the same thing as he grew older. When he was president of Antioch College, he used to stretch out on a couch while interviewing students.

I persuaded a motion-picture director in Hollywood to try a similar technique. He confessed that it worked miracles. I refer to Jack Chertock, who is one of Hollywood's top directors. When he came to see me a few years ago, he was then head of the short-feature department of MGM. Worn out and exhausted, he had tried everything: tonics, vitamins, medicine. Nothing helped much. I suggested that he take a vacation every day. How? By stretching out in his office and relaxing while holding conferences with his staff writers.

When I saw him again, two years later, he said, "A miracle has happened. That is what my own physicians call it. I used to sit up in my chair, tense and taut, while discussing ideas for our short features. Now I stretch out on the office couch during these conferences. I feel better than I have felt in twenty years. Work two hours a day longer, yet I rarely get tired."

How does all this apply to you? If you are a stenographer, you can't take naps in the office as Edison did, and as Sam Goldwyn does; and if you are an accountant, you can't stretch out on the couch while discussing a financial statement with the boss. But if you live in a small city and go home for lunch, you may be able to take a ten-minute nap after lunch. That is what General George C. Marshall used to do. He felt he was so busy directing the U. S. Army in wartime that he *had* to rest at noon. If you are over fifty and feel you are too rushed to do it, then buy immediately all the life insurance you can get. Funerals come high—and suddenly—these days; and the little woman may want to take your insurance money and marry a younger man!

If you can't take a nap at noon, you can at least try to lie down for an hour before the evening meal. It is cheaper than a highball; and, over a long stretch, it is 5467 times more effective. If you can sleep for an hour around five, six, or seven o'clock, you can add one hour a day to your waking life. Why? How? Because an hour's nap before the evening meal plus six hours' sleep at night—a total of seven hours—will do you more good than eight hours of unbroken sleep.

A physical worker can do more work if he takes more time out for rest. Frederick Taylor demonstrated that while working as a scientific-management engineer with the Bethlehem Steel Company. He observed that laboring men were loading approximately 12½ tons of pig iron per man each day on freight cars and that they were exhausted at noon. He made a scientific study of all the fatigue factors involved, and declared that these men should be loading not 12½ tons of pig iron per day, but *forty-seven* tons per day! He figured that they ought to do almost four times as much as they were doing, and not be exhausted. But prove it!

Taylor selected a Mr. Schmidt who was required to work by the stop-watch. Schmidt was told by the man who stood over him with a watch, "Now pick up a 'pig' and walk. ... Now sit down and rest. ... Now walk.... Now rest."

What happened? Schmidt carried forty-seven tons of pig iron each day while the other men carried only 12$$ tons per man. And he practically never failed to work at this pace during the three years that Frederick Taylor was at Bethlehem. Schmidt was able to do this because he rested before he got tired. He worked approximately 26 minutes out of the hour and rested 34 minutes. He rested *more* than he worked—yet he did almost four times as much work as the others! Is this mere hearsay? No, you can read the record yourself on pages 41–62 of *Principles of Scientific Management,* by Frederick Winslow Taylor.

Let me repeat: do what the Army does—take frequent rests. Do what your heart does—rest before you get tired, and you will add one hour a day to your waking life.

"Nothing in the universe can stop you from letting go and starting over."

—Guy Finley

"I believe that you are only in control of so much. So whatever you are not in control of you can't worry about."

—Elizabeth Olsen

14

WHAT MAKES YOU TIRED

Here is an astounding and significant fact: Mental work alone can't make you tired. Sounds absurd. But a few years ago, scientists tried to find out how long the human brain could labor without reaching "a diminished capacity for work," the scientific definition of fatigue. To the amazement of these scientists, they discovered that blood passing through the brain, when it is active, shows no fatigue at all! If you took blood from the veins of a day laborer while he was working, you would find it full of "fatigue toxins" and fatigue products. But if you took a drop of blood from the brain of an Albert Einstein, it would show no fatigue toxins whatever at the end of the day.

So far as the brain is concerned, it can work "as well and as swiftly at the end of eight or even twelve hours of effort as at the beginning." The brain is utterly tireless.... So what makes you tired?

Psychiatrists declare that most of our fatigue derives from our mental and emotional attitudes. One of England's most distinguished psychiatrists, J. A. Hadfield, says in his book *The Psychology of Power* "the greater part of the fatigue from which we suffer is of mental origin; in fact exhaustion of purely physical origin is rare." One of America's most distinguished psychiatrists, Dr. A. A. Brill, goes even further. He declares, "One hundred per cent of the fatigue of the sedentary worker in good health is due to psychological factors, by which we mean emotional factors."

What kinds of emotional factors tire the sedentary (or sitting) worker? Joy? Contentment? No! Never! Boredom, resentment, a feeling of not being appreciated, a feeling of futility, hurry, anxiety, worry—those are the emotional factors that exhaust the sitting worker, make him susceptible to colds, reduce his output, and send him home with a nervous headache. Yes, we get tired because our emotions produce nervous tensions in the body.

The Metropolitan Life Insurance Company pointed that out in a leaflet on fatigue: "Hard work by itself," says this great life-insurance company, "seldom causes fatigue which cannot be cured by a good sleep or rest.... Worry, tenseness, and emotional upsets are three of the biggest causes of fatigue. Often they are to blame when physical or mental work seems to be the cause.... Remember that a tense muscle is a working muscle. Ease up! Save energy for important duties."

Stop now, right where you are, and give yourself a checkup. As you read these lines, are you scowling at the book? Do you feel a strain between the eyes? Are you sitting relaxed in your chair? Or are you hunching up your shoulders? Are the muscles of your face tense? Unless your entire body is as limp and relaxed as an old rag doll, you are at this very moment producing nervous tensions and muscular tensions. *You are producing nervous tensions and nervous fatigue!*

Why do we produce these unnecessary tensions in

doing mental work? Josselyn says, "I find that the chief obstacle ... is the almost universal belief that hard work requires a feeling of effort, else it is not well done." So we scowl when we concentrate. We hunch up our shoulders. We call on our muscles to make the motion of *effort,* which in no way assists our brain in its work.

Here is an astonishing and tragic truth: millions of people who wouldn't dream of wasting dollars go right on wasting and squandering their energy with the recklessness of seven drunken sailors in Singapore.

What is the answer to this nervous fatigue? Relax! Relax! Relax! *Learn to relax while you are doing your work!*

Easy? No. You will probably have to reverse the habits of a lifetime. But it is worth the effort, for it may revolutionize your life! William James said, in his essay "The Gospel of Relaxation": "The American overtension and jerkiness and breathlessness and intensity and agony of expression ...are *bad habits,* nothing more or less." *Tension is a habit. Relaxing is a habit. And bad habits can be broken, good habits formed.*

How do you relax? Do you start with your mind, or do you start with your nerves? You don't start with either. You always begin to *relax with your muscles!*

To show how it is done, start with your eyes. Read this paragraph through, and when you've reached the end, lean back, close your eyes, *and say to your eyes* silently, "Let go. Let go. Stop straining, stop frowning. Let go. Let go." Repeat that over and over very slowly for a minute.

Didn't you notice that after a few seconds the muscles of your eyes *began to obey?* Didn't you feel as though some hand had wiped away the tension? Well, incredible as it seems, you have sampled in that one minute the whole key and secret to the art of relaxing. You can do the same thing with the jaw, with the muscles of the face, with the neck, with the shoulders, the whole of the body. But the most important organ of all is the eye. Dr. Edmund Jacobson of the University of Chicago has gone so far as to say that if you can completely relax the muscles of the eyes, you can forget all your troubles! The reason the eyes are so important in relieving nervous tension is that they burn up one-fourth of all the nervous energies consumed by the body. That is also why so many people with perfectly sound vision suffer from "eyestrain." They are tensing the eyes.

Vicki Baum, the famous novelist, said that when she was a child, she met an old man who taught her one of the most important lessons she ever learned. She had fallen down and cut her knees and hurt her wrist. The old man picked her up; he had once been a circus clown; and, as he brushed her off, he said, "The reason you injured yourself was because you don't know how to relax. You have to pretend you are as limp as a sock, as an old crumpled sock. Come, I'll show you how to do it."

That old man taught Vicki Baum and the other children how to fall, how to do flip-flops, and how to turn somersaults. And always he insisted, "Think of yourself as an old crumpled sock. Then you've *got* to relax!"

You can relax in odd moments, almost anywhere you are. Only don't make an effort to relax. *Relaxation is the absence of all tension and effort.* Think ease and relaxation. Begin by thinking relaxation of the muscles of your eyes and your face, saying over and over, "Let go …let go … let go and relax." Feel the energy flowing out of your facial muscles to the center of your body. Think of yourself as free from tension as a baby.

That is what Galli-Curci, the great soprano, used to do. Helen Jepson told me that she used to see Galli-Curci before a performance, sitting in a chair with all her muscles relaxed and her lower jaw so limp it actually sagged. An excellent practice—it kept her from becoming too nervous before her stage entrance; it prevented fatigue.

Here are suggestions that will help you learn to relax:

Relax in odd moments. Let your body go limp like an old sock. I keep an old, maroon-colored sock on my desk as I work—keep it there as a reminder of how limp I ought to be. If you haven't got a sock, a cat will do. Did you ever pick up a kitten sleeping in the sunshine? If so, both ends sagged like a wet newspaper. Even the yogis in India say that if you want to master the art of relaxation, study the cat. I never saw a tired cat, a cat with a nervous breakdown, or a cat suffering from insomnia, worry, or stomach ulcers. You will probably avoid these disasters if you learn to relax as the cat does.

Work, as much as possible, in a comfortable position. Remember that tensions on the body produce aching shoulders and nervous fatigue.

Check yourself four or five times a day, and say to yourself, "Am I making my work harder than it actually is? Am I using muscles that have nothing to do with the work I am doing?" This will help you form the *habit* of relaxing, and as Dr. David Harold Fink says, "Among those who know psychology best, it is habits two to one."

Test yourself again at the end of the day, by asking yourself, "Just how tired am I? If I am tired, it is not because of the mental work I have done but because of the way I have done it."

"I measure my accomplishments," says Daniel W. Josselyn, "not by how tired I am at the end of the day, but how tired I am not." He says, "When I feel particularly tired at the end of the day, or when irritability proves that my nerves are tired, I know beyond question that it has been an inefficient day both as to quantity and quality." If every businessman in America would learn that same lesson, our death rate from "hypertension" diseases would drop overnight. And we would stop filling up our sanitariums and asylums with men who have been broken by fatigue and worry.

> *"Sometimes people let the same problem make them miserable for years when they could just say, So what. That's one of my favorite things to say. So what."*
> —Andy Warhol

> *"Don't worry about the horse being blind, just load the wagon."*
> —John Madden

15

AVOID FATIGUE AND LOOK YOUNG

One day last autumn, my associate flew up to Boston to attend a session of one of the most unusual medical classes in the world. Medical? Well, yes. It meets once a week at the Boston Dispensary, and the patients who attend it get regular and thorough medical examinations before they are admitted. But actually this class is a psychological clinic. Although it is officially called the Class in Applied Psychology (formerly the Thought Control Class—a name suggested by the first member), its real purpose is to deal with people *who are ill from worry.* And many of these patients are emotionally disturbed housewives.

How did such a class for worriers get started? Well, in 1930, Dr. Joseph H. Pratt—who, by the way, had been a pupil of Sir William Osier—observed that many of the outpatients who came to the Boston Dispensary apparently had nothing wrong with them at all physically; yet they had practically all the symptoms that flesh is heir to. One woman's hands were so crippled with "arthritis" that she had lost all use of them. Another was in agony with all the excruciating symptoms of "cancer of the stomach." Others had backaches, headaches, were chronically tired, or had vague aches and pains. *They actually felt these pains.* But the most exhaustive medical examinations showed that nothing whatever was wrong with these women—in the physical sense. Many old-

fashioned doctors would have said it was all imagination—
"all in the mind."

But Dr. Pratt realized that it was no use to tell these
patients to "go home and forget it." He knew that most of
these women didn't want to be sick; if it was so easy to
forget their ailments, they would do so themselves. So
what could be done?

He opened this class—to a chorus of doubts from the
medical doubters on the sidelines. And the class worked
wonders! In the eighteen years that have passed since it
started, thousands of patients have been "cured" by
attending it. Some of the patients have been coming for
years—as religious in their attendance as though going to
church. My assistant talked to a woman who has hardly
missed a session in more than nine years. She said that
when she first went to the clinic, she was thoroughly
convinced she had a floating kidney and some kind of
heart ailment. She was so worried and tense that she
occasionally lost her eyesight and had spells of blindness.
Yet today she is confident and cheerful and in excellent
health. She looked only about forty, yet she held one of
her grandchildren asleep in her lap. "I used to worry so
much about my family troubles," she said, "that I wished
I could die. But I learned at this clinic the futility of
worrying. I learned to stop it. And I can honestly say now
that my life is serene."

Dr. Rose Hilferding, the medical adviser of the class,
said that she thought one of the best remedies for
lightening worry is "talking your troubles over with
someone you trust. We call it catharsis," she said. "When

patients come here, they can talk their troubles over at length, until they get them off their minds. Brooding over worries alone, and keeping them to oneself, causes great nervous tension. We all have to share our troubles. We have to share worry. We have to feel there is someone in the world who is willing to listen and able to understand."

My assistant witnessed the great relief that came to one woman from talking out her worries. She had domestic worries, and when she first began to talk, she was like a wound-up spring. Then gradually, as she kept on talking, she began to calm down. At the end of the interview, she was actually smiling. Had the problem been solved? No, it wasn't that easy. What caused the change was *talking to someone*, getting a little advice and a little human sympathy. What had really worked the change was the tremendous healing value that lies in—*words!*

Psychoanalysis is based, to some extent, on this healing power of words. Ever since the days of Freud, analysts have known that a patient could find relief from his inner anxieties if he could talk, just talk. Why is this so? Maybe because by talking, we gain a little better insight into our troubles, get a better perspective. No one knows the whole answer. But all of us know that "spitting it out" or "getting it off our chests" brings almost instant relief.

So the next time we have an emotional problem, why don't we look around for someone to talk to? I don't mean, of course, to go around making pests of ourselves by whining and complaining to everyone in sight. Let's decide on someone we can trust, and make an appointment. Maybe a relative, a doctor, a lawyer, a minister, or priest. Then say to that person, "I want your advice. I have a problem, and I wish you would listen while I put it in words. You may be able to advise me. You may see angles to this thing that I can't see myself. But even if you can't, you will help me tremendously if you will just sit and listen while I talk it out."

Talking things out, then, is one of the principle therapies used at the Boston Dispensary Class. But here are some other ideas we picked up at the class—things you, as a housewife, can do in your home.

Keep a notebook or scrapbook for "inspirational" reading. Into this book you can paste all the poems, or short prayers, or quotations, which appeal to you personally and give you a lift. Then, when a rainy afternoon sends your spirits plunging down, perhaps you can find a recipe in this book for dispelling the gloom. Many patients at the Dispensary have kept such notebooks for years. They say it is a spiritual "shot in the arm."

Don't dwell too long on the shortcomings of others! Sure, your husband has faults! If he had been a saint, he never would have married you. Right? One woman at the class who found herself developing into a scolding, nagging, and haggard-faced wife, was brought up short with the question: "What would you do if your husband died?" She was so shocked by the idea that she immediately sat down and drew up a list of all her husband's good points. She made quite a list. Why don't you try the same thing the next time you feel you married a tight-fisted tyrant? Maybe you'll find, after reading his virtues, that he's a man you'd like to meet!

Get interested in your neighbors! Develop a friendly, healthy interest in the people who share the life on your street. One ailing woman who felt herself so "exclusive" that she hadn't any friends, was told to try to make up a story about the next person she met. She began, in the streetcar, to weave backgrounds and settings for the people she saw. She tried to imagine what their lives had been like. First thing you know, she was talking to people everywhere—and today she is happy, alert, and a charming human being, cured of her "pains."

Make up a schedule for tomorrow's work before you go to bed tonight. The class found that many wives feel driven and harassed by the unending round of housework and things they must do. They never got their work finished. They were chased by the clock. To cure this sense of hurry, and worry, the suggestion was made that they draw up a schedule each night for the following day. What happened? More work accomplished; much less fatigue; a feeling of pride and achievement; and time left over to rest and to "primp." (Every woman ought to take some time out in the course of the day to primp and look pretty. My own guess is that when a woman knows she looks pretty, she has little use for "nerves.")

Finally—avoid tension and fatigue. Relax! Relax! Nothing will make you look old sooner than tension and fatigue. Nothing will work such havoc with your freshness and looks! My assistant sat for an hour in the Boston Thought Control Class, while Professor Paul E. Johnson, the director, went over many of the principles we have already discussed—the rules for relaxing. At the end of ten minutes of these relaxing exercises, which my assistant did with the others, she was almost asleep sitting upright in her chair! Why is such stress laid on this physical relaxing? Because the clinic knows—as other doctors know—that if you're going to get the worry-kinks out of people, they've got to relax!

Yes, you, as a housewife, have got to relax! You have one great advantage—you can lie down whenever you want to, and you can lie on the floor! Strangely enough, a good hard floor is better to relax on than an inner-spring bed. It gives more resistance. It is good for the spine.

All right, then, here are some exercises you can do in your home. Try them for a week—and see what you do for your looks and disposition!

Lie flat on the floor whenever you feel tired. Stretch as tall as you can. Roll around if you want to. Do it twice a day.

Close your eyes. You might try saying, as Professor Johnson recommended, something like this: "The sun is shining overhead. The sky is blue and sparkling. Nature is calm and in control of the world—and I, as nature's child, am in tune with the Universe." Or—better still—pray!

If you cannot lie down, because the roast is in the oven and you can't spare the time, then you can achieve almost the same effect sitting down in a chair. A hard, upright chair is the best for relaxing. Sit upright in the chair like a seated Egyptian statue, and let your hands rest, palms down, on the tops of your thighs.

Now, slowly tense your toes—then let them re

Tense the muscles in your legs—and let them relax. Do this slowly upward, with all the muscles of your body, until you get to the neck. Then let your head roll around heavily, as though it were a football. Keep saying to your muscles, "Let go …let go…."

Quiet your nerves with slow, steady breathing. Breathe from deep down. The yogis of India were right: rhythmical breathing is one of the best methods ever discovered for soothing the nerves.

Think of the wrinkles and frowns in your face, and smooth them all out. Loosen up the worry-creases you feel between your brows, and at the sides of your mouth. Do this twice a day, and maybe you won't have to go to a beauty parlor to get a massage. Maybe the lines will disappear from the inside out!

> *"I know but one freedom and that is the freedom of the mind."*
>
> —Antoine de Saint-Exupéry

> *"Instead of fretting about getting everything done, why not simply accept that being alive means having things to do? Then drop into full engagement with whatever you're doing, and let the worry go."*
>
> —Martha Beck

16

FOUR GOOD WORKING HABITS THAT WILL HELP PREVENT FATIGUE AND WORRY

Good Working Habit No. 1: Clear Your Desk of All Papers Except Those Relating to the Immediate Problem at Hand.

Roland L. Williams, President of Chicago and Northwestern Railway, says, "A person with his desk piled high with papers on various matters will find his work much easier and more accurate if he clears that desk of all but the immediate problem on hand. I call this good housekeeping, and it is the number-one step toward efficiency."

If you visit the Library of Congress in Washington, D.C., you will find five words painted on the ceiling—five words written by the poet Pope:

"Order is Heaven's first law."

Order ought to be the first law of business, too. But is it? No, the average businessman's desk is cluttered up with papers that he hasn't looked at for weeks. In fact, the publisher of a New Orleans newspaper once told me that his secretary cleared up one of his desks and found a typewriter that had been missing for two years!

The mere sight of a desk littered with unanswered mail and reports and memos is enough to breed confusion, tension, and worries. It is much worse than that. The constant reminder of "a million things to do and no time to do them" can worry you not only into tension and fatigue, but it can also worry you into high blood pressure, heart trouble, and stomach ulcers.

Dr. John H. Stokes, professor, Graduate School of Medicine, University of Pennsylvania, read a paper before the National Convention of the American Medical Association—a paper entitled "Functional Neuroses as Complications of Organic Disease." In that paper, Dr. Stokes listed eleven conditions under the title: "What to Look for in the Patient's State of Mind." Here is the first item on that list:

"The sense of must or obligation; the unending stretch of things ahead that simply have to be done."

But how can such an elementary procedure as clearing your desk and making decisions help you avoid this high pressure, this sense of *must*, this sense of an "unending stretch of things ahead that simply have to be done"? Dr. William L. Sadler, the famous psychiatrist, tells of a patient who, by using this simple device, avoided a nervous breakdown. The man was an executive in a big Chicago firm. When he came to Dr. Sadler's office, he was tense, nervous, worried. He knew he was heading for a tailspin, but he couldn't quit work. He had to have help.

"While this man was telling me his story," Dr. Sadler says, "my telephone rang. It was the hospital calling; and, instead of deferring the matter, I took time right then to come to a decision. I always settle questions, if possible, right on the spot. I had no sooner hung up than the phone rang again. Again an urgent matter, which I took time to discuss. The third interruption came when a colleague of mine came to my office for advice on a patient who was critically ill. When I had finished with him, I turned to my caller and began to apologize for keeping him waiting. But he had brightened up. He had a completely different look on his face."

"Don't apologize, doctor!" this man said to Sadler. "In the last ten minutes, I think I've got a hunch as to what is wrong with me. I'm going back to my office and revising my working habits…. But before I go, do you mind if I take a look in your desk?"

Dr. Sadler opened up the drawers of his desk. All empty—except for supplies. "Tell me," said the patient, "where do you keep your unfinished business?"

"Finished!" said Sadler.

"And where do you keep your unanswered mail?"

"Answered!" Sadler told him. "My rule is never to lay down a letter until I have answered it. I dictate the reply to my secretary at once."

Six weeks later, this same executive invited Dr. Sadler to come to his office. He was changed—and so was his desk. He opened the desk drawers to show there was no unfinished business inside of the desk. "Six weeks ago," this executive said, "I had three different desks in two different offices—and was snowed under by my work. I was never finished. After talking to you, I came back here and cleared out a wagonload of reports and old papers. Now I work at one desk, settle things as they come up, and don't have a mountain of unfinished business nagging at me and making me tense and worried. But the most astonishing thing is I've recovered completely. There is nothing wrong any more with my health!"

Charles Evans Hughes, former Chief Justice of the United States Supreme Court, said: "Men do not die from overwork. They die from dissipation and worry." Yes, from dissipation of their energies—and worry because they never seem to get their work done.

Good Working Habit No. 2: Do Things in the Order of Their Importance.

Henry L. Doherty, Founder of the nation-wide Cities Service Company, said that regardless of how much salary he paid, there were two abilities he found it almost impossible to find.

Those two priceless abilities are: first, the ability to think. Second, the ability to do things in the order of their importance.

Charles Luckman, the lad who started from scratch and climbed in twelve years to president of the Pepsodent Company, got a salary of a hundred thousand dollars a year, and made a million dollars besides—that lad declares that he owes much of his success to developing the two abilities that Henry L. Doherty said he found almost impossible to find. Charles Luckman said, "As far back as I can remember, I have gotten up at five o'clock in the morning because I can think better then than any other time—I can think better then and plan my day, plan to do things in the order of their importance."

Franklin Bettger, one of America's most successful insurance salesmen, doesn't wait until five o'clock in the morning to plan his day. He plans it the night before—sets a goal for himself—a goal to sell a certain amount of insurance that day. If he fails, that amount is added to the next day—and so on.

I know from long experience that one is not always able to do things in the order of their importance, but I also know that some kind of plan to do first things first is infinitely better than extemporizing as you go along.

If George Bernard Shaw had not made it a rigid rule to do first things first, he would probably have failed as a writer and might have remained a bank cashier all his life. His plan called for writing five pages each day. That plan inspired him to go right on writing five pages a day for nine heartbreaking years, even though he made a total of only thirty dollars in those nine years—about a penny a day. Even Robinson Crusoe wrote out a schedule of what he would do each hour of the day.

Good Working Habit No. 3: When You Face a Problem, Solve It Then and There if You Have the Facts Necessary to Make a Decision. Don't Keep Putting off Decisions.

One of my former students, the late H. P. Howell, told me that when he was a member of the board of directors of U. S. Steel, the meetings of the board were often long-drawn-out affairs—many problems were discussed, few decisions were made. The result: each member of the board had to carry home bundles of reports to study.

Finally, Mr. Howell persuaded the board of directors to take up one problem at a time and come to a decision. No procrastination—no putting off. The decision might be to ask for additional facts; it might be to do something or do nothing. But a decision was reached on each problem before passing on to the next. Mr. Howell told me that the results were striking and salutary: the docket was cleared.

The calendar was clean. No longer was it necessary for each member to carry home a bundle of reports. No longer was there a worried sense of unresolved problems.

A good rule, not only for the board of directors of U. S. Steel, but for you and me.

Good Working Habit No. 4: Learn to Organize, Deputize, and Supervise.

Many a businessman is driving himself to a premature grave because he has never learned to delegate responsibility to others, insists on doing everything himself. Result: details and confusion overwhelm him. He is driven by a sense of hurry, worry, anxiety, and tension. It is hard to learn to delegate responsibilities. I know. It was hard for me, awfully hard. I also know from experience the disasters that can be caused by delegating authority to the wrong people. But difficult as it is to delegate authority, the executive must do it if he is to avoid worry, tension, and fatigue.

The man who builds up a big business, and doesn't learn to organize, deputize, and supervise, usually pops off with heart trouble in his fifties or early sixties—heart trouble caused by tension and worries. Want a specific instance? Look at the death notices in your local paper.

> *"Be soft. Do not let the world make you hard. Do not let pain make you hate. Do not let the bitterness steal your sweetness. Take pride that even though the rest of the world may disagree, you still believe it to be a beautiful place."*
>
> —Kurt Vonnegut

17

HOW TO BANISH BOREDOM

One of the chief causes of fatigue is boredom. To illustrate, let's take the case of Alice, a stenographer who lives on your street. Alice came home one night utterly exhausted. She *acted* fatigued. She *was* fatigued. She had a headache. She had a backache. She was so exhausted she wanted to go to bed without waiting for dinner. Her mother pleaded.... She sat down at the table. The telephone rang. The boyfriend! An invitation to a dance! Her eyes sparkled. Her spirits soared. She rushed upstairs, put on her Alice-blue gown, and danced until three o'clock in the morning; and when she finally did get home, she was not the slightest bit exhausted. She was, in fact, so exhilarated she couldn't fall asleep.

Was Alice really and honestly tired eight hours earlier, when she looked and acted exhausted? Sure she was. She was exhausted because she was bored with her work, perhaps bored with life. There are millions of Alices. You may be one of them.

It is a well-known fact that your emotional attitude usually has far more to do with producing fatigue than has physical exertion. A few years ago, Joseph E. Barmack, Ph.D., published in the *Archives of Psychology* a report of some of his experiments showing how boredom produces fatigue. Dr. Barmack put a group of students through a series of tests in which, he knew, they could have little interest. The result? The students felt tired and sleepy, complained of headaches and eyestrain, felt irritable. In some cases, even their stomachs were upset. Was it all "imagination"? No. Metabolism tests were taken of these students. These tests showed that the blood pressure of the body and the consumption of oxygen actually decrease when a person is bored, and that the whole metabolism picks up immediately as soon as he begins to feel interest and pleasure in his work!

We rarely get tired when we are doing something interesting and exciting. For example, I recently took a vacation in the Canadian Rockies up around Lake Louise. I spent several days trout fishing along Corral Creek, fighting my way through brush higher than my head, stumbling over logs, struggling through fallen timber— yet after eight hours of this, I was not exhausted. Why? Because I was excited, exhilarated. I had a sense of high achievement: six cut-throat trout. But suppose I had been bored by fishing, then how do you think I would have felt? I would have been worn out by such strenuous work at an altitude of seven thousand feet.

Even in such exhausting activities as mountain climbing, boredom may tire you far more than the strenuous work involved. For example, Mr. S. H. Kingman, president of the Farmers and Mechanics Savings Bank of Minneapolis, told me of an incident that is a perfect illustration of that statement. In July, 1943, the Canadian government asked the Canadian Alpine Club to furnish guides to train the members of the Prince of Wales Rangers in mountain climbing. Mr. Kingman was one of the guides chosen to train these soldiers. He told me how he and the other guides—men ranging from forty-two to fifty-nine years of age—took these young army men on long hikes across glaciers and snow fields and up a sheer cliff of forty feet, where they had to climb with ropes and tiny footholds and precarious handholds. They climbed Michael's Peak, the Vice-President Peak, and other unnamed peaks in the Little Yoho Valley in the Canadian Rockies. After fifteen hours of mountain climbing, these young men, who were in the pink of condition (they had just finished a six-week course in tough Commando training), were utterly exhausted.

Was their fatigue caused by using muscles that had not been hardened by Commando training? Any man who had ever been through Commando training would hoot at such a ridiculous question! No, they were utterly exhausted because they were bored by mountain climbing. They were so tired that many of them fell asleep without waiting to eat. But the guides—men who were two and three times as old as the soldiers—were they tired? Yes, but not exhausted. The guides ate dinner and stayed up for hours, talking about the day's experiences. They were not exhausted because they were interested.

When Dr. Edward Thorndike of Columbia was conducting experiments in fatigue, he kept young men awake for almost a week by keeping them constantly interested. After much investigation, Dr. Thorndike is reported to have said, "Boredom is the only real cause of diminution of work."

If you are a mental worker, it is seldom the amount of

work you do that makes you tired. You may be tired by the amount of work you do *not* do. For example, remember the day last week when you were constantly interrupted. No letters answered. Appointments broken. Trouble here and there. Everything went wrong that day. You accomplished nothing whatever, yet you went home exhausted—and with a splitting head.

The next day everything clicked at the office. You accomplished forty times more than you did the previous day. Yet you went home fresh as a snowy-white gardenia. You have had that experience. So have I.

The lesson to be learned? Just this: our fatigue is often caused not by work, but by worry, frustration, and resentment.

While writing this chapter, I went to see a revival of Jerome Kern's delightful musical comedy, *Show Boat*. Captain Andy, captain of the *Cotton Blossom*, says, in one of his philosophical interludes: "The lucky folks arc the ones that get to do the things they enjoy doing." Such folk are lucky because they have more energy, more happiness, less worry, and less fatigue. Where your interests are, there is your energy also. Walking ten blocks with a nagging wife can be more fatiguing than walking ten miles with an adoring sweetheart.

And so what? What can you do about it? Well, here is what one stenographer did about it—a stenographer working for an oil company in Tulsa, Oklahoma. For several days each month, she had one of the dullest jobs imaginable: filling out printed forms for oil leases, inserting figures and statistics. This task was so boring that she resolved, in self-defense, to make it interesting. How? She had a daily contest with herself. She counted the number of forms she filled out each morning, and then tried to excel that record in the afternoon. She counted each day's total and tried to better it the next day. Result? She was soon able to fill out more of these dull printed forms than any other stenographer in her division. And what did all this get her? Praise? No.... Thanks? No.... Promotion? No.... Increased pay? No.... But it did help to prevent the fatigue that is spawned by boredom. It did give her a mental stimulant. Because she had done her best to make a dull job interesting, she had more energy, more zest, and got far more happiness out of her leisure hours.

I happen to know this story is true, because I married that girl.

Here is the story of another stenographer who found it paid to act *as if* her work were interesting. She used to fight her work. But no more. Her name is Miss Vallie G. Golden, and she lives at 473 South Kenilworth Avenue, Elmhurst, Illinois. Here is her story, as she wrote it to me:

"There are four stenographers in my office and each of us is assigned to take letters from several men. Once in a while we get jammed up in these assignments; and one day, when an assistant department head insisted that I do a long letter over, I started to rebel. I tried to point out to him that the letter could be corrected without being retyped—and he retorted that if I didn't do it over, he would find someone else who would! I was absolutely fuming! But as I started to retype this letter, it suddenly occurred to me that there were a lot of other people who would jump at the chance to do the work I was doing. Also, that I was being paid a salary to do just that work. I began to feel better. I suddenly made up my mind to do my work as if I actually enjoyed it—even though I despised it. Then I made this important discovery: if I do my work *as if* I really enjoy it, then I do enjoy it to some extent. I also found I can work faster when I enjoy my work. So there is seldom any need now for me to work overtime. This new attitude of mine gained me the reputation of being a good worker. And when one of the department superintendents needed a private secretary, he asked for me for the job—because, he said, I was willing to do extra work without being sulky! This matter of the power of a changed mental attitude," wrote Miss Golden, "has been a tremendously important discovery to me. It has worked wonders!"

Miss Golden used the wonder-working *"as if"* philosophy of Professor Hans Vaihinger. He taught us to act *"as if"* we were happy—and so on.

If you act *"as if"* you are interested in your job, that bit of acting will tend to make your interest real. It will also tend to decrease your fatigue, your tensions, and your worries.

A few years ago, Harlan A. Howard made a decision that completely altered his life. He resolved to make a dull job interesting—and he certainly had a dull one: washing plates, scrubbing counters, and dishing out ice cream in the high-school lunchroom while the other boys were playing ball or kidding the girls. Harlan Howard despised his job—but since he had to stick to it, he resolved to study ice cream—how it was made, what ingredients were used, why some ice creams were better than others. He studied the chemistry of ice cream, and became a whiz in the high-school chemistry course. He was so interested now in food chemistry that he entered the Massachusetts State College and majored in the field of "food technology." When the New York Cocoa Exchange offered a hundred-dollar prize for the best paper on uses of cocoa and chocolate—a prize open to all college students—who do you suppose won it? ... That's right. Harlan Howard.

When he found it difficult to get a job, he opened a private laboratory in the basement of his home at 750 North Pleasant Street, Amherst, Massachusetts. Shortly after that, a new law was passed. The bacteria in milk had to be counted. Harlan A. Howard was soon counting bacteria for the fourteen milk companies in Amherst— and he had to hire two assistants.

Where will he be twenty-five years from now? Well, the men who are now running the business of food chemistry will be retired then, or dead; and their places will be taken by young lads who are now radiating initiative and enthusiasm. Twenty-five years from now, Harlan A. Howard will probably be one of the leaders in his profession, while some of his classmates to whom he used to sell ice cream over the counter will be sour, unemployed, cussing the government, and complaining that they never had a chance. Harlan A. Howard might never have had a chance, either, if he hadn't resolved to make a dull job interesting.

Years ago, there was another young man who was bored with his dull job of standing at a lathe, turning out bolts in a factory. His first name was Sam. Sam wanted to quit, but he was afraid he couldn't find another job. Since he had to do this dull work, Sam decided he would make it interesting. So he ran a race with the mechanic operating a machine beside him. One of them was to trim off the rough surfaces on his machine, and the other was to trim the bolts down to the proper diameter. They would switch machines occasionally and see who could turn out the most bolts. The foreman, impressed with Sam's speed and accuracy, soon gave him a better job. That was the start of a whole series of promotions. Thirty years later, Sam—Samuel Vauclain—was president of the Baldwin Locomotive Works. But he might have remained a mechanic all his life if he had not resolved to make a dull job interesting.

H. V. Kaltenborn—the famous radio news analyst—once told me how he made a dull job interesting. When he was twenty-two years old, he worked his way across the Atlantic on a cattle boat, feeding and watering the steers. After making a bicycle tour of England, he arrived in Paris, hungry and broke. Pawning his camera for five dollars, he put an ad in the Paris edition of *The New York Herald* and got a job selling stereopticon machines. If you are forty years old, you may remember those old-fashioned stereoscopes that we used to hold up before our eyes to look at two pictures exactly alike. As we looked, a miracle happened. The two lenses in the stereo-scope transformed the two pictures into a single scene with the effect of a third dimension. We saw distance. We got an astounding sense of perspective.

Well, as I was saying, Kaltenborn started out selling these machines from door to door in Paris—and he couldn't speak French. But he earned five thousand dollars in commissions the first year, and made himself one of the highest-paid salesmen in France that year. H. V. Kaltenborn told me that this experience did as much to develop within him the qualities that make for success as did any single year of study at Harvard. Confidence? He told me himself that after that experience, he felt he could have sold The Congressional Record to French housewives.

That experience gave him an intimate understanding of French life that later proved invaluable in interpreting, on the radio, European events.

How did he manage to become an expert salesman when he couldn't speak French? Well, he had his employer write out his sales talk in perfect French, and he memorized it. He would ring a door-bell, a housewife would answer, and Kaltenborn would begin repeating his memorized sales talk with an accent so terrible it was funny. He would show the housewife his pictures, and when she asked a question, he would shrug his shoulders and say, "An American ... an American." He would then take off his hat and point to a copy of the sales talk in perfect French that he had pasted in the top of his hat. The housewife would laugh, he would laugh—and show her more pictures. When H. V. Kaltenborn told me about this, he confessed that the job had been far from easy. He told me that there was only one quality that pulled him through: his determination to make the job interesting. Every morning before he started out, he looked into the mirror and gave himself a pep talk: "Kaltenborn, *you have to do this if you want to eat. Since you have to do it—why not have a good time doing it? Why not imagine every time you ring a doorbell that you are an actor before the footlights and that there's an audience out there looking at you. After all, what you are doing is just as funny as something on the stage. So why not put a lot of zest and enthusiasm into it?*"

Mr. Kaltenborn told me that these daily pep talks helped him transform a task that he had once hated and dreaded into an adventure that he liked and made highly profitable.

When I asked Mr. Kaltenborn if he had any advice to give to the young men of America who are eager to succeed, he said: "Yes, go to bat with yourself every morning. We talk a lot about the importance of physical exercise to wake us up out of the half-sleep in which so many of us walk around. But we need, even more, some spiritual and mental exercises every morning to stir us into action. Give yourself a pep talk every day."

Is giving yourself a pep talk every day silly, superficial, childish? No, on the contrary, it is the very essence of sound psychology. "Our life is what our thoughts make it." Those words are just as true today as they were eighteen centuries ago when Marcus Aurelius first wrote them in his book of *Meditations:* "Our life is what our thoughts make it."

By talking to yourself every hour of the day, you can

direct yourself to think thoughts of courage and happiness, thoughts of power and peace. By talking to yourself about the things you have to be grateful for, you can fill your mind with thoughts that soar and sing.

By thinking the right thoughts, you can make any job less distasteful. Your boss wants you to be interested in your job so that he will make more money. But let's forget about what the boss wants. Think only of what getting interested in your job will do for you. Remind yourself that it may double the amount of happiness you get out of life, for you spend about one half of your waking hours at your work, and if you don't find happiness in your work, you may never find it anywhere. Keep reminding yourself that getting interested in your job will take your mind off your worries, and, in the long run, will probably bring promotion and increased pay. Even if it doesn't do that, it will reduce fatigue to a minimum and help you enjoy your hours of leisure.

"A pessimist sees the difficulty in every opportunity; an optimist sees the opportunity in every difficulty."
—Winston Churchill

"If you're going to worry about what people say, you're never going to make any progress."
—Joseph Murray

18

HOW TO KEEP FROM WORRYING ABOUT INSOMNIA

Do you WORRY when you can't sleep well? Then it may interest you to know that Samuel Untermyer—the famous international lawyer—never got a decent night's sleep in his life.

When Sam Untermyer went to college, he worried about two afflictions—asthma and insomnia. He couldn't seem to cure either, so he decided to do the next best thing—take advantage of his wakefulness. Instead of tossing and turning and worrying himself into a breakdown, he would get up and study. The result? He began ticking off honors in all of his classes, and became one of the prodigies of the College of the City of New York.

Even after he started to practice law, his insomnia continued. But Untermyer didn't worry. "Nature," he said, "will take care of me." Nature did. In spite of the small amount of sleep he was getting, his health kept up and he was able to work as hard as any of the young lawyers of the New York Bar. He even worked harder, for he worked while they slept!

At the age of twenty-one, Sam Untermyer was earning seventy-five thousand dollars a year; and other young attorneys rushed to courtrooms to study his methods. In 1931, he was paid—for handling one case—what was probably the highest lawyer's fee in all history: a cool million dollars—cash on the barrelhead.

Still he had insomnia—read half the night—and then got up at 5 a.m. and started dictating letters. By the time most people were just starting work, his day's work would be almost half done. He lived to the age of eighty-one, this man who had rarely had a sound night's sleep; but if he had fretted and worried about his insomnia, he would probably have wrecked his life.

We spend a third of our lives sleeping—yet nobody knows what sleep really is. We know it is a habit and a state of rest in which nature knits up the raveled sleeve of care, but we don't know how many hours of sleep each individual requires. We don't even know if we *have* to sleep at all!

Fantastic? Well, during the First World War, Paul Kern, a Hungarian soldier, was shot through the frontal lobe of his brain. He recovered from the wound, but, curiously enough, couldn't fall asleep. No matter what the doctors did—and they tried all kinds of sedatives and narcotics, even hypnotism—Paul Kern couldn't be put to sleep or even made to feel drowsy.

The doctors said he wouldn't live long. But he fooled them. He got a job, and went on living in the best of health for years. He would lie down and close his eyes and rest, but he got no sleep whatever. His case was a medical mystery that upset many of our beliefs about sleep.

Some people require far more sleep than others. Toscanini needs only five hours a night, but Calvin Coolidge needed more than twice that much. Coolidge slept eleven hours out of every twenty-four. In other words, Toscanini has been sleeping away approximately one-fifth of his life, while Coolidge slept away almost half of his life.

Worrying about insomnia will hurt you far more than insomnia. For example, one of my students—Ira Sandner, of 173 Overpeck Avenue, Ridgefield Park, New Jersey— was driven nearly to suicide by chronic insomnia.

"I actually thought I was going insane," Ira Sandner told me. "The trouble was, in the beginning, that I was *too sound* a sleeper.

I wouldn't wake up when the alarm clock went off, and the result was that I was getting to work late in the morning. I worried about it—and, in fact, my boss warned me that I would *have* to get to work on time. I knew that if I kept on oversleeping, I would lose my job.

"I told my friends about it, and one of them suggested I concentrate hard on the alarm clock before I went to sleep. That started the insomnia! The tick-tick-tick of that blasted alarm clock became an obsession. It kept me awake, tossing, all night long! When morning came, I was almost ill. I was ill from fatigue and worry. This kept on for eight weeks. I can't put into words the tortures I suffered. I was convinced I was going insane. Sometimes I paced the floor for hours at a time, and I honestly considered jumping out of the window and ending the whole thing!

"At last I went to a doctor I had known all my life. He said: 'Ira, I can't help you. No one can help you because you have brought this thing on yourself. Go to bed nights, and if you can't fall asleep, forget all about it. Just say to yourself, 'I don't care a hang if I don't go to sleep. It's all right with me if I lie awake till morning.' Keep your eyes closed and say, 'As long as I just lie still and don't worry about it, I'll be getting rest, anyway.'

"I did that," says Sandner, "and in two weeks' time I was dropping off to sleep. In less than one month, I was sleeping eight hours, and my nerves were back to normal."

It wasn't insomnia that was killing Ira Sandner; it was his worry about it.

Dr. Nathaniel Kleitman, professor at the University of Chicago, has done more research work on sleep than has any other living man. He is the world's expert on sleep. He declares that he has never known anyone to die from insomnia. To be sure, a man might worry about insomnia until he lowered his vitality and was swept away by germs. But it was the worry that did the damage, not the insomnia itself.

Dr. Kleitman also says that the people who worry about insomnia usually sleep far more than they realize. The man who swears "I never slept a wink last night" may have slept for hours without knowing it. For example, one of the most profound thinkers of the nineteenth century, Herbert Spencer, was an old bachelor, lived in a boardinghouse, and bored everyone with his talk about his insomnia. He even put "stoppings" in his ears to keep out the noise and quiet his nerves. Sometimes he took opium to induce sleep. One night he and Professor Sayce of Oxford shared the same room at a hotel. The next morning Spencer declared he hadn't slept a wink all night.

In reality, it was Professor Sayce who hadn't slept a wink. He had been kept awake all night by Spencer's snoring!

The first requisite for a good night's sleep is a feeling of security. We need to feel that some power greater than ourselves will take care of us until morning. Dr. Thomas Hyslop, of the Great West Riding Asylum, stressed that point in an address before the British Medical Association. He said: "One of the best sleep-producing agents which my years of practice have revealed to me is—*prayer.* I say this purely as a medical man. The exercise of prayer, in those who habitually exert it, must be regarded as the most adequate and normal of all the pacifiers of the mind and calmers of the nerves."

"Let God—and let go."

Jeanette MacDonald told me that when she was depressed and worried and had difficulty in going to sleep, she could always get "a feeling of security" by repeating Psalm XXIII: "The Lord is my shepherd; I shall not want. He maketh me to lie down in green pastures: he leadeth me beside the still waters...."

But if you are not religious, and have to do things the hard way, then learn to relax by physical measures. Dr. David Harold Fink, who wrote *Release from Nervous Tension,* says that the best way to do this is to *talk* to your body. According to Dr. Fink, words are the key to all kinds of hypnosis; and when you consistently can't sleep, it is because you have *talked* yourself into a case of insomnia. The way to undo this is to dehypnotize yourself—and you can do it by saying to the muscles of your body, "Let go, let go—loosen up and relax." We already know that the mind and nerves can't relax while the muscles are tense—so if we want to go to sleep, we start with the muscles. Dr. Fink recommends—and it works out in practice—that we put a pillow under the knees to ease the tension on the legs, and that we tuck small pillows under the arms for the very same reason. Then, by telling the jaw to relax, the eyes, the arms, and the legs, we finally drop off to sleep before we know what has hit us. I've tried it—I know. If you have trouble sleeping, get hold of Dr. Fink's book, *Release from Nervous Tension,* which I have mentioned earlier. It is the only book I know of that is both lively reading and a cure for insomnia.

One of the best cures for insomnia is making yourself physically tired by gardening, swimming, tennis, golf, skiing, or by just plain physically exhausting work. That is what Theodore Dreiser did. When he was a struggling young author, he was worried about insomnia, so he got a job working as a section hand on the New York Central Railway; and after a day of driving spikes and shoveling gravel, he was so exhausted that he could hardly stay awake long enough to eat.

If we get tired enough, nature will force us to sleep even while we are walking. To illustrate, when I was thirteen years old, my father shipped a carload of fat hogs to Saint Joe, Missouri. Since he got two free railroad passes, he took me along with him. Up until that time, I had never been in a town of more than four thousand. When I landed in Saint Joe—a city of sixty thousand—I was agog with excitement. I saw skyscrapers six stories high and—wonder of wonders—I saw a streetcar. I can close my eyes now and still see and hear that streetcar. After the most thrilling and exciting day of my life, Father and I took a train back to Raven-wood, Missouri. Arriving there at two o'clock in the morning, we had to walk four miles home to the farm. And here is the point of the story: I was so exhausted that I slept and dreamed as I walked.

I have often slept while riding horseback. And I am alive to tell it!

When men are completely exhausted they sleep right through the thunder and horror and danger of war. Dr. Foster Kennedy, the famous neurologist, tells me that during the retreat of the Fifth British Army in 1918, he saw soldiers so exhausted that they fell on the ground where they were and fell into a sleep as sound as a coma. They didn't even wake up when he raised their eyelids with his fingers. And he says he noticed that invariably the pupils of the eyes were rolled upward in the sockets. "After that," says Dr Kennedy, "when I had trouble sleeping, I would practice rolling up my eyeballs into this position, and I found that in a few seconds I would begin to yawn and feel sleepy. It was an automatic reflex over which I had no control."

No man ever committed suicide by refusing to sleep and no one ever will. Nature would force a man to sleep in spite of all his will power. Nature will let us go without food or water far longer than she will let us go without sleep.

Speaking of suicide reminds me of a case that Dr.

Henry C. Link describes in his book, *The Rediscovery of Man*. Dr. Link is Vice-president of The Psychological Corporation and he interviews many people who are worried and depressed. In his chapter "On Over-coming Fears and Worries," he tells about a patient who wanted to commit suicide. Dr. Link knew arguing would only make the matter worse, so he said to this man, "If you are going to commit suicide anyway, you might at least do it in a heroic fashion. Run around the block until you drop dead."

He tried it, not once but several times, and each time felt better, in his mind if not in his muscles. By the third night he had achieved what Dr. Link intended in the first place—he was so physically tired (and physically relaxed) that he slept like a log. Later he joined an athletic club and began to compete in competitive sports. Soon he was feeling so good he wanted to live forever!

So, to keep from worrying about insomnia, here are five rules:

If you can't sleep, do what Samuel Untermyer did. Get up and work or read until you do feel sleepy.

Remember that no one was ever killed by lack of sleep. Worrying about insomnia usually causes far more damage than sleeplessness.

Try prayer—or repeat Psalm XXIII, as Jeanette MacDonald does.

Relax your body. Read the book *Release from Nervous Tension*.

Exercise. Get yourself so physically tired you can't awake.

"You'll never find a rainbow if you're looking down."
—Charlie Chaplin

"The Lord is my shepherd; I shall not want. He maketh me to lie down in green pastures: he leadeth me beside the still waters...."
—Psalm XXIII

PART 5

19

REMEMBER THAT NO ONE EVER KICKS
A DEAD DOG

AN EVENT occurred in 1929 that created a national sensation in educational circles. Learned men from all over America rushed to Chicago to witness the affair. A few years earlier, a young man by the name of Robert Hutchins had worked his way through Yale, acting as a waiter, a lumberjack, a tutor, and a clothesline salesman. Now, only eight years later, he was being inaugurated as president of the fourth richest university in America, the University of Chicago. His age? Thirty. Incredible! The older educators shook their heads. Criticism came roaring down upon this "boy wonder" like a rockslide. He was this and he was that—too young, inexperienced—his educational ideas were cockeyed. Even the newspapers joined in the attack.

The day he was inaugurated, a friend said to the father of Robert Maynard Hutchins: "I was shocked this morning to read that newspaper editorial denouncing your son."

"Yes," the elder Hutchins replied, "it was severe, but remember that no one ever kicks a dead dog."

Yes, and the more important a dog is, the more satisfaction people get in kicking him. The Prince of Wales who later became Edward VIII (now Duke of Windsor) had that brought home to him in the seat of his

189

pants. He was attending Dartmouth College in Devonshire at the time—a college that corresponds to our Naval Academy at Annapolis. The Prince was about fourteen. One day one of the naval officers found him crying, and asked him what was wrong. He refused to tell at first, but finally admitted the truth: he was being kicked by the naval cadets. The commodore of the college summoned the boys and explained to them that the Prince had not complained, but he wanted to find out why the Prince had been singled out for this rough treatment.

After much hemming and hawing and toe scraping, the cadets finally confessed that when they themselves became commanders and captains in the King's Navy, they wanted to be able to say that they had kicked the King!

So when you are kicked and criticized, remember that it is often done because it gives the kicker a feeling of importance. It often means that you are accomplishing something and are worthy of attention. Many people get a sense of savage satisfaction out of denouncing those who are better educated than they are or more successful. For example, while I was writing this chapter, I received a letter from a woman denouncing General William Booth, founder of the Salvation Army. I had given a laudatory broadcast about General Booth; so this woman wrote me, saying that General Booth had stolen eight million dollars of the money he had collected to help poor people. The charge, of course, was absurd. But this woman wasn't looking for truth. She was seeking the mean-spirited gratification that she got from tearing down someone far above her. I threw her bitter letter into the wastebasket, and thanked Almighty God that I wasn't married to her. Her letter didn't tell me anything at all about General Booth, but it did tell me a lot about her. Schopenhauer had said it years ago: "Vulgar people take huge delight in the faults and follies of great men."

One hardly thinks of the president of Yale as a vulgar man; yet a former president of Yale, Timothy Dwight, apparently took huge delight in denouncing a man who was running for President of the United States. The president of Yale warned that if this man were elected President, "we may see our wives and daughters the victims of legal prostitution, soberly dishonored, speciously polluted; the outcasts of delicacy and virtue, the loathing of God and man."

Sounds almost like a denunciation of Hitler, doesn't it? But it wasn't. It was a denunciation of Thomas Jefferson. *Which* Thomas Jefferson? Surely not the *immortal* Thomas Jefferson, the author of the Declaration of Independence, the patron saint of democracy? Yea, verily, that was the man.

What American do you suppose was denounced as a "hypocrite," "an impostor," and as "little better than a murderer"? A newspaper cartoon depicted him on a guillotine, the big knife ready to cut off his head. Crowds jeered at him and hissed him as he rode through the streets. Who was he? George Washington.

But that occurred a long time ago. Maybe human nature has improved since then. Let's see. Let's take the case of Admiral Peary—the explorer who startled and thrilled the world by reaching the North Pole with dog sleds on April 6, 1909—a goal that brave men for centuries had suffered and starved and died to attain. Peary himself almost died from cold and starvation; and eight of his toes were frozen so hard they had to be cut off. He was so overwhelmed with disasters that he feared he would go insane. His superior naval officers in Washington were burned up because Peary was getting so much publicity and acclaim. So they accused him of collecting money for scientific expeditions and then "lying around and loafing in the Arctic." And they probably believed it because it is almost impossible not to believe what you want to believe. Their determination to humiliate and block Peary was so violent that only a direct order from President McKinley enabled Peary to continue his career in the Arctic.

Would Peary have been denounced if he had had a desk job in the Navy Department in Washington? No. He wouldn't have been important enough then to have aroused jealousy.

General Grant had an even worse experience than Admiral Peary. In 1862, General Grant won the first great decisive victory that the North had enjoyed—a victory that was achieved in one afternoon, a victory that made Grant a national idol overnight—a victory that had tremendous repercussions even in far-off Europe—a victory that set church bells ringing and bonfires blazing from Maine to the banks of the Mississippi. Yet within six weeks after achieving that great victory, Grant—hero of the North—was *arrested and his army was taken from him. He wept with humiliation and despair.*

Why was General U. S. Grant arrested at the flood tide of his victory? Largely because he had aroused the jealousy and envy of his arrogant superiors.

If we are tempted to be worried about unjust criticism, here is Rule 1:

REMEMBER THAT UNJUST CRITICISM IS OFTEN A DISGUISED COMPLIMENT. REMEMBER THAT NO ONE EVER KICKS A DEAD DOG.

"In this hour, I do not believe that any darkness will endure."

—J.R.R. Tolkien

"Worry is the interest paid by those who borrow trouble."

—George Washington

20

DO THIS—AND CRITICISM CAN'T HURT YOU

I once interviewed Major General Smedley Butler—old "Gimlet-Eye." Old "Hell-Devil" Butler! Remember him? The most colorful, swashbuckling general who ever commanded the United States Marines.

He told me that when he was young, he was desperately eager to be popular, wanted to make a good impression on everyone. In those days the slightest criticism smarted and stung. But he confessed that thirty years in the Marines had toughened his hide. "I have been berated and insulted," he said, "and denounced as a yellow dog, a snake, and a skunk. I have been cursed by the experts. I have been called every possible combination of unprintable cuss words in the English language. Bother me? Huh! When I hear somebody cussing me now, I never turn my head to see who is talking."

Maybe old "Gimlet-Eye" Butler was too indifferent to criticism; but one thing is sure: most of us take the little jibes and javelins that are hurled at us far too seriously. I remember the time, years ago, when a reporter from the *New York Sun* attended a demonstration meeting of my adult-education classes and lampooned me and my work. Was I burned up? I took it as a personal insult. I telephoned Gil Hodges, the Chairman of the Executive Committee of the Sun, and practically demanded that he print an article stating the facts—instead of ridicule. I was determined to make the punishment fit the crime.

I am ashamed now of the way I acted. I realize now that half the people who bought the paper never saw that article. Half of those who read it regarded it as a source of innocent merriment. Half of those who gloated over it forgot all about it in a few weeks.

I realize now that people are not thinking about you and me or caring what is said about us. They are thinking about themselves—before breakfast, after breakfast, and right on until ten minutes past midnight. They would be a thousand times more concerned about a slight headache of their own than they would about the news of your death or mine.

Even if you and I are lied about, ridiculed, double-crossed, knifed in the back, and sold down the river by one out of every six of our most intimate friends—let's not indulge in an orgy of self-pity. Instead, let's remind ourselves that that's precisely what happened to Jesus. One of His twelve most intimate friends turned traitor for a bribe that would amount, in our modern money, to about nineteen dollars. Another one of His twelve most intimate friends openly deserted Jesus the moment He got into trouble, and declared three times that he didn't even know Jesus—and he swore as he said it. One out of six! That is what happened to Jesus. Why should you and I expect a better score?

I discovered years ago that although I couldn't keep people from criticizing me unjustly, I could do something infinitely more important: I could determine whether I would let the unjust condemnation disturb me.

Let's be clear about this: I am not advocating ignoring all criticism. Far from it. I am talking about *ignoring only unjust criticism.* I once asked Eleanor Roosevelt how she handled unjust criticism—and Allah knows she's had a lot of it. She probably has more ardent friends and more violent enemies than any other woman who ever lived in the White House.

She told me that as a young girl she was almost morbidly shy, afraid of what people might say. She was so afraid of criticism that one day she asked her aunt, Theodore Roosevelt's sister, for advice. She said, "Auntie Bye, I want to do so-and-so. But I'm afraid of being criticized."

Teddy Roosevelt's sister looked her in the eye and said, "Never be bothered by what people say, as long as you know in your heart you are right." Eleanor Roosevelt told me that that bit of advice proved to be her Rock of Gibraltar years later, when she was in the White House. She told me that the only way we can avoid all criticism is to be like a Dresden-china figure and stay on a shelf. "Do what you feel in your heart to be right—for you'll be criticized, anyway. You'll be 'damned if you do, and damned if you don't.'" That is her advice.

When the late Matthew C. Brush was President of the American International Corporation at 40 Wall Street, I asked him if he was ever sensitive to criticism; and he replied, "Yes, I was very sensitive to it in my early days. I was eager then to have all the employees in the organization think I was perfect. If they didn't, it worried me. I would try to please first one person who had been sounding off against me; but the very thing I did to patch it up with him would make someone else mad. Then when I tried to fix it up with this person, I would stir up a couple of other bumblebees. I finally discovered that the more I tried to pacify and to smooth over injured feelings in order to escape personal criticism, the more certain I was to increase my enemies. So finally I said to myself, 'If you get your head above the crowd, you're going to be criticized. So get used to the idea.' That helped me tremendously. From that time on I made it a rule to do the very best I could and then put up my old umbrella and let the rain of criticism drain off me instead of run down my neck."

Deems Taylor went a bit further: he let the rain of criticism run down his neck and had a good laugh over it—in public. When he was giving his comments during the intermission of the Sunday-afternoon radio concerts of the New York Philharmonic-Symphony Orchestra, one woman wrote him a letter calling him "a liar, a traitor, a snake, and a moron." Mr. Taylor says in his book, *Of Men and Music:* "I have a suspicion that she didn't care for that talk." On the following week's broadcast, Mr. Taylor read this letter over the radio to millions of listeners—and received another letter from the same lady a few days later, "expressing her unaltered opinion," says Mr. Taylor, "that I was *still* a liar, a traitor, a snake, and a moron." We can't keep from admiring a man who takes criticism like that. We admire his serenity, his unshaken poise, and his sense of humor.

When Charles Schwab was addressing the student

body at Princeton, he confessed that one of the most important lessons he had ever learned was taught to him by an old German who worked in Schwab's steel mill. This old German got involved in a hot wartime argument with the other steelworkers, and they tossed him into the river. "When he came into my office," Mr. Schwab said, "covered with mud and water, I asked him what he had said to the men who had thrown him into the river, and he replied, 'I yust laughed.'"

Mr. Schwab declared that he had adopted that old German's words as his motto: "Yust laugh."

That motto is especially good when you are the victim of unjust criticism. You can answer the man who answers you back, but what can you say to the man who "yust laughs"?

Lincoln might have broken under the strain of the Civil War if he hadn't learned the folly of trying to answer all the vitriolic condemnations hurled at him. His description of how he handled his critics has become a literary gem—a classic. General MacArthur had a copy of it hanging above his headquarters desk during the war; and Winston Churchill has a framed copy of it on the walls of his study at Chartwell. It goes like this: "If I were to try to read, much less to answer, all the attacks made on me, this shop might as well be closed for any other business. I do the very best I know how—the very best I can; and I mean to keep on doing so until the end. If the end brings me out all right, then what is said against me won't matter. If the ends brings me out wrong, then ten angels swearing I was right would make no difference."

When you and I are unjustly criticized, let's remember Rule 2:

DO THE VERY BEST YOU CAN; AND THEN PUT UP YOUR OLD UMBRELLA AND KEEP THE RAIN OF CRITICISM FROM RUNNING DOWN THE BACK OF YOUR NECK.

"Choose to be optimistic, it feels better."
—Dalai Lama XIV

"It's not the work which kills people, it's the worry. It's not the revolution that destroys machinery it's the friction."
—Henry Ward Beecher

21

FOOL THINGS I HAVE DONE

I have a folder in my private filing cabinet marked "FTD"—short for "Fool Things I Have Done." I put in that folder written records of the fool things I have been guilty of. I sometimes dictate these memos to my secretary, but sometimes they are so personal, so stupid, that I am ashamed to dictate them, so I write them out in longhand.

I can still recall some of the criticisms of Dale Carnegie that I put in my "FTD" folders fifteen years ago. If I had been utterly honest with myself, I would now have a filing cabinet bursting out at the seams with these "FTD" memos. I can truthfully repeat what King Saul said thirty centuries ago: "I have played the fool and have erred exceedingly."

When I get out my "FTD" folders and reread the criticisms I have written of myself, they help me deal with the toughest problem I shall ever face: the management of Dale Carnegie.

I used to blame my troubles on other people; but as I have grown older—and wiser, I hope—I have realized that I myself, in the last analysis, am to blame for almost all my misfortunes. Lots of people have discovered that, as they grow older. "No one but myself," said Napoleon at St. Helena, "no one but myself can be blamed for my fall. I have been my own greatest enemy—the cause of my own disastrous fate."

Let me tell you about a man I knew who was an artist when it came to self-appraisal and self-management. His name was H. P. Howell. When the news of his sudden death in the drugstore of the Hotel Ambassador in New York was flashed across the nation on July 31, 1944, Wall Street was shocked, for he was a leader in American finance—chairman of the board of the Commercial National Bank and Trust Company, 56 Wall Street, and a director of several large corporations. He grew up with little formal education, started out in life clerking in a country store, and later became credit manager for U. S. Steel—and was on his way to position and power.

"For years I have kept an engagement book, showing all the appointments I have during the day," Mr. Howell told me when I asked him to explain the reasons for his success. "My family never makes any plans for me on Saturday night, for the family knows that I devote a part of each Saturday evening to self-examination and a review and appraisal of my work during the week. After dinner, I go off by myself, open my engagement book, and think over all the interviews, discussions, and meetings that have taken place since Monday morning. I ask myself: 'What mistakes did I make that time?' 'What did I do that was right—and in what way could I have improved my performance?' 'What lessons can I learn from that experience?' I sometimes find that this weekly review makes me very unhappy. Sometimes I am astonished by my own blunders. Of course, as the years have gone by, these blunders have become less frequent. This system of self-analysis, continued year after year, has done more for me than any other one thing I have ever attempted."

Maybe H. P. Howell borrowed his idea from Ben Franklin. Only Franklin didn't wait until Saturday night. He gave himself a severe going-over *every* night. He discovered that he had thirteen serious faults. Here are three of them: wasting time, stewing around over trifles, arguing and contradicting people. Wise old Ben Franklin realized that, unless he eliminated these handicaps, he wasn't going to get very far. So he battled with one of his shortcomings every day for a week, and kept a record of who had won each day's slugging match. The next week, he would pick out another bad habit, put on the gloves, and when the bell rang, he would come out of his corner fighting. Franklin kept up this battle with his faults every week for more than two years.

No wonder he became one of the best-loved and most influential men this nation ever produced!

Elbert Hubbard said: "Every man is a damn fool for at least five minutes every day. Wisdom consists in not exceeding that limit."

The small man flies into a rage over the slightest criticism, but the wise man is eager to learn from those who have censured him and reproved him and "disputed the passage with him." Walt Whitman put it this way: "Have you learned lessons only of those who admired you, and were tender with you, and stood aside for you? Have you not learned great lessons from those who rejected you, and braced themselves against you, or disputed the passage with you?"

Instead of waiting for our enemies to criticize us or our

work, let's beat them to it. Let's be our own most severe critic. Let's find and remedy all our weaknesses before our enemies get a chance to say a word. That is what Charles Darwin did. In fact, he spent fifteen years criticizing— well, the story goes like this: When Darwin completed the manuscript of his immortal book, *The Origin of Species,* he realized that the publication of his revolutionary concept of creation would rock the intellectual and religious worlds. So he *became his own critic and spent another fifteen years, checking his data, challenging his reasoning, criticizing his conclusions.*

Suppose someone denounced you as "a damn fool"— what would you do? Get angry? Indignant? Here is what Lincoln did: Edward M. Stanton, Lincoln's Secretary of War, once called Lincoln "a damn fool." Stanton was indignant because Lincoln had been meddling in Stanton's affairs. In order to please a selfish politician, Lincoln had signed an order transferring certain regiments. Stanton not only refused to carry out Lincoln's orders, but swore that Lincoln was a damn fool for ever signing such orders. What happened? When Lincoln was told what Stanton had said, Lincoln calmly replied: "If Stanton said I am a damned fool, then I must be, for he is nearly always right. I'll just step over and see for myself."

Lincoln did go to see Stanton. Stanton convinced him that the order was wrong, and Lincoln withdrew it. Lincoln welcomed criticism when he knew it was sincere, founded on knowledge, and given in a spirit of helpfulness.

You and I ought to welcome that kind of criticism, too, for we can't even hope to be right more than three times out of four. At least, that was all Theodore Roosevelt said he could hope for, when he was in the White House. Einstein, the most profound thinker now living, confesses that his conclusions are wrong ninety-nine per cent of the time!

"The opinions of our enemies," said La Rochefoucauld, "come nearer to the truth about us than do our own opinions."

I know that statement may be true many times; yet when anyone starts to criticize me, if I do not watch myself, I instantly and automatically leap to the defensive—even before I have the slightest idea what my critic is going to say. I am disgusted with myself every time I do it. We all tend to resent criticism and lap up praise, regardless of whether either the criticism or the praise is justified. We are not creatures of logic. We are creatures of emotions. Our logic is like a birch-bark canoe tossed about on a deep, dark, stormy sea of emotion.

If we hear that someone has spoken ill of us, let's not try to defend ourselves. Every fool does that. Let's be original—and humble—and brilliant! Let's confound our critic and win applause for ourselves by saying: "If my critic had known about *all my other faults*, he would have criticized me much more severely than he did."

Here is another idea: when your anger is rising because you feel you have been unjustly condemned, why not stop and say: "Just a minute.... I am far from perfect. If Einstein admits he is wrong ninety-nine per cent of the time, maybe I am wrong at least eighty per cent of the time. Maybe I deserve this criticism. If I do, I ought to be thankful for it, and try to profit by it.

Charles Luckman, president of the Pepsodent Company, spends a million dollars a year putting Bop Hope on the air. He doesn't look at the letters praising the program, but he insists on seeing the critical letters. He knows he may learn something from them.

The Ford Company is so eager to find out what is wrong with its management and operations that it recently polled the employees and invited them to criticize the company.

I know a former soap salesman who used even *ask* for criticism. When he first started out selling soap for Colgate, orders came slowly. He worried about losing his job. Since he knew there was nothing wrong with the soap or the price, he figured that the trouble must be himself. When he failed to make a sale, he would often walk around the block trying to figure out what was wrong. Had he been too vague? Did he lack enthusiasm? Sometimes he would go back to the merchant and say: "I haven't come back here to try to sell you any soap. I have come back to get your advice and your criticism. Won't you please tell me what I did that was wrong when I tried to sell you soap a few minutes ago? You are far more experienced and successful than I am. Please give me your criticism. Be frank. Don't pull your punches."

This attitude won him a lot of friends and priceless advice.

What do you suppose ever happened to him? Today, he is president of the Colgate-Palmolive-Peet Soap Company—the world's largest makers of soap. His name is E. H. Little. Last year, only fourteen people in America had a larger income than he had: $240,141.

It takes a big man to do what H. P. Howell, Ben Franklin, and E. H. Little did. And now, while nobody is looking, why not peep into the mirror and ask yourself whether you belong in that kind of company!

To keep from worrying about criticism, here is Rule 3:

LET'S KEEP A RECORD OF THE FOOL THINGS WE HAVE DONE AND CRITICIZE OURSELVES. SINCE WE CAN'T HOPE TO BE PERFECT, LET'S DO WHAT E. H. LITTLE DID: LET'S ASK FOR UNBIASED, HELPFUL, CONSTRUCTIVE CRITICISM.

"Anxiety's like a rocking chair. It gives you something to do, but it doesn't get you very far."
—Jodi Picoult

"People get so in the habit of worry that if you save them from drowning and put them on a bank to dry in the sun with hot chocolate and muffins, they wonder whether they are catching cold."
—John Jay Chapman

22

HOW MY MOTHER AND FATHER
CONQUERED WORRY

As I have said, I was born and brought up on a Missouri farm. Like most farmers of that day, my parents had pretty hard scratching. My mother had been a country schoolteacher and my father had been a farmhand working for twelve dollars a month. Mother made not only my clothes, but also the soap with which we washed our clothes.

We rarely had any cash—except once a year when we sold our hogs. We traded our butter and eggs at the grocery store for flour, sugar, coffee. When I was twelve years old, I didn't have as much as fifty cents a year to spend on myself. I can still remember the day we went to a Fourth-of-July celebration and Father gave me ten cents to spend as I wished. I felt the wealth of the Indies was mine.

I walked a mile to attend a one-room country school. I walked when the snow was deep and the thermometer shivered around twenty-eight degrees below zero. Until I was fourteen, I never had any rubbers or overshoes. During the long, cold winters, my feet were always wet and cold. As a child I never dreamed that anyone had dry, warm feet during the winter.

My parents slaved sixteen hours a day, yet we were constantly oppressed by debts and harassed by hard luck.

One of my earliest memories is watching the flood waters of the 102 River rolling over our corn and hay fields, destroying everything. The floods destroyed our crops six years out of seven. Year after year, our hogs died of cholera and we burned them. I can close my eyes now and recall the pungent odor of burning hog flesh.

One year, the floods didn't come. We raised a bumper corn crop, bought feed cattle, and fattened them with our corn. But the floods might just as well have drowned our corn that year, for the price of fat cattle fell on the Chicago market; and after feeding and fattening the cattle, we got only thirty dollars more for them than what we had paid for them. Thirty dollars for a whole year's work!

No matter what we did, we lost money. I can still remember the mule colts that my father bought. We fed them for three years, hired men to break them, then shipped them to Memphis, Tennessee—and sold them for less than what we had paid for them three years previously.

After ten years of hard, grueling work, we were not only penniless; we were heavily in debt. Our farm was mortgaged. Try as hard as we might, we couldn't even pay the interest on the mortgage. The bank that held the mortgage abused, and insulted my father, and threatened to take his farm away from him. Father was forty-seven years old. After more than thirty years of hard work, he had nothing but debts and humiliation. It was more than he could take. He worried. His health broke. He had no desire for food; in spite of the hard physical work he was doing in the field all day, he had to take medicine to give him an appetite. He lost flesh. The doctor told my mother that he would be dead within six months. Father was so worried that he no longer wanted to live. I have often heard my mother say that when Father went to the barn to feed the horses and milk the cows, and didn't come back as soon as she expected, she would go out to the barn, fearing that she would find his body dangling from the end of a rope. One day as he returned home from Maryville, where the banker had threatened to foreclose the mortgage, he stopped his horses on a bridge crossing the 102 River, got off the wagon, and stood for a long time looking down at the water, debating with himself whether he should jump in and end it all.

Years later, Father told me that the only reason he didn't jump was because of my mother's deep, abiding, and joyous belief that if we loved God and kept His commandments, everything would come out all right. Mother was right. Everything did come out all right in the end. Father lived forty-two happy years longer, and died in 1941, at the age of eighty-nine.

During all those years of struggle and heartache, my mother never worried. She took all her troubles to God in prayer. Every night before we went to bed, Mother would read a chapter from the Bible; frequently Mother or Father would read these comforting words of Jesus: "In my Father's house are many mansions.... I go to prepare a place for you...that where I am, there ye may be also." Then we all knelt down before our chairs in that lonely Missouri farmhouse and prayed for God's love and protection.

When William James was professor of philosophy at Harvard, he said, "Of course, the sovereign cure for worry is religious faith."

You don't have to go to Harvard to discover that. My mother found that out on a Missouri farm. Neither floods nor debts nor disaster could suppress her happy, radiant, and victorious spirit. I can still hear her singing as she worked:

"Peace, peace, wonderful peace,
Flowing down from the Father above,
Sweep over my spirit forever, I pray, in fathomless billows
of love."

My mother wanted me to devote my life to religious work. I thought seriously of becoming a foreign missionary. Then I went away to college; and gradually, as the years passed, a change came over me. I studied biology, science, philosophy, and comparative religions. I read books on how the Bible was written. I began to question many of its assertions. I began to doubt many of the narrow doctrines taught by the country preachers of that day. I was bewildered. Like Walt Whitman, I "felt the curious, abrupt questionings stir within me." I didn't know what to believe. I saw no purpose in life. I stopped praying. I became an agnostic. I believed that all life was planless and aimless. I believed that human beings had no more divine purpose than had the dinosaurs that roamed the earth two hundred million years ago. I felt that someday the human race would perish—just as the dinosaurs had. I knew that science taught that the sun was slowly cooling, and that when its temperature fell even ten per cent, no form of life could exist on earth. I sneered at the idea of a beneficent God who had created man in His own likeness. I believed that the billions upon billions of suns whirling through black, cold, lifeless space had been created by blind force. Maybe they had never been created at all. Maybe they had existed forever—just as time and space have always existed.

Do I profess to know the answers to all those questions now? No. No man has ever been able to explain the mystery of the universe—the mystery of life. We are surrounded by mysteries. The operation of your body is a profound mystery. So is the electricity in your home. So is the flower in the crannied wall. So is the green grass outside your window. Charles F. Kettering, the guiding genius of General Motors Research Laboratories, has been giving Antioch College thirty thousand dollars a year out of his own pocket to try to discover why grass is green. He declares that if we knew how grass is able to transform sunlight, water, and carbon dioxide into food sugar, we could transform civilization.

Even the operation of the engine in your car is a profound mystery. General Motors Research Laboratories have spent years of time and millions of dollars trying to find out how and why a spark in the cylinder sets off an explosion that makes your car run; and they don't know the answer.

The fact that we don't understand the mysteries of our bodies or electricity or a gas engine doesn't keep us from using and enjoying them. The fact that I don't understand the mysteries of prayer and religion, no longer keeps me from enjoying the richer, happier life that religion brings. At long last, I realize the wisdom of Santayana's words: "Man is not made to understand life, but to live it."

I have gone back—well, I was about to say that I had gone *back* to religion; but that would not be accurate. I have gone *forward* to a new concept of religion. I no longer have the faintest interest in the differences in creeds that divide the churches. But I am tremendously interested in what religion does for me, just as I am interested in what electricity and good food and water do for me. They help me to lead a richer, fuller, happier life. But religion does far more than that. It brings me spiritual values. It gives me, as William James put it, "*a new zest for life…more life, a larger, richer, more satisfying life.*" It gives me faith, hope, and courage. It banishes tensions, anxieties, fears, and worries. It gives purpose to my life— and direction. It vastly improves my happiness. It gives me abounding health. It helps me to create for myself "an oasis of peace amidst the whirling sands of life."

Francis Bacon was right when he said, three hundred and fifty years ago: "A little philosophy inclineth man's mind to atheism; but depth in philosophy bringeth men's minds about to religion."

I can remember the days when people talked about the conflict between science and religion. But no more. The newest of all sciences—psychiatry—is teaching what Jesus taught. Why? Because psychiatrists realize that prayer and a strong religious faith will banish the worries, the anxieties, the strains and fears that cause more than half of all our ills. They know, as one of their leaders, Dr. A. A. Brill, said: "Anyone who is truly religious does not develop a neurosis."

If religion isn't true, then life is meaningless. It is a tragic farce.

I interviewed Henry Ford a few years prior to his death. Before I met him, I had expected him to show the strains of the long years he had spent in building up and managing one of the world's greatest businesses. So I was surprised to see how calm, and well and peaceful, he looked at seventy-eight. When I asked him if he ever worried, he replied, "No. I believe God is managing affairs and that He doesn't need any advice from me. With God in charge, I believe that everything will work out for the best in the end. So what is there to worry about?"

Today, even psychiatrists are becoming modern evangelists. They are not urging us to lead religious lives to avoid hell-fires in the next world, but they are urging us to lead religious lives to avoid the hell-fires of this world—the hell-fires of stomach ulcer, angina pectoris, nervous breakdowns, and insanity. As an example of what our psychologists and psychiatrists are teaching, read *The Return to Religion*, by Dr. Henry C. Link. You will probably find a copy in your public library.

Yes, the Christian religion is an inspiring, health-giving activity. Jesus said: "I came that ye might have life and have it more abundantly." Jesus denounced and attacked the dry forms and dead rituals that passed for religion in His day. He was a rebel. He preached a new kind of religion—a religion that threatened to upset the world. That is why He was crucified. He preached that religion should exist for man—not man for religion; that the Sabbath was made for man—not man for the Sabbath. He talked more about fear than He did about sin. *The wrong kind of fear is a sin*—a sin against your health, a sin against the richer, fuller, happier, courageous life that Jesus advocated. Emerson spoke of himself as a "Professor of the Science of Joy." Jesus, too, was a teacher of "the Science of Joy." He commanded His disciples to "rejoice and leap for joy."

Jesus declared that there were only two important things about religion: loving God with all our heart, and our neighbor as ourselves. Any man who does that is religious, regardless of whether he knows it. For example, my father-in-law, Henry Price, of Tulsa, Oklahoma. He tries to live by the golden rule; and he is incapable of doing anything mean, selfish, or dishonest. However, he doesn't attend church, and regards himself as an agnostic. Nonsense! What makes a man a Christian? I'll let John Baillie answer that. He was probably the most distinguished professor who ever taught theology at the University of Edinburgh. He said: "What makes a man a Christian is neither his intellectual acceptance of certain ideas, nor his conformity to a certain rule, but his possession of a certain Spirit, and his participation in a certain Life."

If that makes a man a Christian, then Henry Price is a noble one.

William James—the father of modern psychology—

wrote to his friend, Professor Thomas Davidson, saying that as the years went by, he found himself "less and less able to get along without God."

Earlier in this book I mentioned that when the judges tried to pick the best story on worry sent in by my students, they had so much difficulty in choosing between two outstanding stories that the prize money was split. Here is the second story that tied for first prize—the unforgettable experience of a woman who had to find out the hard way that "she couldn't get along without God."

I am calling this woman Mary Cushman, although that is not her actual name. She has children and grandchildren who might be embarrassed to see her story in print, so I agreed to disguise her identity. However, the woman herself is real—very real. A few months ago, she sat in the armchair beside my desk and told me her story. Here is how it goes:

"During the Depression," she said, "my husband's average salary was eighteen dollars a week. Many times we didn't have even that because he didn't get paid when he was ill—and that was often. He had a series of minor accidents; he also had mumps, scarlet fever, and repeated attacks of flu. We lost the little house that we had built with our own hands. We owed fifty dollars at the grocery store—and had five children to feed. I took in washing and ironing from the neighbors, and bought secondhand clothes from the Salvation Army store and made them over for my children to wear. I made myself ill with worry. One day the grocer, to whom we owed fifty dollars, accused my eleven-year-old boy of stealing a couple of pencils. My son wept as he told me about it. I knew he was honest and sensitive—and I knew that he had been disgraced and humiliated in front of other people. That was the straw that broke my back. I thought of all the misery we had endured; and I couldn't see any hope for the future. I must have become temporarily insane with worry, for I shut off my washing machine, took my little five-year-old daughter into the bedroom, and plugged up the windows and cracks with paper and rags. My little girl said to me, 'Mommy, what are you doing?' and I answered, 'There's a little draft in here.' Then I turned on the gas heater we had in the bedroom—and didn't light it. As I lay down on the bed with my daughter beside me, she said, 'Mommy, this is funny—we just got up a little while ago!' But I said, 'Never mind, we'll take a little nap.' Then I closed my eyes, listening to the gas escape from the heater. I shall never forget the smell of that gas....

"Suddenly I thought I heard music. I listened. I had forgotten to turn the radio off in the kitchen. It didn't matter now. But the music kept on, and presently I heard someone singing an old hymn:

What a friend we have in Jesus,
All our sins and griefs to bear!
What a privilege to carry
Everything to God in prayer,
Oh, what peace we often forfeit
Oh, what needless pains we bear
All because we do not carry
Everything to God in prayer!

"As I listened to that hymn, I realized that I had made a tragic mistake. I had tried to fight all my terrible battles alone. I had not taken everything to God in prayer…. I jumped up, turned off the gas, opened the door, and raised the windows.

"I wept and prayed all the rest of that day. Only I didn't pray for help—instead I poured out my soul in thanksgiving to God for the blessings He had given me: five splendid children—all of them healthy and fine, strong in body and mind. I promised God that never again would I prove so ungrateful. And I have kept that promise.

"Even after we lost our home, and had to move into a little country schoolhouse that we rented for five dollars a month, I thanked God for that schoolhouse; I thanked Him for the fact that I at least had a roof to keep us warm and dry. I thanked God honestly that things were not worse—and I believe that He heard me. For in time things improved—oh, not overnight; but as the depression lightened, we made a little more money. I got a job as a hat-check girl in a large country club, and sold stockings as a side line. To help put himself through college, one of my sons got a job on a farm, milked thirteen cows morning and night. Today my children are grown up and married; I have three fine grand-children. And, as I look back on that terrible day when I turned on the gas, I thank God over and over that I 'woke up' in time. What joys I would have missed if I had carried out that act! How many wonderful years I would have forfeited forever! Whenever I hear now of someone who wants to end his life, I feel like crying out: 'Don't do it! Don't!' The blackest moments we live through can only last a little time—and then comes the future...."

On the average, someone commits suicide in the United States every thirty-five minutes. On the average, someone goes insane every hundred and twenty seconds. Most of these suicides—and probably many of the tragedies of insanity—could have been prevented if these people had only had the solace and peace that are found in religion and prayer.

One of the most distinguished psychiatrists living, Dr. Carl Jung, says on page 264 of his book *Modern Man in Search of a Soul,* "During the past thirty years, people from all the civilized countries of the earth have consulted me. I have treated many hundreds of patients. Among all my patients in the second half of life—that is to say, over thirty-five—there has not been one whose problem in the last resort was not that of finding a religious outlook on life. It is safe to say that every one of them fell ill because he had lost that which the living religions of every age have given to their followers, and none of them has been really healed who did not regain his religious outlook."

That statement is so significant I want to repeat it in *bold type.*

Dr. Carl Jung said:

"During the past thirty years, people from all the civilized countries of the earth have consulted me. I have treated many hundreds of patients. Among all my patients second half of life—that is to say, over thirty-five— has not been one whose problem in the last resort was not that of finding a religious outlook on life. It is safe to say that every one of them fell ill because he had lost that which the living religions of every age have given to their followers, and none of them has been really healed who did not regain his religious outlook."

William James said approximately the same thing: "*Faith* is *one of* the *forces by which men live*," he declared, "*and the total absence of it means collapse.*"

The late Mahatma Gandhi, the greatest Indian leader since Buddha, would have collapsed if he had not been inspired by the sustaining power of prayer. How do I know? Because Gandhi himself said so. "Without prayer," he wrote, "I should have been a lunatic long ago."

Thousands of people could give similar testimony. My own father—well, as I have already said, my own father would have drowned himself had it not been for my mother's prayers and faith. Probably thousands of the tortured souls who are now screaming in our insane asylums could have been saved if they had only turned to a higher power for help instead of trying to fight life's battles alone.

When we are harassed and reach the limit of our own strength, many of us then turn in desperation to God— "There are no atheists in foxholes." But why wait till we are desperate? Why not renew our strength every day? Why wait even until Sunday? For years I have had the habit of dropping into empty churches on *weekday afternoons*. When I feel that I am too rushed and hurried to spare a few minutes to think about spiritual things, I say to myself: "Wait a minute, Dale Carnegie, wait a minute. Why all the feverish hurry and rush, little man? You need to pause and acquire a little perspective." At such times, I frequently drop into the first church that I find open. Although I am a Protestant, I frequently, on weekday afternoons, drop into St. Patrick's Cathedral on Fifth Avenue, and remind myself that I'll be dead in another thirty years, but that the great spiritual truths that all churches teach are eternal. I close my eyes and pray. I find that doing this calms my nerves, rests my body, clarifies my perspective, and helps me revalue my values. May I recommend this practice to you?

During the past six years that I have been writing this book, I have collected hundreds of examples and concrete cases of how men and women conquered fear and worry by prayer. I have in my filing cabinet folders bulging with case histories. Let's take as a typical example the story of a discouraged and disheartened book salesman, John R. Anthony. Mr. Anthony is now an attorney in Houston, Texas, with offices in the Humble Building. Here is his story as he told it to me.

"Twenty-two years ago I closed my private law office to become state representative of an American lawbook company. My specialty was selling a set of lawbooks to lawyers—a set of books that were almost indispensable.

"I was ably and thoroughly trained for the job. I knew all the direct sales talks, and the convincing answers to all possible objections. Before calling on a prospect, I familiarized myself with his rating as an attorney, the nature of his practice, his politics, and hobbies. During my interview, I used that information with ample skill.

Yet, something was wrong. I just couldn't get orders!

"I grew discouraged. As the days and weeks passed, I doubled and redoubled my efforts, but was still unable to close enough sales to pay my expenses. A sense of fear and dread grew within me. I became afraid to call on people. Before I could enter a prospect's office, that feeling of dread flared up so strong that I would pace up and down the hallway outside the door—or go out of the building and circle the block. Then, after losing much valuable time and feigning enough courage by sheer will power to crash the office door, I feebly turned the doorknob with trembling hand—half hoping my prospect would not be in!

"My sales manager threatened to stop my advances if I didn't send in more orders. My wife at home pleaded with me for money to pay the grocery bill for herself and our three children. Worry seized me. Day by day I grew more desperate. I didn't know what to do. As I have already said, I had closed my private law office at home and had given up my clients. Now I was broke. I didn't have the money to pay even my hotel bill. Neither did I have the money to buy a ticket back home; nor did I have the courage to return home a beaten man, even if I had had the ticket. Finally, at the miserable end of another bad day, I trudged back to my hotel room—for the last time, I thought. So far as I was concerned, I was thoroughly beaten. Heartbroken, depressed, I didn't know which way to turn. I hardly cared whether I lived or died. I was sorry I had ever been born. I had nothing but a glass of hot milk that night for dinner. Even that was more than I could afford. I understood that night why desperate men raise a hotel window and jump. I might have done it myself if I had had the courage. I began wondering what was the purpose of life. I didn't know. I couldn't figure it out.

"Since there was no one else to turn to, I turned to God. I began to pray. I implored the Almighty to give me light and understanding and guidance through the dark, dense wilderness of despair that had closed in about me. I asked God to help me get orders for my books, and to give me money to feed my wife and children. After that prayer, I opened my eyes and saw a Gideon Bible that lay on the dresser in that lonely hotel room. I opened it and read those beautiful, immortal promises of Jesus that must have inspired countless generations of lonely, worried, and beaten men throughout the ages—a talk that Jesus gave to His disciples about how to keep from worrying :

"Take no thought for your life, what ye shall eat, or what ye shall drink; nor yet for your body, what ye shall put on. Is not the life more than meat, and the body than raiment? Behold the fowls of the air: for they sow not, neither do they reap, nor gather into barns; yet your heavenly Father feedeth them. Are ye not much better than they?…But seek ye first the kingdom of God, and his righteousness; and all these things shall be added unto you."

"As I prayed and as I read those words, a miracle happened: my nervous tension fell away. My anxieties, fears, and worries were transformed into heart-warming courage and hope and triumphant faith.

"I was happy, even though I didn't have enough money to pay my hotel bill. I went to bed and slept soundly—free from care—as I had not done for many years.

"Next morning, I could hardly hold myself back until the offices of my prospects were open. I approached the office door of my first prospect that beautiful, cold, rainy day with a bold and positive stride. I turned the doorknob with a firm and steady grip. As I entered, I made a beeline for my man, energetically, chin up, and with appropriate dignity, all smiles, and saying, "Good morning, Mr. Smith! I'm John R. Anthony of the All-American Lawbook Company!"

"'Oh, yes, yes,' he replied, smiling, too, as he rose from his chair with outstretched hand. 'I'm glad to see you. Have a seat!'

"I made more sales that day than I had made in weeks. That evening I proudly returned to my hotel like a conquering hero! I felt like a new man. And I *was* a new man, because I had a new and victorious mental attitude. No dinner of hot milk that night. No, sir! I had a steak with all the fixin's. From that day on, my sales zoomed.

"I was born anew that desperate night twenty-two years ago in a little hotel in Amarillo, Texas. My outward situation the next day was the same as it had been through my weeks of failure, but a tremendous thing had happened inside me. I had suddenly become aware of my relationship with God. A mere man alone can easily be defeated, but a man alive with the power of God within him is invincible. I know. I saw it work in my own life.

"'Ask, and it shall be given to you; seek, and ye shall find; knock, and it shall be opened unto you.'"

When Mrs. L. G. Beaird, of 1421 8th Street, Highland, Illinois, was faced with stark tragedy, she discovered that she could find peace and tranquillity by kneeling down and saying, "O Lord, Thy will, not mine, be done."

"One evening our telephone rang," she writes in a letter that I have before me now. "It rang fourteen times before I had the courage to pick up the receiver. I knew it must be the hospital, and I was terrified. I feared that our little boy was dying. He had meningitis. He had already been given penicillin, but it made his temperature fluctuate, and the doctor feared that the disease had traveled to his brain and might cause the development of a brain tumor—and death. The phone call *was* just what I feared. The hospital was calling; the doctor wanted us to come immediately.

"Maybe you can picture the anguish my husband and I went through, sitting in the waiting room. Everyone else had his baby, but we sat there with empty arms, wondering if we would ever hold our little fellow again. When we were finally called into the doctor's private office, the expression on his face filled our hearts with terror. His words brought even more terror. He told us that there was only one chance in four that our baby would live. He said that if we knew another doctor, to please call him in on the case.

"On the way home, my husband broke down and, doubling up his fist, hit the steering wheel, saying, 'Betts, I can't give that little guy up.' Have you ever seen a man cry? It isn't a pleasant experience. We stopped the car and, after talking things over, decided to stop in church and pray that if it was God's will to take our baby, we would resign our will to His. I sank in the pew and said with tears rolling down my cheeks, 'Not my will but Thine be done.'

"The moment I uttered those words, I felt better. A sense of peace that I hadn't felt for a long time came over me. All the way home, I kept repeating, 'O God, Thy will, not mine, be done.' I slept soundly that night for the first time in a week. The doctor called a few days later and said that Bobby had passed the crisis. I thank God for the strong and healthy four-year-old boy we have today."

I know men who regard religion as something for women and children and preachers. They pride themselves on being "he-men" who can fight their battles alone.

How surprised they might be to learn that some of the most famous "he-men" in the world pray every day. For example, "he-man" Jack Dempsey told me that he never goes to bed without saying his prayers. He told me that he never eats a meal without first thanking God for it. He told me that he prayed every day when he was training for a bout, and that when he was fighting, he always prayed just before the bell sounded for each round. "Praying," he said, "helped me fight with courage and confidence."

"He-man" Connie Mack told me that he couldn't go to sleep without saying his prayers.

"He-man" Eddie Rickenbacker told me that he believed his life had been saved by prayer. He prays every day.

"He-man" Edward R. Stettinius, former high official

of General Motors and United States Steel, and former Secretary of State, told me that he prayed for wisdom and guidance every morning and night.

"He-man" J. Pierpont Morgan, the greatest financier of his age, often went alone to Trinity Church, at the head of Wall Street, on Saturday afternoons and knelt in prayer.

When "he-man" Eisenhower flew to England to take supreme command of the British and American forces, he took only one book on the plane with him—the Bible.

"He-man" General Mark Clark told me that he read his Bible every day during the war and knelt down in prayer. So did Chiang Kai-shek, and General Montgomery—"Monty of El Alamein." So did Lord Nelson at Trafalgar. So did General Washington, Robert E. Lee, Stonewall Jackson, and scores of other great military leaders.

These "he-men" discovered the truth of William James's statement: "We and God have business with each other; and in opening ourselves to His influence, our deepest destiny is fulfilled."

A lot of "he-men" are discovering that. Seventy-two million Americans are church members now—an all-time record. As I said before, even the scientists are turning to religion. Take, for example, Dr. Alexis Carrel, who wrote *Man, the Unknown* and won the greatest honour that can be bestowed upon any scientist, the Nobel prize. Dr. Carrel said in a *Reader's Digest* article: "Prayer is the most powerful form of energy one can generate. It is a force as real as terrestrial gravity. As a physician, I have seen men, after all other therapy had failed, lifted out of disease and melancholy by the serene effort of prayer.... Prayer like radium is a source of luminous, self-generating energy.... In prayer, human beings seek to augment their finite energy by addressing themselves to the Infinite source of all energy. When we pray, we link ourselves with the inexhaustible motive power that spins the universe. We pray that a part of this power be apportioned to our needs. Even in asking, our human deficiencies are filled and we arise strengthened and repaired.... Whenever we address God in fervent prayer, we change both soul and body for the better. It could not happen that any man or woman could pray for a single moment without some good result."

Admiral Byrd knows what it means to "link ourselves with the inexhaustible motive power that spins the universe." His ability to do that pulled him through the most trying ordeal of his life. He tells the story in his book *Alone*. In 1934, he spent five months in a hut buried beneath the icecap of Ross Barrier deep in the Antarctic. He was the only living creature south of latitude seventy-eight. Blizzards roared above his shack; the cold plunged down to eighty-two degrees below zero; he was completely surrounded by unending night. And then he found, to his horror, he was being slowly poisoned by carbon monoxide that escaped from his stove! What could he do? The nearest help was 123 miles away, and could not possibly reach him for several months. He tried to fix his stove and ventilating system, but the fumes still escaped. They often knocked him out cold. He lay on the floor completely unconscious. He couldn't eat; he couldn't sleep; he became so feeble that he could hardly leave his bunk. He frequently feared he wouldn't live until morning. He was convinced he would die in that cabin, and his body would be hidden by perpetual snows.

What saved his life? One day, in the depths of his despair, he reached for his diary and tried to set down his philosophy of life. "The human race," he wrote, "is not alone in the universe." He thought of the stars overhead, of the orderly swing of the constellations and planets; of how the everlasting sun would, in its time, return to lighten even the wastes of the South Polar regions. And then he wrote in his diary, "I am not alone."

This realization that he was not alone—not even in a hole in the ice at the end of the earth—was what saved Richard Byrd. "I know it pulled me through," he says. And he goes on to add: "Few men in their lifetime come anywhere near exhausting the resources dwelling within them. There are deep wells of strength that are never used." Richard Byrd learned to tap those wells of strength and use those resources—by turning to God.

Glenn A. Arnold learned amidst the cornfields of Illinois the same lesson that Admiral Byrd learned in the polar icecap. Mr. Arnold, an insurance broker in the Bacon Building, Chillicothe, Illinois, opened his speech on conquering worry like this: "Eight years ago, I turned the key in the lock of my front door for what I believed was the last time in my life. I then climbed in my car and started down for the river. I was a failure," he said. "One month before, my entire little world had come crashing down on my head. My electrical appliance business had gone on the rocks. In my home my mother lay at the point of death. My wife was carrying our second child. Doctors' bills were mounting. We had mortgaged everything we had to start the business—our car and our furniture. I had even taken out a loan on my insurance policies. Now everything was gone. I couldn't take it any longer. So I climbed into my car and started for the river—determined to end the sorry mess.

"I drove a few miles out in the country, pulled off the road, and got out and sat on the ground and wept like a child. Then I really started to think—instead of going around in frightening circles of worry, I tried to think constructively. How bad was my situation? Couldn't it be worse? Was it really hopeless? What could I do to make it better?

"I decided then and there to take the whole problem to the Lord and ask Him to handle it. I prayed. I prayed hard. I prayed as though my very life depended on it—which, in fact, it did. Then a strange thing happened. As soon as I turned all my problems over to a power greater than myself, I immediately felt a peace of mind that I hadn't known in months. I must have sat there for half an hour, weeping and praying. Then I went home and slept like a child.

"The next morning, I arose with confidence. I no longer had anything to fear, for I was depending on God for guidance. That morning I walked into a local department store with my head high; and I spoke with confidence as I applied for a job as salesman in the electrical-appliance department. I knew I would get the job. And I did. I made good at it until the whole appliance business collapsed due to the war. Then I began selling life insurance—still under the management of my Great Guide. That was only five years ago. Now, all my bills are paid; I have a fine family of three bright children; own my own home; have a new car, and own twenty-five thousand dollars in life insurance.

"As I look back, I am glad now that I lost everything and became so depressed that I started for the river—because that tragedy taught me to rely on God; and I now have a peace and confidence that I never dreamed were possible."

Why does religious faith bring us such peace and calm and fortitude? I'll let William James answer that. He says: *"The turbulent billows of the fretful surface leave the deep parts of the ocean undisturbed; and to him who has a hold on vaster and more permanent realities, the hourly vicissitudes of his personal destiny seem relatively insignificant things. The really religious person is accordingly unshakeable and full of equanimity, and calmly ready for any duty that the day may bring forth."*

If we are worried and anxious—why not try God? Why not, as Immanuel Kant said, "accept a belief in God because we need such a belief?" Why not link ourselves now "with the inexhaustible motive power that spins the universe?"

Even if you are not a religious person by nature or training—even if you are an out-and-out skeptic—prayer can help you much more than you believe, for it is a *practical* thing. What do I mean, practical? I mean that prayer fulfills these three very basic psychological needs which all people share, whether they believe in God or not:

Prayer helps us to put into words exactly what is troubling us. Praying, in a way, is very much like writing our problem down on paper. If we ask help for a problem—even from God—we must put it into words.

Prayer gives us a sense of sharing our burdens, of not being alone. Few of us are so strong that we can bear our heaviest burdens, our most agonizing troubles, all by ourselves. Sometimes our worries are of so intimate a nature that we cannot discuss them even with our closest relatives or friends. Then prayer is the answer. Any psychiatrist will tell us that when we are pent-up and tense, and in an agony of spirit, it is therapeutically good to tell someone our troubles. When we can't tell anyone else—we can always tell God.

Prayer puts into force an active principle of *doing*. It's a first step toward *action*. I doubt if anyone can pray for some fulfillment, day after day, without benefiting from it—in other words, without taking some steps to bring it to pass. The world-famous scientist, Dr. Alexis Carrel, said: "Prayer is the most powerful form of energy one can generate." So why not make use of it? Call it God or Allah or Spirit—why quarrel with definitions as long as the mysterious powers of nature take us in hand?

Why not close this book right now, go to your bedroom, shut the door, kneel down, and unburden your heart? If you have lost your faith, beseech Almighty God to renew it; and repeat this beautiful prayer written by

Saint Francis of Assisi seven hundred years ago: "Lord, make me an instrument of Thy Peace. Where there is hatred, let me sow love. Where there is injury, pardon. Where there is doubt, faith. Where there is despair, hope. Where there is darkness, light. Where there is sadness, joy. O Divine Master, grant that I may not so much seek to be consoled as to console; to be understood, as to understand; to be loved, as to love; for it is in giving that we receive, it is in pardoning that we are pardoned, and it is in dying that we are born to Eternal Life."

> *"Some people grumble that roses have thorns; I am grateful that thorns have roses."*
>
> —Alphonse Karr

> *"We never worry about the big things, just the small things."*
>
> —Travis Barker

PART 6

23

EIGHT WORDS THAT CAN
TRANSFORM YOUR LIFE

A few years ago, I was asked to answer this question on a radio program: "What is the biggest lesson you have ever learned?"

That was easy: by far the most vital lesson I have ever learned is the importance of what we think. If I knew what you think, I would know what you are. Our thoughts make us what we are. Our mental attitude is the X factor that determines our fate. Emerson said: "A man is what he thinks about all day long." How could he possibly be anything else?

I now know with a conviction beyond all doubt that the biggest problem you and I have to deal with—in fact, almost the *only* problem we have to deal with—is choosing the right thoughts. If we can do that, we will be on the highroad to solving all our problems. The great philosopher who ruled the Roman Empire, Marcus Aurelius, summed it up in eight words—*eight words that can determine your destiny: "Our life is what our thoughts make it."*

Yes, if we think happy thoughts, we will be happy. If we think miserable thoughts, we will be miserable. If we think fear thoughts, we will be fearful. If we think sickly thoughts, we will probably be ill. If we think failure, we will certainly fail. If we wallow in self-pity, everyone will want to shun us and avoid us. "You are not," said Norman Vincent Peale, "you are not what you think you are; but what you *think*, you are."

Am I advocating a habitual Pollyanna attitude toward all our problems? No, unfortunately, life isn't so simple as all that. But I am advocating that we assume a *positive* attitude instead of a negative attitude. In other words, we need to be concerned about our problems, but not worried. What is the difference between concern and worry? Let me illustrate. Every time I cross the traffic-jammed streets of New York, I am concerned about what I am doing—but not worried. Concern means realizing what the problems are, and calmly taking steps to meet them. Worrying means going around in maddening, futile circles.

A man can be concerned about his serious problems and still walk with his chin up and a carnation in his buttonhole. I have seen Lowell Thomas do just that. I once had the privilege of being associated with Lowell Thomas in presenting his famous films on the Allenby-Lawrence campaigns in World War I. He and his assistants had photographed the war on half a dozen fronts; and, best of all, had brought back a pictorial record of T. E. Lawrence and his colorful Arabian army, and a film record of Allenby's conquest of the Holy Land. His illustrated talks entitled "With Allenby in Palestine and Lawrence in Arabia" were a sensation in London—and around the world. The London opera season was postponed for six weeks so that he could continue telling his tale of high adventure, and showing his pictures at Covent Garden

Royal Opera House. After his sensational success in London came a triumphant tour of many countries. Then he spent two years preparing a film record of life in India and Afghanistan. After a lot of incredibly bad luck, the impossible happened: he found himself broke in London. I was with him at the time. I remember we had to eat cheap meals at the Lyons' Corner House restaurants. We couldn't have eaten even there if Mr. Thomas had not borrowed money from a Scotsman—James McBey, the renowned artist. Here is the point of the story: even when Lowell Thomas was facing huge debts and severe disappointments, he was concerned, but not worried. He knew that if he let his reverses get him down, he would be worthless to everyone, including his creditors. So each morning before he started out, he bought a flower, put it in his buttonhole, and went swinging down Oxford Street with his head high and his step spirited. He thought positive, courageous thoughts and refused to let defeat defeat him. To him, being licked was all a part of the game—the useful training you had to expect if you wanted to get to the top.

Our mental attitude has an almost unbelievable effect even on our physical powers. The famous British psychiatrist, J. A. Hadfield, gives a striking illustration of that fact in his splendid 54-page booklet: *The Psychology of Power.* "I asked three men," he writes, "to submit themselves to test the effect of mental suggestion on their strength, which was measured by gripping a dynamometer." He told them to grip the dynamometer with all their might. He had them do this under three different sets of conditions.

When he tested them under normal waking conditions, their average grip was 101 pounds.

When he tested them after he had hypnotized them and told them that they were very weak, they could grip only 29 pounds—less than a third of their normal strength. (One of these men was a prize fighter; and when he was told under hypnosis that he was weak, he remarked that his arm felt "tiny, just like a baby's.")

When Captain Hadfield then tested these men a third time, telling them under hypnosis that they were very strong, they were able to grip an average of 142 pounds. When their minds were filled with positive thoughts of strength, they increased their actual physical powers almost five hundred per cent.

Such is the incredible power of our mental attitude.

To illustrate the magic power of thought, let me tell you one of the most astounding stories in the annals of America. I could write a book about it; but let's be brief. On a frosty October night, shortly after the close of the Civil War, a homeless, destitute woman, who was little more than a wanderer on the face of the earth, knocked at the door of "Mother" Webster, the wife of a retired sea captain, living in Amesbury, Massachusetts.

Opening the door, "Mother" Webster saw a frail little creature, "scarcely more than a hundred pounds of frightened skin and bones." The stranger, a Mrs. Glover, explained she was seeking a home where she could think and work out a great problem that absorbed her day and night.

"Why not stay here?" Mrs. Webster replied. "I'm all alone in this big house."

Mrs. Glover might have remained indefinitely with "Mother" Webster if the latter's son-in-law, Bill Ellis, hadn't come up from New York for a vacation. When he discovered Mrs. Glover's presence, he shouted: "I'll have no vagabonds in this house;" and he shoved this homeless woman out of the door. A driving rain was falling. She stood shivering in the rain for a few minutes, and then started down the road, looking for shelter.

Here is the astonishing part of the story. That "vagabond" whom Bill Ellis put out of the house was destined to have as much influence on the thinking of the world as any other woman who ever walked this earth. She is now known to millions of devoted followers as Mary Baker Eddy—the founder of Christian Science.

Yet, until this time, she had known little in life except sickness, sorrow, and tragedy. Her first husband had died shortly after their marriage. Her second husband had deserted her and eloped with a married woman. He later died in a poorhouse. She had only one child, a son; and she was forced, because of poverty, illness, and jealousy, to give him up when he was four years old. She lost all track of him and never saw him again for thirty-one years.

Because of her own ill health, Mrs. Eddy had been interested for years in what she called "the science of mind healing." But the dramatic turning point in her life occurred in Lynn, Massachusetts. Walking downtown one cold day, she slipped and fell on the icy pavement—and was knocked unconscious. Her spine was so injured that she was convulsed with spasms. Even the doctor expected her to die. If by some miracle she lived, he declared that she would never walk again.

Lying on what was supposed to be her deathbed, Mary Baker Eddy opened her Bible, and was led, she declared, by divine guidance to read these words from Saint Matthew: "And, behold, they brought to him a man sick of the palsy, lying on a bed: and Jesus…said unto the sick of the palsy; Son, be of good cheer; thy sins be forgiven thee…. Arise, take up thy bed, and go unto thine house. And he arose, and departed to his house."

These words of Jesus, she declared, produced within her such a strength, such a faith, such a surge of healing power, that she "immediately got out of bed and walked."

"That experience," Mrs. Eddy declared, "was the falling apple that led me to the discovery of how to be well myself, and how to make others so…. I gained the scientific certainty that all causation was Mind, and every effect a mental phenomenon."

Such was the way in which Mary Baker Eddy became the founder and high priestess of a new religion: Christian Science—the only great religious faith ever established by a woman—a religion that has encircled the globe.

You are probably saying to yourself by now: "This man, Carnegie, is proselytizing for Christian Science." No. You are wrong. I am not a Christian Scientist. But the longer I live, the more deeply I am convinced of the tremendous power of thought. As a result of thirty-five years spent in teaching adults, I know men and women can banish worry, fear, and various kinds of illnesses, and can transform their lives by changing their thoughts. I know! I know!! I know!!! I have seen such incredible transformations performed hundreds of times. I have seen them so often that I no longer wonder at them.

For example, one of these incredible transformations, which illustrate the power of thought, happened to one of my students. He had a nervous breakdown. What brought it on? Worry. This student told me, "I worried about everything: I worried because I was too thin; because I thought I was losing my hair; because I feared I would never make enough money to get married; because I felt I would never make a good father; because I feared I was losing the girl I wanted to marry; because I felt I was not living a good life. I worried about the impression I was making on other people. I worried because I thought I had stomach ulcers. I could no longer work; I gave up my job. I built up tension inside me until I was like a boiler without a safety valve. The pressure got so unbearable that something had to give—and it did. If you have never had a nervous breakdown, pray God that you never do, for no pain of the body can exceed the excruciating pain of an agonized mind.

"My breakdown was so severe that I couldn't talk even to my own family. I had no control over my thoughts. I was filled with fear. I would jump at the slightest noise. I avoided everybody. I would break out crying for no apparent reason at all.

"Every day was one of agony. I felt that I was deserted by everybody—even God. I was tempted to jump into the river and end it all.

"I decided instead to take a trip to Florida, hoping that a change of scene would help me. As I stepped on the train, my father handed me a letter and told me not to open it until I reached Florida. I landed in Florida during the height of the tourist season. Since I couldn't get in a hotel, I rented a sleeping room in a garage. I tried to get a job on a tramp freighter out of Miami, but had no luck. So I spent my time at the beach. I was more wretched in Florida than I had been at home; so I opened the envelope to see what Dad had written. His note said, 'Son, you are 1500 miles from home, and you don't feel any different, do you? I knew you wouldn't, because you took with you the one thing that is the cause of all your trouble, that is, yourself. There is nothing wrong with either your body or your mind. It is not the situations you have met that have thrown you; it is what you think of these situations. "As a man thinketh in his heart, so is he." When you realize that, son, come home, for you will be cured.'

"Dad's letter made me angry. I was looking for sympathy, not instruction. I was so mad that I decided then and there that I would never go home. That night as I was walking down one of the side streets of Miami, I came to a church where services were going on. Having no place to go, I drifted in and listened to a sermon on the text: 'He who conquers his spirit is mightier than he who taketh a city.' Sitting in the sanctity of the house of God and hearing the same thoughts that my Dad had written in his letter—all this swept the accumulated litter out of my brain. I was able to think clearly and sensibly for the first time in my life. I realized what a fool I had been. I was shocked to see myself in my true light: here I was, wanting to change the whole world and everyone in it—when the only thing that needed changing was the focus of the lens of the camera, which was my mind.

"The next morning I packed and started home. A week later I was back on the job. Four months later I married the girl I had been afraid of losing. We now have a happy family of five children. God has been good to me both materially and mentally. At the time of the breakdown I was a night foreman of a small department handling eighteen people. I am now superintendent of carton manufacture in charge of over four hundred and fifty people. Life is much fuller and friendlier. I believe I appreciate the true values of life now. When moments of uneasiness try to creep in (as they will in everyone's life), I tell myself to get that camera back in focus, and everything is O.K.

"I can honestly say that I am glad I had the breakdown, because I found out the hard way what power our thoughts can have over our mind and our body. Now I can make my thoughts work for me instead of against me. I can see now that Dad was right when he said it wasn't outward situations that had caused all my suffering, but what I thought of those situations. And as soon as I realized that, I was cured—and stayed cured." Such was the experience of this student.

I am deeply convinced that our peace of mind and the joy we get out of living depends not on where we are, or what we have, or who we are, but solely upon our mental attitude. Outward conditions have very little to do with it. For example, let's take the case of old John Brown, who was hanged for seizing the United States arsenal at Harpers Ferry and trying to incite the slaves to rebellion. He rode away to the gallows, sitting on his coffin. The jailer who rode beside him was nervous and worried. But old John Brown was calm and cool. Looking up at the Blue Ridge mountains of Virginia, he exclaimed, "What a beautiful country! I never had an opportunity to really see it before."

Or take the case of Robert Falcon Scott and his companions—the first Englishmen ever to reach the South Pole. Their return trip was probably the cruelest journey ever undertaken by man. Their food was gone—and so was their fuel. They could no longer march because a howling blizzard roared down over the rim of the earth for eleven days and nights—a wind so fierce and sharp that it cut ridges in the polar ice. Scott and his companions knew they were going to die; and they had brought a quantity of opium along for just such an emergency. A big dose of opium, and they could all lie down to pleasant dreams, never to wake again. But they ignored the drug, and died "singing ringing songs of cheer." We know they did because of a farewell letter found with their frozen bodies by a searching party, eight months later.

Yes, if we cherish creative thoughts of courage and calmness, we can enjoy the scenery while sitting on our coffin, riding to the gallows; or we can fill our tents with "ringing songs of cheer," while starving and freezing to death.

Milton in his blindness discovered that same truth

three hundred years ago:

"The mind is its own place, and in itself can make a heaven of hell, a hell of heaven."

Napoleon and Helen Keller are perfect illustrations of Milton's statement: Napoleon had everything men usually crave—glory, power, riches—yet he said at Saint Helena, "I have never known six happy days in my life"; while Helen Keller—blind, deaf, dumb—declared: "I have found life so beautiful."

If half a century of living has taught me anything at all, it has taught me that "nothing can bring you peace but yourself."

I am merely trying to repeat what Emerson said so well in the closing words of his essay on "Self-Reliance": "A political victory, a rise in rents, the recovery of your sick, or the return of your absent friend, or some other quite external event, raises your spirits, and you think good days are preparing for you. Do not believe it. It can never be so. Nothing can bring you peace but yourself."

Epictetus, the great Stoic philosopher, warned that we ought to be more concerned about removing wrong thoughts from the mind than about removing "tumors and abscesses from the body."

Epictetus said that nineteen centuries ago, but modern medicine would back him up. Dr. G. Canby Robinson declared that four out of five patients admitted to John Hopkins Hospital were suffering from conditions brought on in part by emotional strains and stresses. This was often true even in cases of organic disturbances. "Eventually," he declared, "these trace back to maladjustments to life and its problems."

Montaigne, the great French philosopher, adopted these seventeen words as the motto of his life: "A man is not hurt so much by what happens, as by his opinion of what happens." And our *opinion* of what happens is entirely up to us.

What do I mean? Have I the colossal effrontery to tell you to your face—when you are mowed down by troubles, and your nerves are sticking out like wires and curling up at the ends—have I the colossal effrontery to tell you that, under those conditions, you can change your mental attitude by an effort of the will? Yes, I mean precisely that! And that is not all. I am going to show you *how* to do it. It may take a little effort, but the secret is simple.

William James, who has never been topped in his knowledge of practical psychology, once made this observation: *"Action seems to follow feeling, but really action and feeling go together; and by regulating the action, which is under the more direct control of the will, we can indirectly regulate the feeling, which is not."*

In other words, William James tells us that we cannot instantly change our emotions just by "making up our minds to"—but that we *can* change our actions. And that when we change our actions, we will automatically change our feelings.

"Thus," he explains, *"the sovereign voluntary path to cheerfulness, if your cheerfulness be lost, is to sit up cheerfully and to act and speak as if cheerfulness were already there."*

Does that simple trick work? Try it yourself. Put a big, broad, honest-to-God smile on your face; throw back your shoulders; take a good, deep breath; and sing a snatch of song. If you can't sing, whistle. If you can't whistle, hum. You will quickly discover what William James was talking about—that it is *physically impossible* to remain blue or depressed while you are acting out the symptoms of being radiantly happy!

This is one of the little basic truths of nature that can easily work miracles in all of our lives. I know a woman in California—I won't mention her name—who could wipe out all of her miseries in twenty-four hours if only she knew this secret. She's old, and she's a widow—that's sad, I admit—but does she try to act happy? No; if you ask her how she is feeling, she says, "Oh, I'm all right"—but the expression on her face and the whine in her voice say, "Oh, God, if you only knew the troubles I've seen!" She seems to reproach you for being happy in her presence. Hundreds of women are worse off than she is: her husband left her enough insurance to last the rest of her life, and she has married children to give her a home. But I've rarely seen her smile. She complains that all three of her sons-in-law are stingy and selfish—although she is a guest in their homes for months at a time. And she complains that her daughters never give her presents—although she hoards her own money carefully, "for my old age." She is a blight on herself and her unfortunate family! But does it have to be so? That is the pity of it—she could change herself from a miserable, bitter, and unhappy old woman into an honoured and beloved member of the family—if she *wanted* to change. And all she would have to do to work this transformation would be to start acting cheerful; start acting as though she had a little love to give away—instead of squandering it all on her own unhappy and embittered self.

I know a man in Indiana—H. J. Englert, of 1335 11th Street, Tell City, Indiana—who is still alive today because he discovered this secret. Ten years ago Mr. Englert had a case of scarlet fever; and when he recovered, he found he had developed nephritis, a kidney disease. He tried all kinds of doctors, "even quacks," he informs me, but nothing could cure him.

Then, a short time ago, he got other complications. His blood pressure soared. He went to a doctor, and was told that his blood pressure was hitting the top at 214. He was told that it was fatal—that the condition was progressive, and he had better put his affairs in order at once.

"I went home," he says, "and made sure that my insurance was all paid up, then I apologized to my Maker for all my mistakes, and settled down to gloomy meditations. I made everyone unhappy. My wife and family were miserable, and I was buried deep in depression myself. However, after a week of wallowing in self-pity, I said to myself, 'You're acting like a fool! You may not die for a year yet, so why not try to be happy while you're here?'

"I threw back my shoulders, put a smile on my face, and attempted to act as though everything were normal. I admit it was an effort at first—but I forced myself to be pleasant and cheerful; and this not only helped my family, but it also helped me.

"The first thing I knew, I began to *feel* better—almost as well as I pretended to feel! The improvement went on. And today—months after I was supposed to be in my grave—I am not only happy, well, and alive, but my blood pressure is down! I know one thing for certain: the doctor's prediction would certainly have come true if I had gone on thinking 'dying' thoughts of defeat. But I gave my body a chance to heal itself, by nothing in the world but a change of mental attitude!"

Let me ask you a question: If merely acting cheerful and thinking positive thoughts of health and courage could save this man's life, why should you and I tolerate for one minute more our minor glooms and depressions? Why make ourselves, and everyone around us, unhappy and blue, when it is possible for us to start creating happiness by merely acting cheerful?

Years ago, I read a little book that had a lasting and profound effect on my life. It was called *As a Man Thinketh,* by James Allen, and here's what it said:

"A man will find that as he alters his thoughts towards things and other people, things and other people will alter towards him…. Let a man radically alter his thoughts, and he will be astonished at the rapid transformation it will effect in the material conditions of his life. Men do not attract that which they want, but that which they are…. The divinity that shapes our ends is in ourselves. It is our very self…. All that a man achieves is the direct result of his own thoughts…. A man can only rise, conquer and achieve by lifting up his thoughts. He can only remain weak and abject and miserable by refusing to lift up his thoughts."

According to the book of Genesis, the Creator gave man dominion over the whole wide earth. A mighty big present. But I am not interested in any such superroyal prerogatives. All I desire is dominion over myself— dominion over my thoughts; dominion over my fears; dominion over my mind and over my spirit. And the wonderful thing is that I know that I can attain this dominion to an astonishing degree, any time I want to, by merely controlling my actions—which in turn control my reactions.

So let us remember these words of William James: *"Much of what we call Evil...can often be converted into a bracing and tonic good by a simple change of the sufferer's inner attitude from one of fear to one of fight."*

Let's *fight* for our happiness!

Let's fight for our happiness by following a daily program of cheerful and constructive thinking. Here is such a program. It is entitled "Just for Today." I found this program so inspiring that I gave away hundreds of copies. It was written thirty-six years ago by the late Sibyl F. Partridge. If you and I follow it, we will eliminate most of our worries and increase immeasurably our portion of what the French call *la joie de vivre*.

JUST FOR TODAY

Just for today I will be happy. This assumes that what Abraham Lincoln said is true, that "most folks are about as happy as they make up their minds to be." Happiness within; it is not a matter of externals.

Just for today I will try to adjust myself to what is, and not try to adjust everything to my own desires. I will take my family, my business, and my luck as they come and fit myself to them.

Just for today I will take care of my body. I will exercise it, care for it, nourish it, not abuse it nor neglect it, so that it will be a perfect machine for my bidding.

Just for today I will try to strengthen my mind. I will learn something useful. I will not be a mental loafer. I will read something that requires effort, thought and concentration.

Just for today I will exercise my soul in three ways; I will do somebody a good turn and not get found out. I will do at least two things I don't want to do, as William James suggests, just for exercise.

Just for today I will be agreeable. I will look as well as I can, dress as becomingly as possible, talk low, act courteously, be liberal with praise, criticize not at all, nor find fault with anything and not try to regulate nor improve anyone.

Just for today I will try to live through this day only, not to tackle my whole life problem at once. I can do things for twelve hours that would appall me if I had to keep them up for a lifetime.

Just for today I will have a program. I will write down what I expect to do every hour. I may not follow it exactly, but I will have it. It will eliminate two pests, hurry and indecision.

Just for today I will have a quiet half-hour all by myself and relax. In this half-hour sometimes I will think of

God, so as to get a little more perspective into my life.

Just for today I will be unafraid, especially I will not be afraid to be happy, to enjoy what is beautiful, to love, and to believe that those I love, love me.

If we want to develop a mental attitude that will bring us peace and happiness, here is Rule 1:

THINK AND ACT CHEERFULLY, AND YOU WILL FEEL CHEERFUL

"I am so far from being a pessimist...on the contrary, in spite of my scars, I am tickled to death at life."
—Eugene O'Neill

"If you look into your own heart, and you find nothing wrong there, what is there to worry about? What is there to fear?"
—Confucius

24

THE HIGH COST OF GETTING EVEN

One night, years ago, as I was traveling through Yellowstone Park, I sat with other tourists on bleachers facing a dense growth of pine and spruce. Presently the animal which we had been waiting to see, the terror of the forests, the grizzly bear, strode out into the glare of the lights and began devouring the garbage that had been dumped there from the kitchen of one of the park hotels. A forest ranger, Major Martindale, sat on a horse and talked to the excited tourists about bears. He told us that the grizzly bear can whip any other animal in the Western world, with the possible exception of the buffalo and the Kadiak bear; yet I noticed that night that there was one animal, and only one, that the grizzly permitted to come out of the forest and eat with him under the glare of the lights: a skunk. The grizzly knew that he could liquidate a skunk with one swipe of his mighty paw. Why didn't he do it? Because he had found from experience that it didn't pay.

I found that out, too. As a farm boy, I trapped four-legged skunks along the hedgerows in Missouri; and, as a man, I encountered a few two-legged skunks on the sidewalks of New York. I have found from sad experience that it doesn't pay to stir up either variety.

When we hate our enemies, we are giving them power over us: power over our sleep, our appetites, our blood pressure, our health, and our happiness. Our enemies would dance with joy if only they knew how they were worrying us, lacerating us, and getting even with us! Our hate is not hurting them at all, but our hate is turning our own days and nights into a hellish turmoil.

Who do you suppose said this: "If selfish people try to take advantage of you, cross them off your list, but don't try to get even. When you try to get even, you hurt yourself more than you hurt the other fellow?" ...Those words sound as if they might have been uttered by some starry-eyed idealist. But they weren't. Those words appeared in a bulletin issued by the Police Department of Milwaukee.

How will trying to get even hurt you? In many ways. According to *Life* magazine, it may even wreck your health. "The chief personality characteristic of persons with hypertension [high blood pressure] is resentment," said *Life*. "When resentment is chronic, chronic hypertension and heart trouble follow."

So you see that when Jesus said, "Love your enemies," He was not only preaching sound ethics. He was also preaching twentieth-century medicine. When He said, "Forgive seventy times seven," Jesus was telling you and me how to keep from having high blood pressure, heart trouble, stomach ulcers, and many other ailments.

A friend of mine recently had a serious heart attack. Her physician put her to bed and ordered her to refuse to get angry about anything, no matter what happened. Physicians know that if you have a weak heart, a fit of anger *can* kill you. Did I say, *can* kill you? A fit of anger *did* kill a restaurant owner, in Spokane, Washington, a few years ago. I have in front of me now a letter from Jerry Swartout, chief of the police department, Spokane, Washington, saying: "A few years ago, William Falkaber, a man of sixty-eight who owned a café here in Spokane, killed himself by flying into a rage because his cook insisted on drinking coffee out of his saucer. The café owner was so indignant that he grabbed a revolver and started to chase the cook and fell dead from heart failure—with his hand still gripping the gun. The coroner's report declared that anger had caused the heart failure."

When Jesus said, "Love your enemies," He was also telling us how to improve our looks. I know women—and so do you—whose faces have been wrinkled and hardened by hate and disfigured by resentment. All the beauty treatments in Christendom won't improve their looks half so much as would a heart full of forgiveness, tenderness, and love.

Hatred destroys our ability to enjoy even our food. The Bible puts it this way: "Better is a dinner of herbs where love is, than a stalled ox and hatred therewith."

Wouldn't our enemies rub their hands with glee if they knew that our hate for them was exhausting us, making us tired and nervous, ruining our looks, giving us heart trouble, and probably shortening our lives?

Even if we can't love our enemies, let's at least love ourselves. Let's love ourselves so much that we won't permit our enemies to control our happiness, our health, and our looks. As Shakespeare put it:

"Heat not a furnace for your foe so hot

That it do singe yourself."

When Jesus said that we should forgive our enemies "seventy times seven," He was also preaching sound business. For example, I have before me as I write a letter I received from George Rona, Fradegata'n 24, Uppsala, Sweden. For years, George Rona was an attorney in Vienna; but during the Second World War, he fled to Sweden. He had no money, needed work badly. Since he could speak and write several languages, he hoped to get a position as correspondent for some firm engaged in importing or exporting. Most of the firms replied that they had no need of such services because of the war, but they would keep his name on file...and so on. One man, however, wrote George Rona a letter saying: "What you imagine about my business is not true. You are both wrong and foolish. I do not need any correspondent. Even if I did need one, I wouldn't hire you because you can't even write good Swedish. Your letter is full of mistakes."

When George Rona read that letter, he was as mad as Donald Duck. What did this Swede mean by telling him he couldn't write the language! Why, the letter that this Swede himself had written was full of mistakes! So George Rona wrote a letter that was calculated to burn this man up. Then he paused. He said to himself, "Wait a minute, now. How do I know this man isn't right? I have studied Swedish, but it's not my native language, so maybe I do make mistakes I don't know anything about. If I do, then I certainly have to study harder if I ever hope to get a job. This man has possibly done me a favor, even though he didn't mean to. The mere fact that he expressed himself in disagreeable terms doesn't alter my debt to him. Therefore, I am going to write him and *thank* him for what he has done."

So George Rona tore up the scorching letter he had already written, and wrote another that said: "It was kind of you to go to the trouble of writing to me, especially when you do not need a correspondent. I am sorry I was mistaken about your firm. The reason that I wrote to you was that I made inquiry and your name was given to me as a leader in your field. I did not know I had made grammatical errors in my letter. I am sorry and ashamed of myself. I will now apply myself more diligently to the study of the Swedish language and try to correct my mistakes. I want to thank you for helping me get started on the road to self-improvement."

Within a few days, George Rona got a letter from this man, asking Rona to come to see him. Rona went—and got a job. George Rona discovered for himself that "a soft answer turneth away wrath."

We may not be saintly enough to love our enemies, but, for the sake of our own health and happiness, let's at least forgive them and forget them. That is the smart thing to do. "To be wronged or robbed," said Confucius, "is nothing unless you continue to remember it." I once asked General Eisenhower's son, John, if his father ever nourished resentments. "No," he replied, "Dad never wastes a minute thinking about people he doesn't like."

There is an old saying that a man is a fool who can't be angry, but a man is wise who won't be angry.

That was the policy of William J. Gaynor, former Mayor of New York. Bitterly denounced by the yellow press, he was shot by a maniac and almost killed. As he lay in the hospital, fighting for his life, he said: "Every night, I forgive everything and everybody." Is that too idealistic? Too much sweetness and light? If so, let's turn for counsel to the great German philosopher, Schopenhauer, author of *Studies in Pessimism.* He regarded life as a futile and painful adventure. Gloom dripped from him as he walked; yet out of the depths of his despair, Schopenhauer cried: "If possible, no animosity should be felt for anyone."

I once asked Bernard Baruch—the man who was the trusted adviser to six Presidents: Wilson, Harding, Coolidge, Hoover, Roosevelt, and Truman—whether he was ever disturbed by the attacks of his enemies. "No man can humiliate me or disturb me," he replied. "I won't let him."

No one can humiliate or disturb you and me, either— *unless* we *let him.*

Sticks and stones may break my bones,
But words can never hurt me.

Throughout the ages, mankind has burned its candles before those Christ-like individuals who bore no malice against their enemies. I have often stood in the Jasper National Park, in Canada, and gazed upon one of the most beautiful mountains in the Western world—a mountain named in honor of Edith Cavell, the British nurse who went to her death like a saint before a German firing squad on October 12, 1915. Her crime? She had hidden and fed and nursed wounded French and English soldiers in her Belgian home, and had helped them escape into Holland. As the English chaplain entered her cell in the military prison in Brussels that October morning, to prepare her for death, Edith Cavell uttered two sentences that have been preserved in bronze and granite: "I realize that patriotism is not enough. I must have no hatred or bitterness toward anyone." Four years later, her body was removed to England and memorial services were held in Westminster Abbey. I once spent a year in London; I have often stood before the statue of Edith Cavell opposite the National Portrait Gallery and read her immortal words carved in granite: "I realize that patriotism is not enough. I must have no hatred or bitterness toward anyone." One sure way to forgive and forget our enemies is to become absorbed in some cause infinitely bigger than ourselves. Then the insults and the enmities we encounter won't matter because we will be oblivious of everything but our *cause*. As an example, let's take an intensely dramatic event that was about to take place in the pine woods of Mississippi back in 1918. A lynching! Laurence Jones, a coloured teacher and preacher, was about to be lynched. A few years ago, I visited the school that Laurence Jones founded—the Piney Woods Country School—and I spoke before the student body. That school is nationally known today, but the incident I am going to relate occurred long before that. It occurred back in the highly emotional days of the First World War. A rumor had spread through central Mississippi that the Germans were arousing the Negroes and inciting them to rebellion.

Laurence Jones, the man who was about to be lynched, was, as I have already said, a Negro himself and was accused of helping to arouse his race to insurrection. A group of white men—pausing outside the church—had heard Laurence Jones shouting to his congregation: "Life is a battle in which every Negro must gird on his armor and *fight* to survive and succeed."

"Fight!" "Armor!" Enough! Galloping off into the night, these excited young men recruited a mob, returned to the church, put a rope around the preacher, dragged him for a mile up the road, stood him on a heap of faggots, lighted matches, and were ready to hang him and burn him at the same time, when someone shouted: "Let's make the blankety-blank-blank talk before he burns. Speech! Speech!" Laurence Jones, standing on the faggots, spoke with a rope around his neck, spoke for his life and his *cause*. He had been graduated from the University of Iowa in 1907. His sterling character, his scholarship, and his musical ability had made him popular with both the students and the faculty. Upon graduation, he had turned down the offer of a hotel man to set him up in business, and had turned down the offer of a wealthy man to finance his musical education. Why? Because he was on fire with a vision. Reading the story of Booker T. Washington's life, he had been inspired to devote his own life to educating the poverty-stricken, illiterate members of his race. So he went to the most backward belt he could find in the South—a spot twenty-five miles south of Jackson, Mississippi. Pawning his watch for $1.65, he started his school in the open woods with a stump for a desk. Laurence Jones told these angry men who were waiting to lynch him of the struggle he had had to educate these unschooled boys and girls and to train them to be good farmers, mechanics, cooks, housekeepers. He told of the white men who had helped him in his struggle to establish Piney Woods Country School—white men who had given him land, lumber, and pigs, cows and money, to help him carry on his educational work.

When Laurence Jones was asked afterward if he didn't hate the men who had dragged him up the road to hang him and burn him, he replied that he was *"too busy with his cause* to hate—too *absorbed in something bigger than himself."* *"I have no time to quarrel,"* he said, *"no time for regrets, and no man can force me to stoop low enough to hate him."*

As Laurence Jones talked with sincere and moving eloquence, as he pleaded, not for himself, but his cause, the mob began to soften. Finally, an old Confederate veteran in the crowd said: "I believe this boy is telling the truth. I know the white men whose names he has mentioned. He is doing a fine work. We have made a mistake. We ought to help him instead of hang him." The Confederate veteran passed his hat through the crowd and raised a gift of fifty-two dollars and forty cents from the very men who had gathered there to hang the founder of Piney Woods Country School—the man who said: "I have no time to quarrel, no time for regrets, and no man can force me to stoop low enough to hate him."

Epictetus pointed out nineteen centuries ago that we

reap what we sow and that somehow fate almost always makes us pay for our malefactions. "In the long run," said Epictetus, "every man will pay the penalty for his own misdeeds. The man who remembers this will be angry with no one, indignant with no one, revile no one, blame no one, offend no one, hate no one."

Probably no other man in American history was ever more denounced and hated and double-crossed than Lincoln. Yet Lincoln, according to Herndon's classic biography, "never judged men by his like or dislike for them. If any given act was to be performed, he could understand that his enemy could do it just as well as anyone. If a man had maligned him or been guilty of personal ill-treatment, and was the fittest man for the place, Lincoln would give him that place, just as soon as he would give it to a friend…. I do not think he ever removed a man because he was his enemy or because he disliked him."

Lincoln was denounced and insulted by some of the very men he had appointed to positions of high power— men like McClellan, Seward, Stanton, and Chase. Yet Lincoln believed, according to Herndon, his law partner, that "no man was to be eulogized for what he did; or censured for what he did or did not do," because "all of us are the children of conditions, of circumstances, of environment, of education, of acquired habits and of heredity, molding men as they are and will forever be."

Perhaps Lincoln was right. If you and I had inherited the same physical, mental, and emotional characteristics that our enemies have inherited, and if life had done to us what it has done to them, we would act exactly as they do. We couldn't possibly do anything else. Let's be charitable enough to repeat the prayer of the Sioux Indians: "O Great Spirit, keep me from ever judging and criticizing a man until I have walked in his moccasins for two weeks." So instead of hating our enemies, let's pity them and thank God that life has not made us what they are. Instead of heaping condemnation and revenge upon our enemies, let's give them our understanding, our sympathy, our help, our forgiveness, and our prayers.

I was brought up in a family which read the Scriptures or repeated a verse from the Bible each night and then knelt down and said "family prayers." I can still hear my father, in a lonely Missouri farmhouse, repeating these words of Jesus—words that will continue to be repeated as long as man cherishes his ideals: "Love your enemies, bless them that curse you, do good to them that hate you, and pray for them which despitefully use you, and persecute you."

My father tried to live those words of Jesus; and they gave him an inner peace that the captains and the kings of earth have often sought for in vain.

To cultivate a mental attitude that will bring you peace and happiness, remember that Rule 2 is:

LET'S NEVER TRY TO GET EVEN WITH OUR ENEMIES, BECAUSE IF WE DO WE WILL HURT OURSELVES FAR MORE THAN WE HURT THEM. LET'S DO AS GENERAL EISENHOWER DOES: LET'S NEVER WASTE A MINUTE THINKING ABOUT PEOPLE WE DON'T LIKE.

"How wonderful it is that nobody need wait a single moment before starting to improve the world."
                                                    —Anne Frank

"Sticks and stones may break my bones, but words can never hurt me."

25

NEVER WORRY ABOUT INGRATITUDE

I recently met a businessman in Texas who was burned up with indignation. I was warned that he would tell me about it within fifteen minutes after I met him. He did. The incident he was angry about had occurred eleven months previously, but he was still burned up about it. He couldn't talk of anything else. He had given his thirty-four employees ten thousand dollars in Christmas bonuses—approximately three hundred dollars each—and no one had thanked him. "I am sorry," he complained bitterly, "that I ever gave them a penny!"

"An angry man," said Confucius, "is always full of poison." This man was so full of poison that I honestly pitied him. He was about sixty years old. Now, life-insurance companies figure that, on the average, we will live slightly more than two thirds of the difference between our present age and eighty. So this man—if he was lucky—probably had about fourteen or fifteen years to live. Yet he had already wasted almost one of his few remaining years by his bitterness and resentment over an event that was past and gone. I pitied him.

Instead of wallowing in resentment and self-pity, he might have asked himself *why* he didn't get any appreciation. Maybe he had underpaid and overworked his employees. Maybe they considered a Christmas bonus not a gift, but something they had earned. Maybe he was so critical and unapproachable that no one dared or cared to thank him. Maybe they felt he gave the bonus because most of the profits were going for taxes anyway.

On the other hand, maybe the employees were selfish, mean, and ill-mannered. Maybe this. Maybe that. I don't know any more about it than you do. But I do know that Dr. Samuel Johnson said:

"Gratitude is a fruit of great cultivation. You do not find it among gross people."

Here is the point I am trying to make: *this man made the human and distressing mistake of expecting gratitude.* He just didn't know human nature.

If you saved a man's life, would you expect him to be grateful? You might—but Samuel Leibowitz, who was a famous criminal lawyer before he became a judge, saved *seventy-eight* men from going to the electric chair! How many of these men, do you suppose, stopped to thank Samuel Leibowitz, or ever took the trouble to send him a Christmas card? How many? Guess.... That's right—none.

Christ healed ten lepers in one afternoon—but how many of those lepers even stopped to thank Him? Only one. Look it up in Saint Luke. When Christ turned around to His disciples and asked, "Where are the other nine?" they had all run away. Disappeared without thanks! Let me ask you a question: Why should you and I—or this businessman in Texas—expect more thanks for our small favors than was given to Jesus Christ?

And when it comes to money matters! Well, that is even more hopeless. Charles Schwab told me that he had once saved a bank cashier who had speculated in the stock market with funds belonging to the bank. Schwab put up the money to save this man from going to the penitentiary. Was the cashier grateful? Oh, yes, for a little while. Then he turned against Schwab and reviled him and denounced him—the very man who had kept him out of jail!

If you gave one of your relatives a million dollars, would you expect him to be grateful? Andrew Carnegie did just that. But if Andrew Carnegie had come back from the grave a little while later, he would have been shocked to find this relative cursing him! Why? Because Old Andy had left 365 million dollars to public charities—and had "cut him off with one measly million," as he put it.

That's how it goes. Human nature has always been human nature—and it probably won't change in your lifetime. So why not accept it? Why not be as realistic about it as was old Marcus Aurelius, one of the wisest men who ever ruled the Roman Empire. He wrote in his diary one day: "I am going to meet people today who talk too much—people who are selfish, egotistical, ungrateful. But I won't be surprised or disturbed, for I couldn't imagine a world without such people."

That makes sense, doesn't it? If you and I go around grumbling about ingratitude, who is to blame? Is it human nature—or is it our ignorance of human nature? Let's not expect gratitude. Then, if we get some occasionally, it will come as a delightful surprise. If we don't get it, we won't be disturbed.

Here is the first point I am trying to make in this chapter: *It is natural for people to forget to be grateful; so, if we go around expecting gratitude, we are headed straight for a lot of heartaches.*

I know a woman in New York who is always complaining because she is lonely. Not one of her relatives wants to go near her—and no wonder. If you visit her, she will tell you for hours what she did for her nieces when they were children: she nursed them through the measles and the mumps and the whooping cough; she boarded them for years; she helped to send one of them through business school, and she made a home for the other until she got married.

Do the nieces come to see her? Oh, yes, now and then, out of a spirit of duty. But they dread these visits. They know they will have to sit and listen for hours to half-veiled reproaches. They will be treated to an endless litany of bitter complaints and self-pitying sighs. And when this woman can no longer bludgeon, browbeat, or bully her nieces into coming to see her, she has one of her "spells." She develops a heart attack.

Is the heart attack real? Oh, yes. The doctors say she has "a nervous heart," suffers from palpitations. But the doctors also say they can do nothing for her—her trouble is emotional.

What this woman really wants is love and attention. But she calls it "gratitude." And she will never get gratitude or love, because she demands it. She thinks it's her due.

There are thousands of women like her, women who are ill from "ingratitude," loneliness, and neglect. They long to be loved; but the only way in this world that they can ever hope to be loved is to stop asking for it and to start pouring out love without hope of return.

Does that sound like sheer, impractical, visionary idealism? It isn't. It is just horse sense. It is a good way for you and me to find the happiness we long for. I know. I have seen it happen right in my own family. My own mother and father gave for the joy of helping others. We were poor—always overwhelmed by debts. Yet, poor as we were, my father and mother always managed to send money every year to an orphans' home. The Christian Home in Council Bluffs, Iowa. Mother and Father never visited that home. Probably no one thanked them for their gifts—except by letter—but they were richly repaid, for they had the joy of helping little children—without wishing for or expecting any gratitude in return.

After I left home, I would always send Father and Mother a check at Christmas and urge them to indulge in a few luxuries for themselves. But they rarely did. When I came home a few days before Christmas, Father would tell me of the coal and groceries they had bought for some "widder woman" in town who had a lot of children and no money to buy food and fuel. What joy they got out of these gifts—the joy of giving without expecting anything whatever in return!

I believe my father would almost have qualified for Aristotle's description of the ideal man—the man most worthy of being happy. "The ideal man," said Aristotle, "takes joy in doing favours for others; but he feels ashamed to have others do favours for him. For it is a mark of superiority to confer a kindness; but it is a mark of inferiority to receive it."

Here is the second point I am trying to make in this chapter: *If we want to find happiness, lets stop thinking about gratitude or ingratitude and give for the inner joy of giving.*

Parents have been tearing their hair about the ingratitude of children for ten thousand years.

Even Shakespeare's King Lear cried out, "How sharper than a serpent's tooth it is to have a thankless child!"

But why should children be thankful—unless we train them to be? Ingratitude is natural—like weeds. Gratitude is like a rose. It has to be fed and watered and cultivated and loved and protected.

If our children are ungrateful, who is to blame? Maybe we are. If we have never taught them to express gratitude to others, how can we expect them to be grateful to us?

I know a man in Chicago who has cause to complain of the ingratitude of his stepsons. He slaved in a box factory, seldom earning more than forty dollars a week. He married a widow, and she persuaded him to borrow money and send her two grown sons to college. Out of his salary of forty dollars a week, he had to pay for food, rent, fuel, clothes, and also for the payments on his notes. He did this for four years, working like a coolie, and never complaining.

Did he get any thanks? No; his wife took it all for granted—and so did her sons. They never imagined that they owed their step-father anything—not even thanks!

Who was to blame? The boys? Yes; but the mother was

even more to blame. She thought it was a shame to burden their young lives with "a sense of obligation." She didn't want her sons to "start out under debt." So she never dreamed of saying: "What a prince your stepfather is to help you through college!" Instead, she took the attitude: "Oh, that's the least he can do."

She thought she was sparing her sons, but, in reality, she was sending them out into life with the dangerous idea that the world owed them a living. And it *was* a dangerous idea—for one of those sons tried to "borrow" from an employer, and ended up in jail!

We must remember that our children are very much what we make them. For example, my mother's sister— Viola Alexander, of 144 West Minnehaha Parkway, Minneapolis—is a shining example of a woman who has never had cause to complain about the "ingratitude" of children. When I was a boy, Aunt Viola took her own mother into her home to love and take care of; and she did the same thing for her husband's mother. I can still close my eyes and see those two old ladies sitting before the fire in Aunt Viola's farmhouse. Were they any "trouble" to Aunt Viola? Oh, often, I suppose. But you would never have guessed it from her attitude. She *loved* those old ladies—so she pampered them, and spoiled them, and made them feel at home. In addition, Aunt Viola had six children of her own; but it never occurred to her that she was doing anything especially noble, or deserved any halos for taking these old ladies into her home. To her, it was the natural thing, the right thing, the thing she wanted to do.

Where is Aunt Viola today? Well, she has now been a widow for twenty-odd years, and she has five grown-up children—five separate households—all clamouring to share her, and to have her come and live in their homes! Her children adore her; they never get enough of her. Out of "gratitude"? Nonsense! It is love—*sheer love*. Those children breathed in warmth and radiant human-kindness all during their childhoods. Is it any wonder that, now that the situation is reversed, they *give back* love?

So let us remember that to raise grateful children, we have to *be* grateful. Let us remember "little pitchers have big ears"—and watch what we say. To illustrate—the next time we are tempted to belittle someone's kindness in the presence of our children, let's stop. Let's never say: "Look at these dishcloths Cousin Sue sent for Christmas. She knit them herself. They didn't cost her a cent!" The remark may seem trivial to us—but the children are listening. So, instead, we had better say: "Look at the hours Cousin Sue spent making these for Christmas! Isn't she nice? Let's write her a thank-you note right now." And our children may unconsciously absorb the habit of praise and appreciation.

To avoid resentment and worry over ingratitude, here is Rule 3:

INSTEAD OF WORRYING ABOUT INGRATITUDE, LET'S EXPECT IT. LET'S REMEMBER THAT JESUS HEALED TEN LEPERS IN ONE DAY—AND ONLY ONE THANKED HIM. WHY SHOULD WE EXPECT MORE GRATITUDE THAN JESUS GOT?

LET'S REMEMBER THAT THE ONLY WAY TO FIND HAPPINESS
IS NOT TO EXPECT GRATITUDE, BUT TO GIVE FOR THE JOY
OF GIVING.

LET'S REMEMBER THAT GRATITUDE IS A "CULTIVATED" TRAIT;
SO IF WE WANT OUR CHILDREN TO BE GRATEFUL, WE
MUST TRAIN THEM TO BE GRATEFUL.

"Don't let your mind bully your body into believing it must carry the burden of its worries."

—Astrid Alauda

"Worry and reasoning are two of Satan's most successful tools."

—Joyce Meyer

26

WOULD YOU TAKE A MILLION DOLLARS
FOR WHAT YOU HAVE?

I have known Harold Abbott for years. He lives at 820 South Madison Avenue, Webb City, Missouri. He used to be my lecture manager. One day he and I met in Kansas City and he drove me down to my farm at Belton, Missouri. During that drive, I asked him how he kept from worrying; and he told me an inspiring story that I shall never forget.

"I used to worry a lot," he said, "but one spring day in 1934, I was walking down West Dougherty Street in Webb City when I saw a sight that banished all my worries. It all happened in ten seconds, but during those ten seconds I learned more about how to live than I had learned in the previous ten years. For two years I had been running a grocery store in Webb City," Harold Abbott said, as he told me the story. "I had not only lost all my savings, but I had incurred debts that took me seven years to pay back. My grocery store had been closed the previous Saturday; and now I was going to the Merchants and Miners Bank to borrow money so I could go to Kansas City to look for a job. I walked like a beaten man. I had lost all my fight and faith. Then suddenly I saw coming down the street a man who had no legs. He was sitting on a little wooden platform equipped with wheels from roller skates. He propelled himself along the street with a block of wood in each hand. I met him just after he had crossed the street and was starting to lift himself up a few inches over the curb to the sidewalk. As he tilted his little wooden platform to an angle, his eyes met mine. He greeted me with a grand smile. 'Good morning, sir. It is a fine morning, isn't it?' he said with spirit. As I stood looking at him, I realized how rich I was. I had two legs. I could walk. I felt ashamed of my self-pity. I said to myself if he can be happy, cheerful, and confident without legs, I certainly can with legs. I could already feel my chest lifting. I had intended to ask the Merchants and Miners Bank for only one hundred dollars. But now I had courage to ask for *two* hundred. I had intended to say that I wanted to go to Kansas City to *try* to get a job. But now I announced confidently that I wanted to go to Kansas City to *get* a job. I got the loan; and I got the job.

"I now have the following words pasted on my bathroom mirror, and I read them every morning as I shave:

I had the blues because I had no shoes,
Until upon the street, I met a man who had no feet.

I once asked Eddie Rickenbacker what was the biggest lesson he had learned from drifting about with his companions in life rafts for twenty-one days, hopelessly lost in the Pacific. "The biggest lesson I learned from that experience," he said, "was that if you have all the fresh water you want to drink and all the food you want to eat, you ought never to complain about anything."

Time ran an article about a sergeant who had been wounded on Guadalcanal. Hit in the throat by a shell fragment, this sergeant had had seven blood transfusions. Writing a note to his doctor, he asked: "Will I live?" The doctor replied: "Yes." He wrote another note, asking: "Will I be able to talk?" Again the answer was yes. He then wrote another note, saying: *"Then what in the hell am I worrying about?"*

Why don't you stop right now and ask yourself: "What in the hell am I worrying about?" You will probably find that it is comparatively unimportant and insignificant.

About ninety per cent of the things in our lives are right and about ten per cent are wrong. If we want to be happy, all we have to do is to concentrate on the ninety per cent that are right and ignore the ten per cent that are wrong. If we want to be worried and bitter and have stomach ulcers, all we have to do is to concentrate on the ten per cent that are wrong and ignore the ninety per cent that are glorious.

The words "Think and Thank" are inscribed in many of the Cromwellian churches of England. These words ought to be inscribed on our hearts, too: "Think and Thank." Think of all we have to be grateful for, and thank God for all our boons and bounties.

Jonathan Swift, author of *Gulliver's Travels,* was the most devastating pessimist in English literature. He was so sorry that he had been born that he wore black and fasted on his birthdays; yet, in his despair, this supreme pessimist of English literature praised the great health-giving powers of cheerfulness and happiness. "The best doctors in the world," he declared, "are Doctor Diet, Doctor Quiet, and Doctor Merryman."

You and I may have the services of "Doctor Merryman" free every hour of the day by keeping our attention fixed on all the incredible riches we possess—riches exceeding by far the fabled treasures of Ali Baba. Would you sell both your eyes for a billion dollars? What would you take for your two legs? Your hands? Your hearing? Your children? Your family? Add up your assets, and you will find that you won't sell what you have for all the gold ever amassed by the Rockefellers, the Fords, and the Morgans combined.

But do we appreciate all this? Ah, no. As Schopenhauer said: "We seldom think of what we have but always of what we lack." Yes, the tendency to "seldom think of what we have but always of what we lack" is the greatest tragedy on earth. It has probably caused more misery than all the wars and diseases in history.

It caused John Palmer to turn "from a regular guy into an old grouch," and almost wrecked his home. I know because he told me so.

Mr. Palmer lives at 30, 19th Avenue, Paterson, New Jersey. "Shortly after I returned from the Army," he said, "I started in business for myself. I worked hard day and night. Things were going nicely. Then trouble started. I couldn't get parts and materials. I was afraid I would have to give up my business. I worried so much that I changed from a regular guy into an old grouch. I became so sour and cross that—well, I didn't know it then; but I now realize that I came very near to losing my happy home. Then one day a young, disabled veteran who works for me said, 'Johnny, you ought to be ashamed of yourself.

You take on as if you were the only person in the world with troubles. Suppose you do have to shut up shop for a while—so what? You can start up again when things get normal. You've got a lot to be thankful for. Yet you are always growling. Boy, how I wish I were in your shoes! Look at me. I've got only one arm, and half of my face is shot away, and yet, I am not complaining. If you don't stop your growling and grumbling, you will lose not only your business, but also your health, your home, and your friends!'

"Those remarks stopped me dead in my tracks. They made me realize how well off I was. I resolved then and there that I would change and be my old self again—and I did."

A friend of mine, Lucile Blake, had to tremble on the edge of tragedy before she learned to be happy about what she had instead of worrying over what she lacked.

I met Lucile years ago, when we were both studying short-story writing in the Columbia University School of Journalism. Nine years ago, she got the shock of her life. She was living then in Tucson, Arizona. She had—well, here is the story as she told it to me:

"I had been living in a whirl: studying the organ at the University of Arizona, conducting a speech clinic in town, and teaching a class in musical appreciation at the Desert Willow Ranch, where I was staying. I was going in for parties, dances, horseback rides under the stars. One morning I collapsed. My heart! 'You will have to lie in bed for a year of complete rest,' the doctor said. He didn't encourage me to believe I would ever be strong again.

"In bed for a year! To be an invalid—perhaps to die! I was terrorstricken! Why did all this have to happen to me? What had I done to deserve it? I wept and wailed. I was bitter and rebellious. But I did go to bed as the doctor advised. A neighbour of mine, Mr. Rudolf, an artist, said to me, 'You think now that spending a year in bed will be a tragedy. But it won't be. You will have time to think and get acquainted with yourself. You will make more spiritual growth in these next few months than you have made during all your previous life.' I became calmer, and tried to develop a new sense of values. I read books of inspiration. One day I heard a radio commentator say: 'You can express only what is in your own consciousness.' I had heard words like these many times before, but now they reached down inside me, and took root. I resolved to think only the thoughts I wanted to live by: thoughts of joy, happiness, health. I forced myself each morning, as soon as I awoke, to go over all the things I had to be grateful for. No pain. A lovely young daughter. My eyesight. My hearing. Lovely music on the radio. Time to read.

Good food. Good friends. I was so cheerful and had so many visitors that the doctor put up a sign saying that only one visitor at a time would be allowed in my cabin— and only at certain hours.

"Nine years have passed since then, and I now lead a full, active life. I am deeply grateful now for that year I spent in bed. It was the most valuable and the happiest year I spent in Arizona. The habit I formed then of counting my blessings each morning still remains with me. It is one of my most precious possessions. I am ashamed to realize that I never really learned to live until I feared I was going to die."

My dear Lucile Blake, you may not realize it, but you learned the same lesson that Dr. Samuel Johnson learned two hundred years ago. "The habit of looking on the best side of every event," said Dr. Johnson, "is worth more than a thousand pounds a year."

Those words were uttered, mind you, not by a professional optimist, but by a man who had known anxiety, rags, and hunger for twenty years—and finally became one of the most eminent writers of his generation and the most celebrated conversationalist of all time.

Logan Pearsall Smith packed a lot of wisdom into a few words when he said: "There are two things to aim at in life: first, to get what you want; and, after that, to enjoy it. Only the wisest of mankind achieve the second."

Would you like to know how to make even dishwashing at the kitchen sink a thrilling experience? If so, read an inspiring book of incredible courage by Borghild Dahl. It is called *I Wanted to See.* You may borrow it from your public library or purchase it from your local bookstore or from the publisher, The Macmillan Company, 60 Fifth Avenue, New York City.

This book was written by a woman who was practically blind for half a century. "I had only one eye," she writes, "and it was so covered with dense scars that I had to do all my seeing through one small opening in the left of the eye. I could see a book only by holding it up close to my face and by straining my one eye as hard as I could to the left."

But she refused to be pitied, refused to be considered "different." As a child, she wanted to play hopscotch with other children, but she couldn't see the markings. So after the other children had gone home, she got down on the ground and crawled along with her eyes near to the marks. She memorized every bit of the ground where she and her friends played and soon became an expert at running games. She did her reading at home, holding a book of large print so close to her eyes that her eyelashes brushed the pages. She earned two college degrees: an A.B. from the University of Minnesota and a Master of Arts from Columbia University.

She started teaching in the tiny village of Twin Valley, Minnesota, and rose until she became professor of journalism and literature at Augustana College in Sioux Falls, South Dakota. She taught there for thirteen years, lecturing before women's clubs and giving radio talks about books and authors. "In the back of my mind," she writes, "there had always lurked a fear of total blindness. In order to overcome this, I had adopted a cheerful, almost hilarious, attitude toward life."

Then in 1943, when she was fifty-two years old, a miracle happened: an operation at the famous Mayo Clinic. She could now see forty times as well as she had ever been able to see before.

A new and exciting world of loveliness opened before her. She now found it thrilling even to wash dishes in the kitchen sink. "I begin to play with the white fluffy suds in the dishpan," she writes. "I dip my hands into them and I pick up a ball of tiny soap bubbles. I hold them up against the light, and in each of them I can see the brilliant colours of a miniature rainbow."

As she looked through the window above the kitchen sink, she saw "the flapping gray-black wings of the sparrows flying through the thick, falling snow."

She found such ecstasy looking at the soap bubbles and sparrows that she closed her book with these words: "'Dear Lord,' I whisper, 'Our Father in Heaven, I thank Thee. I thank Thee.'"

Imagine thanking God because you can wash dishes and see rainbows in bubbles and sparrows flying through the snow!

You and I ought to be ashamed of ourselves. All the days of our years we have been living in a fairyland of beauty, but we have been too blind to see, too satiated to enjoy.

If we want to stop worrying and start living, rule 4 is:

COUNT YOUR BLESSINGS—NOT YOUR TROUBLES!

"I promise you, nothing is as chaotic as it seems. Nothing is worth your health. Nothing is worth poisoning yourself into stress, anxiety, and fear."
—Steve Maraboli

"There is nothing that wastes the body like worry, and one who has any faith in God should be ashamed to worry about anything whatsoever."
—Mahatma Gandhi

27

FIND YOURSELF AND BE YOURSELF: REMEMBER THERE IS NO ONE ELSE ON EARTH LIKE YOU

I have a letter from Mrs. Edith Allred, of Mount Airy, North Carolina: "As a child, I was extremely sensitive and shy," she says in her letter. "I was always overweight and my cheeks made me look even fatter than I was. I had an old-fashioned mother who thought it was foolish to make clothes look pretty. She always said: 'Wide will wear while narrow will tear'; and she dressed me accordingly. I never went to parties; never had any fun; and when I went to school, I never joined the other children in outside activities, not even athletics. I was morbidly shy. I felt I was 'different' from everybody else, and entirely undesirable.

"When I grew up, I married a man who was several years my senior. But I didn't change. My in-laws were a poised and self-confident family. They were everything I should have been but simply was not. I tried my best to be like them, but I couldn't. Every attempt they made to draw me out of myself only drove me further into my shell. I became nervous and irritable. I avoided all friends. I got so bad, I even dreaded the sound of the doorbell ringing! I was a failure. I knew it; and I was afraid my husband would find it out. So, whenever we were in public, I tried to be gay, and overacted my part. I knew I overacted; and I would be miserable for days afterwards.

At last I became so unhappy that I could see no point in prolonging my existence. I began to think of suicide."

What happened to change this unhappy woman's life? Just a chance remark!

"A chance remark," Mrs. Allred continued, "transformed my whole life. My mother-in-law was talking one day of how she brought her children up, and she said, 'No matter what happened, I always insisted on their being themselves.' 'On being them-selves.' That remark is what did it! In a flash, I realized I had brought all this misery on myself by trying to fit myself into a pattern to which I did not conform.

"I changed overnight! I started being myself. I tried to make a study of my own personality. Tried to find out *what I was.* I studied my strong points. I learned all I could about colours and styles, and dressed in a way that I felt was becoming to me. I reached out to make friends. I joined an organization—a small one at first—and was petrified with fright when they put me on a program. But each time I spoke, I gained a little courage. It took a long while—but today I have more happiness than I ever dreamed possible. In rearing my own children, I have always taught them the lesson I had to learn from such bitter experience: *No matter what happens, always be yourself!*"

This problem of being willing to be yourself is "as old as history," says Dr. James Gordon Gilkey, "and as universal as human life." This problem of being unwilling to be yourself is the hidden spring behind many neuroses and psychoses and complexes. Angelo Patri has written thirteen books and thousands of syndicated newspaper articles on the subject of child training, and he says: "Nobody is so miserable as he who longs to be somebody and something other than the person he is in body and mind."

This craving to be something you are not is especially rampant in Hollywood. Sam Wood, one of Hollywood's best-known directors, says the greatest headache he has with aspiring young actors is exactly this problem: to make them be themselves. They all want to be second-rate Lana Turners or third-rate Clark Gables. "The public has already had that flavour," Sam Wood keeps telling them; "now it wants something else."

Before he started directing such pictures as *Goodbye, Mr. Chips* and *For Whom the Bell Tolls,* Sam Wood spent years in the real-estate business, developing sales personalities. He declares that the same principles apply in the business world as in the world of moving pictures. You won't get anywhere playing the ape. You can't be a parrot. "Experience has taught me," says Sam Wood, "that it is safest to drop, as quickly as possible, people who pretend to be what they aren't."

I recently asked Paul Boynton, employment director for the Socony-Vacuum Oil Company, what is the biggest mistake people make in applying for jobs. He ought to know: he has interviewed more than sixty thousand job seekers; and he has written a book entitled *6 Ways to Get a Job.* He replied: "The biggest mistake people make in applying for jobs is in not being themselves. Instead of taking their hair down and being completely frank, they often try to give you the answers they think you want." But it doesn't work, because nobody wants a phony. Nobody ever wants a counterfeit coin.

A certain daughter of a streetcar conductor had to learn that lesson the hard way. She longed to be a singer. But her face was her misfortune. She had a large mouth and protruding buck teeth. When she first sang in public—in a New Jersey night club—she tried to pull down her upper lip to cover her teeth. She tried to act "glamorous." The result? She made herself ridiculous. She was headed for failure.

However, there was a man in this night club who heard the girl sing and thought she had talent. "See here," he said bluntly, "I've been watching your performance and I know what it is you're trying to hide. You're ashamed of your teeth!" The girl was embarrassed, but the man continued, "What of it? Is there any particular crime in having buck teeth? Don't try to hide them! Open your mouth, and the audience will love you when they see you're not ashamed. Besides," he said shrewdly, "those teeth you're trying to hide may make your fortune!"

Cass Daley took his advice and forgot about her teeth. From *that time* on, she thought only about her audience. She opened her mouth wide and sang with such gusto and enjoyment that she became a top star in movies and radio. Other comedians are now trying to copy *her!*

The renowned William James was speaking of men who had never found themselves when he declared that the average man develops only ten per cent of his latent mental abilities. "Compared to what we ought to be," he wrote, "we are only half awake. We are making use of only a small part of our physical and mental resources. Stating the thing broadly, the human individual thus lives far within his limits. He possesses powers of various sorts which he habitually fails to use."

You and I have such abilities, so let's not waste a second worrying because we are not like other people. You are something new in this world. Never before, since the beginning of time, has there ever been anybody exactly like you; and never again throughout all the ages to come will there ever be anybody exactly like you again. The new science of genetics informs us that you are what you are largely as a result of twenty-four chromosomes contributed by your father and twenty-four chromosomes contributed by your mother. These forty-eight chromosomes comprise everything that determines what you inherit. In each chromosome there may be, says Amran Scheinfeld, "anywhere from scores to hundreds of genes—with a single gene, in some cases, able to change the whole life of an individual." Truly, we are "fearfully and wonderfully" made.

Even after your mother and father met and mated, there was only one chance in 300,000 billion that the person who is specifically you would be born! In other words, if you had 300,000 billion brothers and sisters, they might have all been different from you. Is all this guesswork? No. It is a scientific fact. If you would like to read more about it, go to your public library and borrow a book entitled *You and Heredity*, by Amran Scheinfeld.

I can talk with conviction about this subject of being

yourself because I feel deeply about it. I know what I am talking about. I know from bitter and costly experience. To illustrate: when I first came to New York from the cornfields of Missouri, I enrolled in the American Academy of Dramatic Arts. I aspired to be an actor. I had what I thought was a brilliant idea, a short cut to success, an idea so simple, so foolproof, that I couldn't understand why thousands of ambitious people hadn't already discovered it. It was this: I would study how the famous actors of that day—John Drew, Walter Hampden, and Otis Skinner—got their effects. Then I would imitate the best points of each one of them and make myself into a shining, triumphant combination of all of them. How silly! How absurd! I had to waste years of my life imitating other people before it penetrated through my thick Missouri skull that I had to be myself, and that I couldn't possibly be anyone else.

That distressing experience ought to have taught me a lasting lesson. But it didn't. Not me. I was too dumb. I had to learn it all over again. Several years later, I set out to write what I hoped would be the best book on public speaking for businessmen that had ever been written. I had the same foolish idea about writing this book that I had formerly had about acting: I was going to *borrow* the ideas of a lot of other writers and put them all in one book—a book that would have everything. So I got scores of books on public speaking and spent a year incorporating their ideas into my manuscript. But it finally dawned on me once again that I was playing the fool. This hodgepodge of other men's ideas that I had written was so synthetic, so dull, that no businessman would ever plod through it. So I tossed a year's work into the wastebasket, and started all over again. This time I said to myself: "You've got to be Dale Carnegie, with all his faults and limitations. You can't possibly be anybody else." So I quit trying to be a combination of other men, and rolled up my sleeves and did what I should have done in the first place: I wrote a textbook on public speaking out of my own experiences, observations, and convictions as a speaker and a teacher of speaking. I learned—for all time, I hope—the lesson that Sir Walter Raleigh learned. (I am *not* talking about the Sir Walter who threw his coat in the mud for the Queen to step on. I am talking about the Sir Walter Raleigh who was professor of English literature at Oxford back in 1904.) "I can't write a book commensurate with Shakespeare," he said, "but I can write a book by me."

Be yourself. Act on the sage advice that Irving Berlin gave the late George Gershwin. When Berlin and Gershwin first met, Berlin was famous but Gershwin was a struggling young composer working for thirty-five dollars a week in Tin Pan Alley. Berlin, impressed by Gershwin's ability, offered Gershwin a job as his musical secretary at almost three times the salary he was then getting. "But don't take the job," Berlin advised. "If you do, you may develop into a second-rate Berlin. But if you insist on being yourself, someday you'll become a first-rate Gershwin."

Gershwin heeded that warning and slowly transformed himself into one of the significant American composers of his generation.

Charlie Chaplin, Will Rogers, Mary Margaret McBride, Gene Autry, and millions of others had to learn the lesson I am trying to hammer home in this chapter. They had to learn the hard way—just as I did.

When Charlie Chaplin first started making films, the director of the pictures insisted on Chaplin's imitating a popular German comedian of that day. Charlie Chaplin got nowhere until he acted himself. Bob Hope had a similar experience: spent years in a singing-and-dancing act—and got nowhere until he began to wisecrack and be himself. Will Rogers twirled a rope in vaudeville for years without saying a word. He got nowhere until he discovered his unique gift for humour and began to talk as he twirled his rope.

When Mary Margaret McBride first went on the air, she tried to be an Irish comedian and failed. When she tried to be just what she was—a plain country girl from Missouri—she became one of the most popular radio stars in New York.

When Gene Autry tried to get rid of his Texas accent and dressed like city boys and claimed he was from New York, people merely laughed behind his back. But when he started twanging his banjo and singing cowboy ballads, Gene Autry started out on a career that made him the world's most popular cowboy, both in pictures and on the radio.

You are something new in this world. Be glad of it. Make the most of what nature gave you. In the last analysis, all art is autobiographical. You can sing only what you are. You can paint only what you are. You must be what your experiences, your environment, and your heredity have made you. For better or for worse, you must cultivate your own little garden. For better or for worse, you must play your own little instrument in the orchestra of life.

As Emerson said in his essay on "Self-Reliance:" "There is a time in every man's education when he arrives at the conviction that envy is ignorance; that imitation is suicide; that he must take himself for better, for worse, as his portion; that though the wide universe is full of good, no kernel of nourishing corn can come to him but through his toil bestowed on that plot of ground which is given him to till. The power which resides in him is new in nature, and none but he knows what that is which he can do, nor does he know until he has tried."

That is the way Emerson said it. But here is the way a poet—the late Douglas Malloch—said it:

> "If you can't be a pine on the top of the hill,
> Be a scrub in the valley—but be the best little scrub by the side of the rill;
> Be a bush, if you can't be a tree.
> If you can't be a bush, be a bit of the grass,
> And some highway happier make;
> If you can't be a muskie, then just be a bass—
> But the liveliest bass in the lake!
> We can't all be captains, we've got to be crew,
> There's something for all of us here.
> There's big work to do and there's lesser to do,
> And the task we must do is the near.

If you can't be a highway, then just be a trail,
If you can't be the sun, be a star;
It isn't by size that you win or you fail—
Be the best of whatever you are!'

To cultivate a mental attitude that will bring us peace and freedom from worry, here is Rule 5:

LET'S NOT IMITATE OTHERS.
LET'S FIND OURSELVES AND BE OURSELVES

"There must be quite a few things that a hot bath won't cure, but I don't know many of them."
—Sylvia Plath

"There is something at work that's bigger than us. It's about having a trust in life and being at peace that things are happening the way they should. You do what you do as well as you can do it, and then you don't worry or agonize about the outcome."
—Sherilyn Fenn

28

IF YOU HAVE A LEMON, MAKE LEMONADE

While writing this book, I dropped in one day at the University of Chicago and asked the Chancellor, Robert Maynard Hutchins, how he kept from worrying. He replied, "I have always tried to follow a bit of advice given to me by the late Julius Rosenwald, President of Sears, Roebuck and Company: 'When you have a lemon, make lemonade.'"

That is what a great educator does. But the fool does the exact opposite. If he finds that life has handed him a lemon, he gives up and says, "I'm beaten. It is fate. I haven't got a chance." Then he proceeds to rail against the world and indulge in an orgy of self-pity. But when the wise man is handed a lemon, he says: "What lesson can I learn from this misfortune? How can I improve my situation? How can I turn this lemon into lemonade?"

After spending a lifetime studying people and their hidden reserves of power, the great psychologist, Alfred Adler, declared that one of the wonder-filled characteristics of human beings is "their power to turn a minus into a plus."

Here is an interesting and stimulating story of a woman I know who did just that. Her name is Thelma Thompson, and she lives at 100 Morningside Drive, New York City. "During the war," she said, as she told me of her experience, "during the war, my husband was stationed at an Army training camp near the Mojave Desert, in California. I went to live there in order to be near him. I hated the place. I loathed it. I had never before been so miserable. My husband was ordered out on maneuvers in the Mojave Desert, and I was left in a tiny shack alone. The heat was unbearable—125 degrees in the shade of a cactus. Not a soul to talk to but Mexicans and Indians, and they couldn't speak English. The wind blew incessantly, and all the food I ate, and the very air I breathed, were filled with sand, sand, sand!

"I was so utterly wretched, so sorry for myself, that I wrote to my parents. I told them I was giving up and coming back home. I said I couldn't stand it one minute longer. I would rather be in jail! My father answered my letter with just two lines—two lines that will always sing in my memory—two lines that completely altered my life:

> *Two men looked out from prison bars,*
> *One saw the mud, the other saw the stars.*

"I read those two lines over and over. I was ashamed of myself. I made up my mind I would find out what was good in my present situation; I would look for the stars.

"I made friends with the natives, and their reaction amazed me. When I showed interest in their weaving and pottery, they gave me presents of their favorite pieces which they had refused to sell to tourists. I studied the fascinating forms of the cactus and the yuccas and the Joshua trees. I learned about prairie dogs, watched for the desert sunsets, and hunted for seashells that had been left there millions of years ago when the sands of the desert had been an ocean floor.

"What brought about this astonishing change in me? The Mojave Desert hadn't changed. The Indians hadn't changed. But I had. I had changed my attitude of mind. And by doing so, I transformed a wretched experience into the most exciting adventure of my life. I was stimulated and excited by this new world that I had discovered. I was so excited I wrote a book about it—a novel that was published under the title *Bright Ramparts*.... *I* had looked out of my self-created prison and found the stars."

Thelma Thompson, you discovered an old truth that the Greeks taught five hundred years before Christ was born: "The best things are the most difficult."

Harry Emerson Fosdick repeated it again in the twentieth century: "Happiness is not mostly pleasure; it is mostly victory. Yes, the victory that comes from a sense of achievement, of triumph, of turning our lemons into lemonades.

I once visited a happy farmer down in Florida who turned even a poison lemon into lemonade. When he first got this farm, he was discouraged. The land was so wretched he could neither grow fruit nor raise pigs. Nothing thrived there but scrub oaks and rattlesnakes. Then he got his idea. He would turn his liability into an asset: he would make the most of these rattlesnakes. To everyone's amazement, he started canning rattlesnake meat. When I stopped to visit him a few years ago, I found that tourists were pouring in to see his rattlesnake farm at the rate of twenty thousand a year. His business was thriving. I saw poison from the fangs of his rattlers being shipped to laboratories to make antivenom toxin; I saw rattlesnake skins being sold at fancy prices to make women's shoes and handbags. I saw canned rattlesnake meat being shipped to customers all over the world. I bought a picture postcard of the place and mailed it at the local post office of the village, which had been re-christened "Rattlesnake, Florida," in honor of a man who had turned a poison lemon into a sweet lemonade.

As I have traveled up and down and back and forth across this nation time after time, it has been my privilege to meet dozens of men and women who have demonstrated "their power to turn a minus into a plus."

The late William Bolitho, author of *Twelve Against the Gods*, put it like this: "The most important thing in life is not to capitalize on your gains. Any fool can do that. The really important thing is to profit from your losses. That requires intelligence; and it makes the difference between a man of sense and a fool."

Bolitho uttered those words after he had lost a leg in a railway accident. But I know a man who lost both legs and turned his minus into a plus. His name is Ben Fortson. I met him in a hotel elevator in Atlanta, Georgia. As I stepped into the elevator, I noticed this cheerful-looking man, who had both legs missing, sitting in a wheel chair in a corner of the elevator. When the elevator stopped at his floor, he asked me pleasantly if I would step to one corner, so he could manage his chair better. "So sorry," he said, "to inconvenience you"—and a deep, heart-warming smile lighted his face as he said it.

When I left the elevator and went to my room, I could think of nothing but this cheerful cripple. So I hunted him up and asked him to tell me his story.

"It happened in 1929," he told me with a smile. "I had gone out to cut a load of hickory poles to stake the beans in my garden. I had loaded the poles on my Ford and started back home. Suddenly one pole slipped under the car and jammed the steering apparatus at the very moment I was making a sharp turn. The car shot over an embankment and hurled me against a tree. My spine was hurt. My legs were paralyzed.

"I was twenty-four when that happened, and I have never taken a step since."

Twenty-four years old, and sentenced to a wheel chair for the rest of his life! I asked him how he managed to take it so courageously, and he said, "I didn't." He said he raged and rebelled. He fumed about his fate. But as the years dragged on, he found that his rebellion wasn't getting him anything except bitterness. "I finally realized," he said, "that other people were kind and courteous to me. So the least I could do was to be kind and courteous to them."

I asked if he still felt, after all these years, that his accident had been a terrible misfortune, and he promptly said, "No." He said, "I'm almost glad now that it happened." He told me that after he got over the shock and resentment, he began to live in a different world. He began to read and developed a love for good literature. In fourteen years, he said, he had read at least fourteen hundred books; and those books had opened up new horizons for him and made his life richer than he ever thought possible. He began to listen to good music; and he is now thrilled by great symphonies that would have bored him before. But the biggest change was that he had time to think. "For the first time in my life," he said, "I was able to look at the world and get a real sense of values. I began to realize that most of the things I had been striving for before weren't worthwhile at all."

As a result of his reading, he became interested in politics, studied public questions, made speeches from his wheel chair! He got to know people and people got to know him. Today Ben Fortson—still in his wheelchair—is Secretary of State for the state of Georgia!

During the last thirty-five years, I have been conducting adult-education classes in New York City, and I have discovered that one of the major regrets of many adults is that they never went to college. They seem to think that not having a college education is a great handicap. I know that this isn't necessarily true because I have known thousands of successful men who never went beyond high school. So I often tell these students the story of a man I knew who had never finished even grade school. He was brought up in blighting poverty. When his father died, his father's friends had to chip in to pay for the coffin in which he was buried. After his father's death, his mother worked in an umbrella factory ten hours a day and then brought piecework home and worked until eleven o'clock at night.

The boy brought up in these circumstances went in for

amateur dramatics put on by a club in his church. He got such a thrill out of acting that he decided to take up public speaking. This led him into politics. By the time he reached thirty, he was elected to the New York State legislature. But he was woefully unprepared for such a responsibility. In fact, he told me that frankly he didn't know what it was all about. He studied the long, complicated bills that he was supposed to vote on—but, as far as he was concerned, those bills might as well have been written in the language of the Choctaw Indians. He was worried and bewildered when he was made a member of the committee on forests before he had ever set foot in a forest. He was worried and bewildered when he was made a member of the State Banking Commission before he had ever had a bank account. He himself told me that he was so discouraged that he would have resigned from the legislature if he hadn't been ashamed to admit defeat to his mother. In despair, he decided to study sixteen hours a day and turn his lemon of ignorance into a lemonade of knowledge. By doing that, he transformed himself from a local politician into a national figure and made himself so outstanding that *The New York Times* called him "the best-loved citizen of New York."

I am talking about Al Smith.

Ten years after Al Smith set out on his program of political self-education, he was the greatest living authority on the government of New York State. He was elected Governor of New York for four terms—a record never attained by any other man. In 1928, he was the Democratic candidate for President. Six great universities—including Columbia and Harvard—conferred honorary degrees upon this man who had never gone beyond grade school.

Al Smith himself told me that none of these things would ever have come to pass if he hadn't worked hard sixteen hours a day to turn his minus into a plus.

Nietzsche's formula for the superior man was "not only to bear up under necessity but to love it."

The more I have studied the careers of men of achievement the more deeply I have been convinced that a surprisingly large number of them succeeded because they started out with handicaps that spurred them on to great endeavor and great rewards. As William James said: "Our very infirmities help us unexpectedly."

Yes, it is highly probable that Milton wrote better poetry because he was blind and that Beethoven composed better music because he was deaf.

Helen Keller's brilliant career was inspired and made possible because of her blindness and deafness.

If Tchaikovsky had not been frustrated—and driven almost to suicide by his tragic marriage—if his own life had not been pathetic, he probably would never have been able to compose his immortal "Symphonie Pathétique."

If Dostoevsky and Tolstoy had not led tortured lives, they would probably never have been able to write their immortal novels.

"If I had not been so great an invalid," wrote the man who changed the scientific concept of life on earth—"if I had not been so great an invalid, I should not have done so much work as I have accomplished." That was Charles Darwin's confession that his infirmities had helped him unexpectedly.

The same day that Darwin was born in England, another baby was born in a log cabin in the forests of Kentucky. He, too, was helped by his infirmities. His name was Lincoln—Abraham Lincoln. If he had been reared in an aristocratic family and had had a law degree from Harvard and a happy married life, he would probably never have found in the depths of his heart the haunting words that he immortalized at Gettysburg, nor the sacred poem that he spoke at his second inauguration— the most beautiful and noble phrases ever uttered by a ruler of men: "With malice toward none; with charity for all…"

Harry Emerson Fosdick says in his book, *The Power to See it Through*, "There is a Scandinavian saying which some of us might well take as a rallying cry for our lives: 'The north wind made the Vikings.' Wherever did we get the idea that secure and pleasant living, the absence of difficulty, and the comfort of ease, ever of themselves made people either good or happy? Upon the contrary, people who pity themselves go on pitying themselves even when they are laid softly on a cushion, but always in history character and happiness have come to people in all sorts of circumstances, good, bad, and indifferent, when they shouldered their personal responsibility. So, repeatedly the north wind has made the Vikings."

Suppose we are so discouraged that we feel there is no hope of our ever being able to turn our lemons into lemonade—then here are two reasons why we ought to try, anyway—two reasons why we have everything to gain and nothing to lose.

Reason one: We may succeed.

Reason two: Even if we don't succeed, the mere attempt to turn our minus into a plus will cause us to look forward instead of backward; it will replace negative thoughts with positive thoughts; it will release creative energy and spur us to get so busy that we won't have either the time or the inclination to mourn over what is past and forever gone.

Once when Ole Bull, the world-famous violinist, was giving a concert in Paris, the A string on his violin suddenly snapped. But Ole Bull simply finished the melody on three strings. "That is life," says Harry Emerson Fosdick, "to have your A string snap and finish on three strings."

That is not only life. It is more than life. *It is life triumphant!*

If I had the power to do so, I would have these words of William Bolitho carved in eternal bronze and hung in every schoolhouse in the land:

The most important thing in life is not to capitalize on your gains. Any fool can do that. The really important thing is to profit from your losses. That requires intelligence; and it makes the difference between a man of sense and a fool.

So, to cultivate a mental attitude that will bring us peace and happiness, let's do something about Rule 6:

WHEN FATE HANDS US A LEMON,
LET'S TRY TO MAKE LEMONADE.

"People have a hard time letting go of their suffering. Out of a fear or the unknown, they prefer suffering that is familiar."

—Thich Nhat Hanh

"Worry does not empty tomorrow of its sorrow. It empties today of its strength."

—Corrie Ten Boom

29

HOW TO CURE MELANCHOLY
IN FOURTEEN DAYS

When i started writing this book, I offered a two-hundred-dollar prize for the most helpful and inspiring true story on "How I Conquered Worry."

The three judges for this contest were: Eddie Rickenbacker, president, Eastern Air Lines; Dr. Stewart W. McClelland, president, Lincoln Memorial University; H. V. Kaltenborn, radio news analyst. However, we received two stories so superb that the judges found it impossible to choose between them. So we divided the prize. Here is one of the stories that tied for first prize—the story of C. R. Burton (who works for Whizzer Motor Sales of Missouri, Inc.), 1067 Commercial Street, Springfield, Missouri.

"I lost my mother when I was nine years old, and my father when I was twelve," Mr. Burton wrote me. "My father was killed, but my mother simply walked out of the house one day nineteen years ago; and I have never seen her since. Neither have I ever seen my two little sisters that she took with her. She never even wrote me a letter until after she had been gone seven years. My father was killed in an accident three years after Mother left. He and a partner had bought a café in a small Missouri town; and while Father was away on a business trip, his partner sold the café for cash and skipped out. A friend wired

Father to hurry back home; and in his hurry, Father was killed in a car accident at Salinas, Kansas. Two of my father's sisters, who were poor and old and sick, took three of the children into their homes. Nobody wanted me and my little brother. We were left at the mercy of the town. We were haunted by the fear of being called orphans and treated as orphans. Our fears soon materialized, too. I lived for a little while with a poor family in town. But times were hard and the head of the family lost his job, so they couldn't afford to feed me any longer. Then Mr. and Mrs. Loftin took me to live with them on their farm eleven miles from town. Mr. Loftin was seventy years old, and sick in bed with shingles. He told me I could stay there 'as long as I didn't lie, didn't steal, and did as I was told.' Those three orders became my Bible. I lived by them strictly. I started to school, but the first week found me at home, bawling like a baby. The other children picked on me and poked fun at my big nose and said I was dumb and called me an 'orphan brat.' I was hurt so badly that I wanted to fight them; but Mr. Loftin, the farmer who had taken me in, said to me: 'Always remember that it takes a bigger man to walk away from a fight than it does to stay and fight.' I didn't fight until one day a kid picked up some chicken manure from the schoolhouse yard and threw it in my face. I beat the hell out of him; and made a couple of friends. They said he had it coming to him.

"I was proud of a new cap that Mrs. Loftin had bought me. One day one of the big girls jerked it off my head and filled it with water and ruined it. She said she filled it with water so that 'the water would wet my thick skull and keep my popcorn brains from popping.'

"I never cried at school, but I used to bawl it out at home. Then one day Mrs. Loftin gave me some advice that did away with all troubles and worries and turned my enemies into friends. She said, 'Ralph, they won't tease you and call you an 'orphan brat' any more if you will get interested in them and see how much you can do for them.' I took her advice. I studied hard; and though I soon headed the class, I was never envied because I went out of my way to help them.

"I helped several of the boys write their themes and essays. I wrote complete debates for some of the boys. One lad was ashamed to let his folks know that I was helping him. So he used to tell his mother he was going possum hunting. Then he would come to Mr. Loftin's farm and tie his dogs up in the barn while I helped him with his lessons. I wrote book reviews for one lad and I spent several evenings helping one of the girls on her math.

"Death struck our neighborhood. Two elderly farmers died and one woman was deserted by her husband. I was the only male in four families. I helped these widows for two years. On my way to and from school, I stopped at their farms, cut wood for them, milked their cows, and fed and watered their stock. I was now blessed instead of cursed. I was accepted as a friend by everyone. They showed me their real feelings when I returned home from the Navy. More than two hundred farmers came to see me the first day I was home. Some of them drove as far as eighty miles, and their concern for me was really sincere. Because I have been busy and happy trying to help other people, I have few worries; and I haven't been called an 'orphan brat' now for thirteen years."

Hooray for C. R. Burton! He knows how to win friends! And he also knows how to conquer worry and enjoy life.

So did the late Dr. Frank Loope, of Seattle, Washington. He was an invalid for twenty-three years. Arthritis. Yet Stuart Whithouse of the *Seattle Star* wrote me, saying, "I interviewed Dr. Loope many times; and *I have never known a man more unselfish* or a *man who got more out of life.*"

How did this bed-ridden invalid get so much out of life? I'll give you two guesses. Did he do it by complaining and criticizing? No... By wallowing in self-pity and demanding that he be the center of attention and everyone cater to him? No.... Still wrong. He did it by adopting as his slogan the motto of the Prince of Wales: "*Ich dien—I serve.*" He accumulated the names and addresses of other invalids and cheered both them and himself by writing happy, encouraging letters. In fact, he organized a letter-writing club for invalids and got them writing letters to one another. Finally, he formed a national organization called The Shut-in Society.

As he lay in bed, he wrote an average of fourteen hundred letters a year and brought joy to thousands of invalids by getting radios and books for shut-ins.

What was the chief difference between Dr. Loope and a lot of other people? Just this: Dr. Loope had the inner glow of a man with a purpose, a mission. He had the joy of knowing that he was being used by an idea far nobler and more significant than himself, instead of being, as Shaw put it, "a self-centered, little clod of ailments and grievances complaining that the world would not devote itself to making him happy."

Here is the most astonishing statement that *I* ever read from the pen of a great psychiatrist. This statement was made by Alfred Adler. He used to say to his melancholia patients: "You can be cured in fourteen days if you follow this prescription. Try to think every day how you can please someone."

That statement sounds so incredible that I feel I ought to try to explain it by quoting a couple of pages from Dr. Adler's splendid book, *What Life Should Mean to You.*

"Melancholia," says Adler on page 258 of *What Life Should Mean to You:*

> Melancholia is like a long-continued rage and reproach against others, though for the purpose of gaining care, sympathy and support, the patient seems only to be dejected about his own guilt. A melancholiac's first memory is generally something like this: "I remember I wanted to lie on the couch, but my brother was lying there. I cried so much that he had to leave."

Melancholiacs are often inclined to revenge themselves by committing suicide, and the doctor's first care is to avoid giving them an excuse for suicide. I myself try to relieve the whole tension by proposing to them, as the first rule in treatment, "Never do anything you don't like." This seems to be very modest, but I believe that it goes to the root of the whole trouble. If a melancholiac is able to do anything he wants, whom can he accuse? What has he got to revenge himself for? "If you want to go to the theater," I tell him, "or to go on a holiday, do it. If you find on the way that you don't want to, stop it." It is the best situation any one could be in. It gives a satisfaction to his striving for superiority. He is like God and can do what he pleases. On the other hand, it does not fit very easily into his style of life. He wants to dominate and accuse others and if they agree with him there is no way of dominating them. This rule is a great relief and I have never had a suicide among my patients.

Generally the patient replies, "But there is nothing I like doing." I have prepared for this answer, because I have heard it so often. "Then refrain from doing anything you dislike," I say. Sometimes, however, he will reply, "I should like to stay in bed all day." I know that, if I allow it, he will no longer want to do it. I know that, if I hinder him, he will start a war. I always agree.

This is one rule. Another attacks their style of life still more directly. I tell them, "You can *be* cured in fourteen days if you follow this prescription. Try to think every day *how* you can please some one." See what this means to them. They are occupied with the thought, "How can I worry some one." The answers are very interesting. Some say, "This will be very easy for me. I have done it all my life." They have never done it. I ask them to think it over. They do not think it over. I tell them, "You can make use of all the time you spend when you are unable to go to sleep by thinking how you can please some one, and it will be a big step forward in your health." When I see them next day, I ask them, "Did you think over what I suggested?" They answer, "Last night I went to sleep as soon as I got into bed. All this must be done, of course, in a modest, friendly manner, without a hint of superiority.

Others will answer, "I could never do it. "I am so worried." I tell them, "Don't stop worrying; but at the same time you can think now and then of others". I want to direct their interest always towards their fellows. Many say, "Why should I please others? Others do not try to please me." "You must think of your health," I answer. "The others will suffer later on." It is extremely rare that I have found a patient who said, "I have thought over what you suggested." All my efforts are devoted towards increasing the social interest of the patient. I know that the real reason for his malady is his lack of co-operation and I want him to see it too. As soon as he can connect himself with his fellow men on an equal and co-operative footing, he is cured…. The most important task imposed by religion has always been "Love thy neighbor."… It is the individual who is not interested in his fellow man who has the greatest difficulties in life and provides the greatest injury to others. It is from among such individuals that all human failures spring…. All that we demand of a human being, and the highest praise we can give him, is that he should be a good fellow worker, a friend to all other men, and a true partner in love and marriage.

Dr. Adler urges us to do a good deed every day. And

what is a good deed? "A good deed," said the prophet Mohammed, "is one that brings a smile of joy to the face of another."

Why will doing a good deed every day produce such astounding effects on the doer? Because trying to please others will cause us to stop thinking of ourselves: the very thing that produces worry and fear and melancholia.

Mrs. William T. Moon, who operates the Moon Secretarial School, 521 Fifth Avenue, New York, didn't have to spend two weeks thinking how she could please someone in order to banish her melancholy. She went Alfred Adler one better—no, she went Adler *thirteen* better. She banished her melancholy, not in fourteen days, but in *one* day, by thinking how she could please a couple of orphans.

It happened like this: "In December, five years ago," said Mrs. Moon, "I was engulfed in a feeling of sorrow and self-pity. After several years of happy married life, I had lost my husband. As the Christmas holidays approached, my sadness deepened. I had never spent a Christmas alone in all my life; and I dreaded to see this Christmas come. Friends had invited me to spend Christmas with them. But I did not feel up to any gaiety. I knew I would be a wet blanket at any party. So, I refused their kind invitations. As Christmas Eve approached, I was more and more overwhelmed with self-pity. True, I should have been thankful for many things, as all of us have many things for which to be thankful. The day before Christmas, I left my office at three o'clock in the afternoon and started walking aimlessly up Fifth Avenue, hoping that I might banish my self-pity and melancholy. The avenue was jammed with gay and happy crowds—scenes that brought back memories of happy years that were gone. I just couldn't bear the thought of going home to a lonely and empty apartment. I was bewildered. I didn't know what to do. I couldn't keep the tears back. After walking aimlessly for an hour or so, I found myself in front of a bus terminal. I remembered that my husband and I had often boarded an unknown bus for adventure, so I boarded the first bus I found at the station. After crossing the Hudson River and riding for some time, I heard the bus conductor say, 'Last stop, lady.' I got off. I didn't even know the name of the town. It was a quiet, peaceful little place. While waiting for the next bus home, I started walking up a residential street. As I passed a church, I heard the beautiful strains of 'Silent Night.' I went in. The church was empty except for the organist. I sat down unnoticed in one of the pews. The lights from the gaily decorated Christmas tree made the decorations seem like myriads of stars dancing in the moonbeams. The long-drawn cadences of the music—and the fact that I had forgotten to eat since morning—made me drowsy. I was weary and heavy-laden, so I drifted off to sleep.

"When I awoke, I didn't know where I was. I was terrified. I saw in front of me two small children who had apparently come in to see the Christmas tree. One, a little girl, was pointing at me and saying 'I wonder if Santa Claus brought her.' These children were also frightened when I awoke. I told them that I wouldn't hurt them. They were poorly dressed. I asked them where their mother and daddy were. 'We ain't got no mother and daddy,' they said.

"Here were two little orphans much worse off than I had ever been. They made me feel ashamed of my sorrow and self-pity. I showed them the Christmas tree and then took them to a drugstore and we had some refreshments, and I bought them some candy and a few presents. My loneliness vanished as if by magic. These two orphans gave me the only real happiness and self-forgetfulness that I had had in months. As I chatted with them, I realized how lucky I had been. I thanked God that all my Christmases as a child had been bright with parental love and tenderness. Those two little orphans did far more for me than I did for them. That experience showed me again the necessity of making other people happy in order to be happy ourselves. I found that happiness is contagious. By giving, we receive. By helping someone and giving out love, I had conquered worry and sorrow and self-pity, and felt like a new person. And I was a new person—not only then, but in the years that followed."

I could fill a book with stories of people who forgot themselves into health and happiness. For example, let's take the case of Margaret Tayler Yates, one of the most popular women in the United States Navy.

Mrs. Yates is a writer of novels, but none of her mystery stories is half so interesting as the true story of what happened to her that fateful morning when the Japanese struck our fleet at Pearl Harbor. Mrs. Yates had been an invalid for more than a year: bad heart. She spent twenty-two out of every twenty-four hours in bed. The longest journey that she undertook was a walk into the garden to take a sunbath. Even then, she had to lean on the maid's arm as she walked. She herself told me that in those days she expected to be an invalid for the balance of her life. "I would never have really lived again," she told me, "if the Japs had not struck Pearl Harbor and jarred me out of my complacency.

"When this happened," Mrs. Yates said, as she told her story, "everything was chaos and confusion. One bomb struck so near my home, the concussion threw me out of bed. Army trucks rushed out to Hickam Field, Scofield Barracks, and Kaneohe Bay Air Station, to bring Army and Navy wives and children to the public schools. There the Red Cross telephoned those who had extra rooms to take them in. The Red Cross workers knew that I had a telephone beside my bed, so they asked me to be a clearinghouse of information. So I kept track of where Army and Navy wives and children were being housed, and all Navy and Army men were instructed by the Red Cross to telephone me to find out where their families were.

"I soon discovered that my husband, Commander Robert Raleigh Yates, was safe. I tried to cheer up the wives who did not know whether their husbands had been killed; and I tried to give consolation to the widows whose husbands had been killed—and they were many. Two thousand, one hundred and seventeen officers and enlisted men in the Navy and Marine Corps were killed and 960 were reported missing.

"At first I answered these phone calls while lying in

bed. Then I answered them sitting up in bed. Finally, I got so busy, so excited, that I forgot all about my weakness and got out of bed and sat by a table. By helping others who were much worse off than I was, I forgot all about myself; and I have never gone back to bed again except for my regular eight hours of sleep each night. I realize now that if the Japs had not struck at Pearl Harbor, I would probably have remained a semi-invalid all my life. I was comfortable in bed. I was constantly waited on, and I now realize that I was unconsciously losing my will to rehabilitate myself.

"The attack on Pearl Harbor was one of the greatest tragedies in American history, but as far as I was concerned, it was one of the best things that ever happened to me. That terrible crisis gave me strength that I never dreamed I possessed. It took my attention off myself and focused it on others. It gave me something big and vital and important to live for. I no longer had time to think about myself or care about myself."

A third of the people who rush to psychiatrists for help could probably cure themselves if they would only do as Margaret Yates did: get interested in helping others. My idea? No, that is approximately what Carl Jung said. And he ought to know—if anybody does. He said: "About one third of my patients are suffering from no clinically definable neurosis, but from the senselessness and emptiness of their lives." To put it another way, they are trying to thumb a ride through life—and the parade passes them by. So they rush to a psychiatrist with their petty, senseless, useless lives.

Having missed the boat, they stand on the wharf, blaming everyone except themselves and demanding that the world cater to their self-centered desires.

You may be saying to yourself now: "Well, I am not impressed by these stories. I myself could get interested in a couple of orphans I met on Christmas Eve; and if I had been at Pearl Harbor, I would gladly have done what Margaret Tayler Yates did. But with me things are different: I live an ordinary humdrum life. I work at a dull job eight hours a day. Nothing dramatic ever happens to me. How can I get interested in helping others? And why should I? What is there in it for me?"

A fair question. I'll try to answer it. However humdrum your existence may be, you surely meet *some* people every day of your life. What do you do about them? Do you merely stare through them, or do you try to find out what it is that makes them tick? How about the postman, for example—he walks hundreds of miles every year, delivering mail to your door; but have you ever taken the trouble to find out where he lives, or ask to see a snapshot of his wife and his kids? Did you ever ask him if his feet get tired, or if he ever gets bored?

What about the grocery boy, the newspaper vendor, the chap at the corner who polishes your shoes? These people are human—bursting with troubles, and dreams, and private ambitions. They are also bursting for the chance to share them with someone. But do you ever let them? Do you ever show an eager, honest interest in them or their lives? That's the sort of thing I mean. You don't have to become a Florence Nightingale or a social reformer to help improve the world—your own private world; you can start tomorrow morning with the people you meet!

What's in it for you? Much greater happiness! Greater satisfaction, and pride in yourself! Aristotle called this kind of attitude "enlightened selfishness." Zoroaster said, "Doing good to others is not a duty. It is a joy, for it increases your own health and happiness." And Benjamin Franklin summed it up very simply—"When you are good to others," said Franklin, "you are best to yourself."

"No discovery of modern psychology," writes Henry C. Link, director of the Psychological Service Center in New York, "no discovery of modern psychology is, in my opinion, so important as its scientific proof of the necessity of self-sacrifice or discipline to self-realization and happiness."

Thinking of others will not only keep you from worrying about yourself; it will also help you to make a lot of friends and have a lot of fun. How? Well, I once asked Professor William Lyon Phelps, of Yale, how he did it; and here is what he said:

"I never go into a hotel or a barbershop or a store without saying something agreeable to everyone I meet. I try to say something that treats them as an individual— not merely a cog in a machine. I sometimes compliment the girl who waits on me in the store by telling her how beautiful her eyes are—or her hair. I will ask a barber if he doesn't get tired standing on his feet all day. I'll ask him how he came to take up barbering—how long he has been at it and how many heads of hair he has cut. I'll help him figure it out. I find that taking an interest in people makes them beam with pleasure. I frequently shake hands with a redcap who has carried my grip. It gives him a new lift and freshens him up for the whole day. One extremely hot summer day, I went into a dining car of the New Haven Railway to have lunch. The crowded car was almost like a furnace and the service was slow. When the steward finally got around to handing me the menu, I said: 'The boys back there cooking in that hot kitchen certainly must be suffering today.' The steward began to curse. His tones were bitter. At first, I thought he was angry. 'Good God Almighty,' he exclaimed, 'people come in here and complain about the food. They kick about the slow service and growl about the heat and the prices. I have listened to their criticisms for nineteen years and you are the first person and the only person that has ever expressed any sympathy for the cooks back there in the boiling kitchen. I wish to God we had more passengers like you.'

"The steward was astounded because I had thought of the colored cooks as human beings, and not merely as a cog in the organization of a great railway. What people want," continued Professor Phelps, "is a little attention as human beings. When I meet a man on the street with a beautiful dog, I always comment on the dog's beauty. As I walk on and glance back over my shoulder, I frequently see the man petting and admiring the dog. My appreciation has renewed his appreciation.

"One time in England, I met a shepherd, and expressed my sincere admiration for his big, intelligent sheep dog. I asked him to tell me how he trained the dog. As I walked away, I glanced back over my shoulder and saw the dog standing with his paws on the shepherd's shoulders and the shepherd was petting him. By taking a little interest in the shepherd and his dog, I made the shepherd happy. I made the dog happy and I made myself happy."

Can you imagine a man who goes around shaking hands with porters and expressing sympathy for the cooks in the hot kitchen—and telling people how much he admires their dogs—can you imagine a man like that being sour and worried and needing the services of a psychiatrist? You can't, can you? No, of course not. A Chinese proverb puts it this way: "A bit of fragrance always clings to the hand that gives you roses."

You didn't have to tell that to Billy Phelps of Yale. He knew it. He lived it.

If you are a man, skip this paragraph. It won't interest you. It tells how a worried, unhappy girl got several men to propose to her. The girl who did that is a grandmother now. A few years ago, I spent the night in her and her husband's home. I had been giving a lecture in her town; and the next morning she drove me about fifty miles to catch a train on the main line of the New York Central. We got to talking about winning friends, and she said: "Mr. Carnegie, I am going to tell you something that I have never confessed to anyone before—not even to my husband." (By the way, this story isn't going to be half so interesting as you probably imagine.) She told me that she had been reared in a social-register family in Philadelphia. "The tragedy of my girlhood and young woman-hood," she said, "was our poverty. We could never entertain the way the other girls in my social set entertained. My clothes were never of the best quality. I outgrew them and they didn't fit and they were often out of style. I was so humiliated, so ashamed, that I often cried myself to sleep. Finally, in sheer desperation, I hit upon the idea of always asking my partner at dinner parties to tell me about his experience, his ideas, and his plans for the future. I didn't ask these questions because I was especially interested in the answers. I did it solely to keep my partner from looking at my poor clothes. But a strange thing happened: as I listened to these young men talk and learned more about them, I really became interested in listening to what they had to say. I became so interested that I myself sometimes forgot about my clothes. But the astounding thing to me was this: since I was a good listener and encouraged the boys to talk about themselves, I gave them happiness and I gradually became the most popular girl in our social group and three of these men proposed marriage to me."

(There you are, girls: that is the way it is done.)

Some people who read this chapter are going to say: "All this talk about getting interested in others is a lot of damn nonsense! Sheer religious pap! None of that stuff for me! I am going to put money in my purse. I am going to grab all I can get—and grab it now—and to hell with the other dumb clucks!"

Well, if that is your opinion, you are entitled to it; but if you are right, then all the great philosophers and teachers since the beginning of recorded history—Jesus,

Confucius, Buddha, Plato, Aristotle, Socrates, Saint Francis—were all wrong. But since you may sneer at the teachings of religious leaders, let's turn for advice to a couple of atheists. First, let's take the late A. E. Housman, professor at Cambridge University, and one of the most distinguished scholars of his generation. In 1936, he gave an address at Cambridge University on "The Name and Nature of Poetry." In that address, he declared that "the greatest truth ever uttered and the most profound moral discovery of all time were these words of Jesus: 'He that findeth his life shall lose it: and he that loseth his life for my sake shall find it.'"

We have heard preachers say that all our lives. But Housman was an atheist, a pessimist, a man who contemplated suicide; and yet he felt that the man who thought only of himself wouldn't get much out of life. He would be miserable. But the man who forgot himself in service to others would find the joy of living.

If you are not impressed by what A. E. Housman said, let's turn for advice to the most distinguished American atheist of the twentieth century: Theodore Dreiser. Dreiser ridiculed all religions as fairy tales and regarded life as "a tale told by an idiot, full of sound and fury, signifying nothing." Yet Dreiser advocated the one great principle that Jesus taught—service to others. "If he [man] is to extract any joy out of his span," Dreiser said, "he must think and plan to make things better not only for himself but for others, since joy for himself depends upon his joy in others and theirs in him." If we are going "to make things better for others"—as Dreiser advocated—

let's be quick about it. Time is a-wastin'. "I shall pass this way but once. Therefore any good that I can do or any kindness that I can show—let me do it now. Let me not defer nor neglect it, for I shall not pass this way again."

So if you want to banish worry and cultivate peace and happiness, here is Rule 7:

FORGET YOURSELF BY BECOMING INTERESTED IN OTHERS. DO EVERY DAY A GOOD DEED THAT WILL PUT A SMILE OF JOY ON SOMEONE'S FACE.

"Worry never robs tomorrow of its sorrow, it only saps today of its joy."

—Leo Buscaglia

"All right, every day ain't going to be the best day of your life, don't worry about that. If you stick to it you hold the possibility open that you will have better days."

—Wendell Berry

30

ONE OF THE TWO MAJOR DECISIONS OF YOUR LIFE

If you are under eighteen, you will probably soon be called upon to make the two most important decisions of your life—decisions that will profoundly alter all the days of your years; decisions that may have far-reaching effects upon your happiness, your income, your health; decisions that may make or break you.

What are these two tremendous decisions?

First: *How are you going to make a living?* Are you going to be a farmer, a mail carrier, a chemist, a forest ranger, a stenographer, a horse doctor, a college professor, or are you going to run a ham-burger stand?

Second: Whom are you going to select to be the father or mother of your children?

Both of those great decisions are frequently gambles. "Every boy," says Harry Emerson Fosdick in his book, *The Power to See It Through*, "every boy is a gambler when he chooses a vocation. He must stake his life on it."

How can you reduce the gamble in selecting a vocation? Read on; we will tell you as best we can. First, try, if possible, to find work that you enjoy. I once asked David M. Goodrich, Chairman of the Board, B. F. Goodrich Company—tire manufacturers—what he considered the first requisite of success in business, and he replied— "Having a good time at your work. If you enjoy what you are doing," he said, "you may work long hours, but it won't seem like work at all. It will seem like play."

Edison was a good example of that. Edison—the unschooled newsboy who grew up to transform the industrial life of America—Edison, the man who often ate and slept in his laboratory and toiled there for eighteen hours a day. But it wasn't toil to him. "I never did a day's work in my life," he exclaimed. "It was all fun."

No wonder he succeeded!

I once heard Charles Schwab say much the same thing. He said: "A man can succeed at almost anything for which he has unlimited enthusiasm."

But how can you have enthusiasm for a job when you haven't the foggiest idea of what you want to do? "The greatest tragedy I know of," said Mrs. Edna Kerr, who once hired thousands of employees for the Dupont Company, and is now assistant director of industrial relations for the American Home Products Company—"The greatest tragedy I know of," she told me, "is that so many young people never discover what they really want to do. I think no one else is so much to be pitied as the person who gets nothing at all out of his work but his pay." Mrs. Kerr reports that even college graduates come to her and say, "I have a B.A. degree from Dartmouth [or an M.A. from Cornell]. Have you some kind of work I can do for your firm?" They don't know themselves what they are able to do, or even what they would like to do. Is it any wonder that so many men and women who start out in life with competent minds and rosy dreams end up at forty in utter frustration and even with a nervous breakdown? In fact, finding the right occupation is important even for your health. When Dr. Raymond Pearl, of Johns Hopkins, made a study, together with some insurance companies, to discover the factors that make for a long life, he placed "the right occupation" high on the list. He might have said, with Thomas Carlyle, "Blessed is the man who has found his work. Let him ask no other blessedness."

I recently spent an evening with Paul W. Boynton, employment supervisor for the Socony-Vacuum Oil Company. During the last twenty years he has interviewed more than seventy-five thousand people looking for jobs, and he has written a book entitled *6 Ways to Get a Job*. I asked him: "What is the greatest mistake young people make today in looking for work?" "They don't know what they want to do," he said. "It is perfectly appalling to realize that a man will give more thought to buying a suit of clothes that will wear out in a few years than he will give to choosing the career on which his whole future depends—on which his whole future happiness and peace of mind are based!"

And so what? What can you do about it? You can take advantage of a new profession called *vocational guidance*. It may help you—or harm you—depending on the ability and character of the counselor you consult. This new profession isn't even within gunshot of perfection yet. It hasn't even reached the Model T stage. But it has a great future. How can you make use of this science? By finding out where, in your community, you can get vocational tests and vocational advice. All the larger cities and thousands of smaller communities throughout the United States have this kind of service. If you are a veteran, the Veterans Administration will tell you where to apply. If you're not a veteran, then ask your public library or your local board of education where you may get vocational guidance. Hundreds of high schools and colleges have vocational-guidance bureaus. If you live in the country, write to your State Supervisor, Occupational Information and Guidance Service, in care of your state capitol. Many states have supervisors to give this sort of advice. In addition to the public agencies, a number of nation-wide organizations, such as the YMCA, YWCA, American Red Cross, B'nai B'rith, Boys' Clubs of America, Kiwanis Clubs, and the Salvation Army, have counselors to help you solve your vocational problems.

They can only suggest. You have to make the decisions. Remember that these counselors are far from infallible. They don't always agree with one another. They sometimes make ridiculous mistakes. For example, a vocational-guidance counselor advised one of my students to become a writer solely because she had a large vocabulary. How absurd! It isn't as simple as that. Good writing is the kind that transfers your thoughts and emotions to the reader— and to do that, you don't need a large vocabulary, but you do need ideas, experience, convictions, and excitement. The vocational counselor who advised this girl with a large vocabulary to become an author succeeded in doing only one thing: he turned an erstwhile happy stenographer into a frustrated, would-be novelist.

The point I am trying to make is that vocational-guidance experts, even as you and I, are not infallible. Perhaps you had better consult several of them—and then interpret their findings in the sunlight of common sense.

You may think it strange that I am including a chapter like this in a book devoted to worry. But it isn't strange at all, when you understand how many of our worries, regrets, and frustrations are spawned by work we despise. Ask your father about it—or your neighbor or your boss. No less an intellectual giant than John Stuart Mill declared that industrial misfits are "among the heaviest losses of society." Yes, and among the unhappiest people on this earth are those same "industrial misfits" who hate their daily work!

Do you know the kind of man who "cracked up" in the Army? The man who was misplaced! I'm not talking about battle casualties, but about the men who cracked up in ordinary service. Dr. William Menninger, one of our greatest living psychiatrists, was in charge of the Army's neuropsychiatric division during the war, and he says: "We learned much in the Army as to the importance of selection and of placement, of putting the right man in the right job…. A conviction of the importance of the job at hand was extremely important. *Where a man had no interest, where he felt he was misplaced, where he thought he was not appreciated, where he believed his talents were being misused, invariably we found a potential if not an actual psychiatric casualty.*"

Yes—and for the same reasons, a man may "crack up" in industry. If he despises his business, he can crack it up, too.

Take, for example, the case of Phil Johnson. Phil Johnson's father owned a laundry, so he gave his son a job, hoping the boy would work into the business. But Phil hated the laundry, so he dawdled, loafed, did what he had to do and not a lick more. Some days he was "absent." His father was so hurt to think he had a shiftless, ambitionless son that he was actually ashamed before his employees.

One day Phil Johnson told his father he wanted to be a mechanic—work in a machine shop. What? Go back to overalls? The old man was shocked. But Phil had his way. He worked in greasy dungarees. He did much harder work than was required at the laundry. He worked longer hours, and he whistled at his job! He took up engineering, learned about engines, puttered with machines—and when Philip Johnson died, in 1944, he was president of the Boeing Aircraft Company, and was making the Flying Fortresses that helped to win the war! If he had stuck with the laundry, what would have happened to him and the laundry—especially after his father's death? My guess is he would have ruined the business—cracked it up and run it into the ground.

Even at the risk of starting family rows, *I* would like to say to young people: *Don't feel compelled to enter a business or trade just because your family wants you to do it!* Don't enter a career unless you want to do it! However, consider carefully the advice of your parents. They have probably lived twice as long as you have. They have gained the kind of wisdom that comes only from much experience and the passing of many years. But, in the last analysis, you are the one who has to make the final decision. You are the one who is going to be either happy or miserable at your work.

Now, having said this, let me give you the following suggestions—some of them warnings—about choosing your work:

Read and study the following five suggestions about selecting a vocational-guidance counselor. These suggestions are right from the horse's mouth. They were made by one of America's leading vocational-guidance experts, Professor Harry Dexter Kitson.

"Don't go to anyone who tells you that he has a magic system that will indicate your 'vocational aptitude.' In this group are phrenologists, astrologers, 'character analysts,' handwriting experts. Their 'systems' do not work."

"Don't go to anyone who tells you that he can give you a test that will indicate what occupation you should choose. Such a person violates the principle that a vocational counselor must take into account the physical, social, and economic conditions surrounding the counselee; and he should render his service in the light of the occupational opportunities open to the counselee."

"Seek a vocational counselor who has an adequate library of information about occupations and uses it in the counseling process."

"A thorough vocational-guidance service generally requires more than one interview."

"Never accept vocational guidance by mail."

Keep out of business and professions that are already jam-

packed and overflowing! There are more than twenty thousand different ways of making a living in America. Think of it! Over twenty thousand. But do young people know this? Not unless they hire a swami to gaze into a crystal ball. The result? In one school, two thirds of the boys confined their choices to five occupations—five out of twenty thousand—and four fifths of the girls did the same. Small wonder that a few businesses and professions are overcrowded—small wonder that insecurity, worry, and "anxiety neuroses" are rampant at times among the white-collar fraternity! Beware especially of trying to elbow your way into such overcrowded fields as law, journalism, radio, motion pictures, and the "glamour occupations."

Stay out of activities where the chances are only one out of ten of your being able to make a living. As an example, take selling life insurance. Each year countless thousands of men—frequently unemployed men—start out trying to sell life insurance without bothering to find out in advance what is likely to happen to them! Here is *approximately what does happen*, according to Franklin L. Bettger, Real Estate Trust Building, Philadelphia. For twenty years Mr. Bettger was one of the outstandingly successful insurance salesmen in America. He declares that ninety per cent of the men who start selling life insurance get so heartsick and discouraged that they give it up within a year. Out of the ten who remain, one man will sell ninety per cent of all the insurance sold by the ten and the remaining nine men will sell only ten per cent of the insurance. To put it another way: if you start selling life insurance, the chances are nine to one that you will fail and quit within twelve months; and the chances are only one in a hundred that you will make ten thousand a year out of it. Even if you remain at it, the chances are only one out of ten that you will be able to do anything more than barely scratch out a living.

Spend weeks—even months, if necessary—finding out all you can about an occupation before deciding to devote your life to it! How? By interviewing men and women who have already spent ten, twenty, or forty years in that occupation.

These interviews may have a profound effect on your future. I know that from my own experience. When I was in my early twenties, I sought the vocational advice of two older men. As I look back now, I can see that those two interviews were turning points in my career. In fact, it would be difficult for me even to imagine what my life would have been like had I not had those two interviews.

How can you get these vocational-guidance interviews? To illustrate, let's suppose that you are thinking about studying to be an architect. Before you make your decision, you ought to spend weeks interviewing the architects in your city and in adjoining cities. You can get their names and addresses out of a classified telephone directory. You can call at their offices either with or without an appointment. If you wish to make an appointment, write them something like this:

Won't you please do me a little favor? I want your advice. I am eighteen years old, and I am thinking about studying to be an architect. Before I make up my mind, I would like to ask your advice.

If you are too busy to see me at your office, I would be most grateful if you would grant me the privilege of seeing you for half an hour at your home.

Here is a list of questions I would like to ask you:

If you had your life to live over, would you become an architect again?

After you have sized me up, I want to ask you whether you think I have what it takes to succeed as an architect.

Is the profession of architecture overcrowded?

If I studied architecture for four years, would it be difficult for me to get a job? What kind of job would I have to take at first?

If I had average ability, how much could I hope to earn during the first five years?

What are the advantages and disadvantages of being an architect?

If I were your son, would you advise me to become an architect?

If you are timid, and hesitate to face a "big shot" alone, here are two suggestions that will help.

First, get a lad of your own age to go with you. The two of you will bolster up one another's confidence. If you haven't someone of your own age to go with you, ask your father to go with you.

Second, remember that by asking his advice you are paying this man a compliment. He may feel flattered by your request. Remember that adults like to give advice to young men and women. The architect will probably enjoy the interview.

If you hesitate to write letters asking for an appointment, then go to a man's office without an appointment and tell him you would be most grateful if he would give you a bit of advice.

Suppose you call on five architects and they are all too busy to see you (which isn't likely), call on five more. Some of them will see you and give you priceless advice—advice that may save you years of lost time and heartbreak.

Remember that you are making one of the two most vital and far-reaching decisions of your life. So, take time to get the facts before you act. If you don't, you may spend half a lifetime regretting it.

If you can afford to do so, offer to pay a man for a half-hour of his time and advice.

Get over the mistaken belief that you are fitted for only a single occupation! Every normal person can succeed at a number of occupations, and every normal person would probably fail in many occupations. Take myself, for example: if I had studied and prepared myself for the following occupations, I believe I would have had a good chance of achieving some small measure of success—and also of enjoying my work. I refer to such occupations as farming, fruit growing, scientific agriculture, medicine, selling, advertising, editing a country newspaper, teaching, and forestry. On the other hand, I am sure I would have been unhappy, and a failure, at bookkeeping, accounting, engineering, operating a hotel or a factory, architecture, all mechanical trades, and hundreds of other activities.

"A day of worry is more exhausting than a week of work."

—John Lubbock

"If you ask what is the single most important key to longevity, I would have to say it is avoiding worry, stress and tension. And if you didn't ask me, I'd still have to say it."

—George Burns

HOW TO ENJOY YOUR LIFE AND YOUR JOB

PART I

WIN FRIENDS AND INFLUENCE PEOPLE

1

HOW TO MAKE PEOPLE LIKE YOU INSTANTLY

I was waiting in line to register a letter in the post office at Thirty-third Street and Eighth Avenue in New York. I noticed that the clerk appeared to be bored with the job—weighing envelopes, handing out stamps, making change, issuing receipts—the same monotonous grind year after year. So I said to myself: "I am going to try to make that clerk like me. Obviously, to make him like me, I must say something nice, not about myself, but about him." So I asked myself, "What is there about him that I can honestly admire?" That is sometimes a hard question to answer, especially with strangers; but, in this case, it happened to be easy. I instantly saw something I admired no end.

So while he was weighing my envelope, I remarked with enthusiasm: "I certainly wish I had your head of hair."

He looked up, half-startled, his face beaming with smiles. "Well, it isn't as good as it used to be," he said modestly. I assured him that although it might have lost some of its pristine glory, nevertheless it was still magnificent. He was immensely pleased. We carried on a pleasant little conversation and the last thing he said to me was: "Many people have admired my hair."

I'll bet that person went out to lunch that day walking on air. I'll bet he went home that night and told his wife about it. I'll bet he looked in the mirror and said: "It is a beautiful head of hair."

I told this story once in public and a man asked me afterward: "What did you want to get out of him?"

What did I want to get out of him!!! What did I want to get out of him!!!

If we are so contemptibly selfish that we can't radiate a little happiness and pass on a bit of honest appreciation without trying to get something out of the other person in return—if our souls are no bigger than sour crab apples, we shall meet with the failure we so richly deserve.

Oh yes, I did want something out of that chap. I wanted something priceless. And I got it. I got the feeling that I had done something for him without his being able to do anything whatever in return for me. That is a feeling that flows and sings in your memory long after the incident is past.

There is one all-important law of human conduct. If we obey that law, we shall almost never get into trouble. In fact, that law, if obeyed, will bring us countless friends and constant happiness. But the very instant we break the law, we shall get into endless trouble. The law is this: *Always make the other person feel important.* John Dewey said that the desire to be important is the deepest urge in human nature; and William James said: "The deepest principle in human nature is the craving to be appreciated." As I have already pointed out, it is this urge that differentiates us from the animals. It is this urge that has been responsible for civilization itself.

Philosophers have been speculating on the rules of human

relationships for thousands of years, and out of all that speculation, there has evolved only one important precept. It is not new. It is as old as history. Zoroaster taught it to his followers in Persia twenty-five hundred years ago. Confucius preached it in China twenty-four centuries ago. Lao-tse, the founder of Taoism, taught it to his disciples in the Valley of the Han twenty-five centuries ago. Buddha preached it on the bank of the Holy Ganges five hundred years before Christ. The sacred books of Hinduism taught it a thousand years before that. Jesus taught it among the stony hills of Judea nineteen centuries ago. Jesus summed it up in one thought—probably the most important rule in the world: "Do unto others as you would have others do unto you."

You want the approval of those with whom you come in contact. You want recognition of your true worth. You want a feeling that you are important in your little world. You don't want to listen to cheap, insincere flattery, but you do crave sincere appreciation. You want your friends and associates to be, as Charles Schwab put it, "hearty in their approbation and lavish in their praise." All of us want that.

So let's obey the Golden Rule, and give unto others what we would have others give unto us.

How? When? Where? The answer is: All the time, everywhere.

David G. Smith of Eau Claire, Wisconsin, told one of our classes how he handled a delicate situation when he was asked to take charge of the refreshment booth at a charity concert.

"The night of the concert I arrived at the park and

found two elderly ladies in a very bad humor standing next to the refreshment stand. Apparently each thought that she was in charge of this project. As I stood there pondering what to do, one of the members of the sponsoring committee appeared and handed me a cash box and thanked me for taking over the project. She introduced Rose and Jane as my helpers and then ran off.

"A great silence ensued. Realizing that the cash box was a symbol of authority (of sorts), I gave the box to Rose and explained that I might not be able to keep the money straight and that if she took care of it I would feel better. I then suggested to Jane that she show two teenagers who had been assigned to refreshments how to operate the soda machine, and I asked her to be responsible for that part of the project.

"The evening was very enjoyable, with Rose happily counting the money, Jane supervising the teenagers, and me enjoying the concert."

You don't have to wait until you are ambassador to France or chairman of the Clambake Committee of your lodge before you use this philosophy of appreciation. You can work magic with it almost every day.

If, for example, the waitress brings us mashed potatoes when we have ordered French fries, let's say: "I'm sorry to trouble you, but I prefer French fries." She'll probably reply, "No trouble at all" and will be glad to change the potatoes, because we have shown respect for her.

Little phrases such as "I'm sorry to trouble you," "Would you be so kind as to?" "Won't you please?" "Would you mind?" "Thank you"—little courtesies like these relieve the monotonous grind of everyday life—and, incidentally, they are the hallmark of good breeding.

The unvarnished truth is that almost all the people you meet feel themselves superior to you in some way, and a sure way to their hearts is to let them realize in some subtle way that you recognize their importance, and recognize it sincerely.

Remember what Emerson said: "Every man I meet is my superior in some way. In that, I learn of him."

And the pathetic part of it is that frequently those who have the least justification for a feeling of achievement bolster their egos by a show of tumult and conceit that is truly nauseating. As Shakespeare put it: "...man, proud man / Drest in a little brief authority / ...Plays such fantastic tricks before high heaven / As make the angels weep."

I am going to tell you how business people in my own courses have applied these principles with remarkable results. Let's take the case of a Connecticut attorney (because of his relatives he prefers not to have his name mentioned).

Shortly after joining the course, Mr. R—drove to Long Island with his wife to visit some of her relatives. She left him to chat with an old aunt of hers and then rushed off by herself to visit some of the younger relatives. Since he soon had to give a speech professionally on how he applied the principles of appreciation, he thought he would gain some worthwhile experience talking with the elderly lady. So he looked around the house to see what he could honestly admire.

"This house was built about 1890, wasn't it?" he inquired.

"Yes," she replied, "that is precisely the year it was built."

"It reminds me of the house I was born in," he said. "It's beautiful. Well built. Roomy. You know, they don't build houses like this anymore."

"You're right," the old lady agreed. "The young folks nowadays don't care for beautiful homes. All they want is a small apartment, and then they go off gadding about in their automobiles.

"This is a dream house," she said in a voice vibrating with tender memories. "This house was built with love. My husband and I dreamed about it for years before we built it. We didn't have an architect. We planned it all ourselves."

She showed Mr. R about the house, and he expressed his hearty admiration for the beautiful treasures she had picked up in her travels and cherished over a lifetime— paisley shawls, an old English tea set, Wedgwood china, French beds and chairs, Italian paintings, and silk draperies that had once hung in a French château.

After showing Mr. R—through the house, she took him out to the garage. There, jacked up on blocks, was a Packard car—in mint condition.

"My husband bought that car for me shortly before he passed on," she said softly. "I have never ridden in it since his death... You appreciate nice things, and I'm going to give this car to you."

"Why, Aunty," he said, "you overwhelm me. I appreciate your generosity, of course; but I couldn't possibly accept it. I'm not even a relative of yours. I have a new car, and you have many relatives who would like to have that Packard."

"Relatives!" she exclaimed. "Yes, I have relatives who are just waiting till I die so they can get that car. But they are not going to get it."

"If you don't want to give it to them, you can very easily sell it to a secondhand dealer," he told her.

"Sell it!" she cried. "Do you think I would sell this car? Do you think I could stand to see strangers riding up and down the street in that car—that car that my husband bought for me? I wouldn't dream of selling it. I'm going to give it to you. You appreciate beautiful things."

He tried to get out of accepting the car, but he couldn't without hurting her feelings.

This lady, left all alone in a big house with her paisley shawls, her French antiques, and her memories, was starving for a little recognition. She had once been young and beautiful and sought-after. She had once built a house warm with love and had collected things from all over Europe to make it beautiful. Now, in the isolated loneliness of old age, she craved a little human warmth, a little genuine appreciation—and no one gave it to her. And when she found it, like a spring in the desert, her gratitude couldn't adequately express itself with anything less than the gift of her cherished Packard.

Let's take another case: Donald M. McMahon, who was superintendent of Lewis and Valentine, nurserymen and landscape architects in Rye, New York, related this incident:

"Shortly after I attended the talk on 'How to Win Friends and Influence People,' I was landscaping the estate of a famous judge. The owner came out to give me a few instructions about where he wished to plant a mass of rhododendrons and azaleas.

"I said, 'Judge, you have a lovely hobby. I've been admiring your beautiful dogs. I understand you win a lot of blue ribbons every year at the show in Madison Square Garden.'

"The effect of this little expression of appreciation was striking.

"'Yes,' the judge replied, 'I do have a lot of fun with my dogs. Would you like to see my kennel?'

"He spent almost an hour showing me his dogs and the prizes they had won. He even brought out their pedigrees and explained about the bloodlines responsible for such beauty and intelligence.

"Finally, turning to me, he asked: 'Do you have any small children?'

"'Yes, I do,' I replied. 'I have a son.'

"'Well, wouldn't he like a puppy?' the judge inquired.

"'Oh, yes, he'd be tickled pink.'

"'All right, I'm going to give him one,' the judge announced.

"He started to tell me how to feed the puppy. Then he paused. 'You'll forget it if I tell you. I'll write it out.' So the judge went in the house, typed out the pedigree and feeding instructions, and gave me a puppy worth several hundred dollars and one hour and fifteen minutes of his valuable time largely because I had expressed my honest admiration for his hobby and achievements."

George Eastman, of Kodak fame, invented the transparent film that made motion pictures possible, amassed a fortune of a hundred million dollars, and made himself one of the most famous businessmen on earth. Yet in spite of all these tremendous accomplishments, he craved a little recognition even as you and I.

To illustrate: When Eastman was building the Eastman School of Music and also Kilbourn Hall in Rochester, James Adamson, then president of the Superior Seating Company of New York, wanted to get the order to supply the theater chairs for these buildings. Phoning the architect, Mr. Adamson made an appointment to see Mr. Eastman in Rochester.

When Adamson arrived, the architect said: "I know you want to get this order, but I can tell you right now that you won't stand a ghost of a show if you take more than five minutes of George Eastman's time. He is a strict disciplinarian. He is very busy. So tell your story quickly and get out."

Adamson was prepared to do just that.

When he was ushered into the room he saw Mr. Eastman bending over a pile of papers at his desk. Presently, Mr. Eastman looked up, removed his glasses, and walked toward the architect and Mr. Adamson, saying: "Good morning, gentlemen, what can I do for you?"

The architect introduced them, and then Mr. Adamson said: "While we've been waiting for you, Mr. Eastman, I've been admiring your office. I wouldn't mind working in a room like this myself. I'm in the interior-woodworking business, and I never saw a more beautiful office in all my life.

George Eastman replied: "You remind me of something I had almost forgotten. It is beautiful, isn't it? I enjoyed it a great deal when it was first built. But I come down here now with a lot of other things on my mind and sometimes don't even see the room for weeks at a time."

Adamson walked over and rubbed his hand across a panel. "This is English oak, isn't it? A little different in texture from Italian oak."

"Yes," Eastman replied. "Imported English oak. It was selected for me by a friend who specializes in fine woods."

Then Eastman showed him about the room, commenting on the proportions, the coloring, the hand carving, and other efforts he had helped to plan and execute.

While drifting about the room, admiring the woodwork, they paused before a window, and George Eastman, in his modest, soft-spoken way, pointed out some of the institutions through which he was trying to help humanity: the University of Rochester, the General Hospital, the Homeopathic Hospital, the Friendly Home, the Children's Hospital. Mr. Adamson congratulated him warmly on the idealistic way he was using his wealth to alleviate the sufferings of humanity. Presently, George Eastman unlocked a glass case and pulled out the first camera he had ever owned—an invention he had bought from an Englishman.

Adamson questioned him at length about his early

struggles to get started in business, and Mr. Eastman spoke with real feeling about the poverty of his childhood, telling how his widowed mother had kept a boardinghouse while he clerked in an insurance office. The terror of poverty haunted him day and night, and he resolved to make enough money so that his mother wouldn't have to work. Mr. Adamson drew him out with further questions and listened, absorbed, while he related the story of his experiments with dry photographic plates. He told how he had worked in an office all day, and sometimes experimented all night, taking only brief naps while the chemicals were working and sleeping in his clothes for seventy-two hours at a stretch.

James Adamson had been ushered into Eastman's office at ten-fifteen and had been warned that he must not take more than five minutes; but an hour passed, then two hours passed. And they were still talking.

Finally, George Eastman turned to Adamson and said, "The last time I was in Japan I bought some chairs, brought them home, and put them in my sun porch. But the sun peeled the paint, so I went downtown the other day and bought some paint and painted the chairs myself. Would you like to see what sort of a job I can do painting chairs?

All right. Come up to my home and have lunch with me and I'll show you."

After lunch, Mr. Eastman showed Adamson the chairs he had brought from Japan. They weren't worth more than a few dollars, but George Eastman, now a multimillionaire, was proud of them because he himself had painted them.

The order for the seats amounted to ninety thousand dollars. Who do you suppose got the order—James Adamson or one of his competitors? From the time of this story until Mr. Eastman's death, he and James Adamson were close friends.

Claude Marais, a restaurant owner in Rouen, France, used this principle and saved his restaurant the loss of a key employee. This woman had been in his employ for five years and was a vital link between M. Marais and his staff of twenty-one people. He was shocked to receive a registered letter from her advising him of her resignation.

M. Marais reported: "I was very surprised and, even more, disappointed, because I was under the impression that I had been fair to her and receptive to her needs. Inasmuch as she was a friend as well as an employee, I probably had taken her too much for granted and maybe was even more demanding of her than of other employees.

"I could not, of course, accept this resignation without some explanation. I took her aside and said, 'Paulette, you must understand that I cannot accept your resignation. You mean a great deal to me and to this company, and you are as important to the success of this restaurant as I am.' I repeated this in front of the entire staff, and I invited her to my home and reiterated my confidence in her with my family present.

"Paulette withdrew her resignation, and today I can rely on her as never before. I frequently reinforce this by expressing my appreciation for what she does and showing her how important she is to me and to the restaurant."

"Talk to people about themselves," said Disraeli, one

of the shrewdest men who ever ruled the British Empire. "Talk to people about themselves and they will listen for hours."

Always Make the Other Person Feel Important

> *Inaction breeds doubt and fear. Action breeds confidence and courage. If you want to conquer fear, do not sit home and think about it. Go out and get busy.*
>
> —Dale Carnegie

2

DO THIS AND YOU'LL BE WELCOME ANYWHERE

Why read this book to find out how to win friends? Why not study the technique of the greatest winner of friends the world has ever known? Who is he? You may meet him tomorrow coming down the street. When you get within ten feet of him, he will begin to wag his tail. If you stop and pat him, he will almost jump out of his skin to show you how much he likes you. And you know that behind this show of affection on his part, there are no ulterior motives: he doesn't want to sell you any real estate, and he doesn't want to marry you.

Did you ever stop to think that a dog is the only animal that doesn't have to work for a living? A hen has to lay eggs, a cow has to give milk, and a canary has to sing. But a dog makes his living by giving you nothing but love.

When I was five years old, my father bought a little yellow-haired pup for fifty cents. He was the light and joy of my childhood. Every afternoon about four-thirty, he would sit in the front yard with his beautiful eyes staring steadfastly at the path, and as soon as he heard my voice or saw me swinging my dinner pail through the buck brush, he was off like a shot, racing breathlessly up the hill to greet me with leaps of joy and barks of sheer ecstasy.

Tippy was my constant companion for five years. Then

one tragic night—I shall never forget it—he was killed within ten feet of me, killed by lightning. Tippy's death was the tragedy of my boyhood.

You never read a book on psychology, Tippy. You didn't need to. You knew by some divine instinct that you can make more friends in two months by becoming genuinely interested in other people than you can in two years by trying to get other people interested in you. Let me repeat that. You can make more friends in two months by becoming interested in other people than you can in two years by trying to get other people interested in you.

Yet I know and you know people who blunder through life trying to wigwag other people into becoming interested in them.

Of course, it doesn't work. People are not interested in you. They are not interested in me. They are interested in themselves—morning, noon, and after dinner.

The New York Telephone Company made a detailed study of telephone conversations to find out which word is the most frequently used. You have guessed it: it is the personal pronoun "I." "I." "I." It was used 3,900 times in 500 telephone conversations. "I." "I." "I." "I."

When you see a group photograph that you are in, whose picture do you look for first?

If we merely try to impress people and get people interested in us, we will never have many true, sincere friends. Friends, real friends, are not made that way.

Napoleon tried it, and in his last meeting with Josephine he said: "Josephine, I have been as fortunate as any man ever was on this earth; and yet, at this hour, you are the only person in the world on whom I can rely." And historians doubt that he could rely even on her.

I once took a course in short-story writing at New York University, and during that course the editor of a leading magazine talked to our class. He said he could pick up any one of the dozens of stories that drifted across his desk every day and after reading a few paragraphs he could feel whether or not the author liked people. "If the author doesn't like people," he said, "people won't like his or her stories."

This hard-boiled editor stopped twice in the course of his talk on fiction writing and apologized for preaching a sermon. "I am telling you," he said, "the same things your preacher would tell you, but remember, you have to be interested in people if you want to be a successful writer of stories."

If that is true of writing fiction, you can be sure it is true of dealing with people face-to-face.

I spent an evening in the dressing room of Howard Thurston the last time he appeared on Broadway— Thurston was the acknowledged dean of magicians. For forty years he had traveled all over the world, time and again, creating illusions, mystifying audiences, and making people gasp with astonishment. More than 60 million people had paid admission to his show, and he had made almost $2 million in profit.

I asked Mr. Thurston to tell me the secret of his success. His schooling certainly had nothing to do with it, for he ran away from home as a small boy, became a hobo, rode in boxcars, slept in haystacks, begged his food from door to door, and learned to read by looking out of boxcars at signs along the railway.

Did he have a superior knowledge of magic? No, he told me hundreds of books had been written about legerdemain and scores of people knew as much about it as he did. But he had two things that the others didn't have. First, he had the ability to put his personality across the footlights. He was a master showman. He knew human nature. Everything he did, every gesture, every intonation of his voice, every lifting of an eyebrow had been carefully rehearsed, and his actions were timed to split seconds. But, in addition to that, Thurston had a genuine interest in people. He told me that many magicians would look at the audience and say to themselves, "Well, there is a bunch of suckers out there, a bunch of hicks; I'll fool them all right." But Thurston's method was totally different. He told me that every time he went on stage he said to himself: "I am grateful because these people came to see me. They make it possible for me to make my living in a very agreeable way. I'm going to give them the very best I possibly can."

He declared he never stepped in front of the footlights without first saying to himself over and over: "I love my audience. I love my audience." Ridiculous? Absurd? You are privileged to think anything you like. I am merely passing it on to you without comment as a recipe used by one of the most famous magicians of all time.

George Dyke of North Warren, Pennsylvania, was forced to retire from his service station business after thirty years when a new highway was constructed over the site of his station. It wasn't long before the idle days of retirement began to bore him, so he started filling in his time trying to play music on his old fiddle. Soon he was traveling the area to listen to music and talk with many of the accomplished fiddlers. In his humble and friendly way he became generally interested in learning the background and interests of every musician he met. Although he was not a great fiddler himself, he made many friends in this pursuit. He attended competitions and soon became known to the country music fans in the eastern part of the United States as "Uncle George, the Fiddle Scraper from Kinzua County." When we heard Uncle George, he was seventy-two and enjoying every minute of his life. By having a sustained interest in other people, he created a new life for himself at a time when most people consider their productive years over.

That, too, was one of the secrets of Theodore Roosevelt's astonishing popularity. Even his servants loved him. His valet, James E. Amos, wrote a book about him entitled *Theodore Roosevelt, Hero to His Valet*. In that book Amos relates this illuminating incident:

> My wife one time asked the President about a bobwhite. She had never seen one and he described it to her fully. Sometime later, the telephone at our cottage rang. [Amos and his wife lived in a little cottage on the Roosevelt estate at Oyster Bay.] My wife answered it and it was Mr. Roosevelt himself. He had called her, he said, to tell her that there was

a bobwhite outside her window and that if she would look out she might see it. Little things like that were so characteristic of him. Whenever he went by our cottage, even though we were out of sight, we would hear him call out: "Oo-oo-oo, Annie?" or "Oo-oo-oo, James!" It was just a friendly greeting as he went by.

How could employees keep from liking a man like that? How could anyone keep from liking him?

Roosevelt called at the White House one day when the President and Mrs. Taft were away. His honest liking for humble people was shown by the fact that he greeted all the old White House servants by name, even the scullery maids.

"When he saw Alice, the kitchen maid," writes Archie Butt, "he asked her if she still made corn bread. Alice told him that she sometimes made it for the servants, but no one ate it upstairs.

"'They show bad taste,' Roosevelt boomed, 'and I'll tell the President so when I see him.'

"Alice brought a piece to him on a plate, and he went over to the office eating it as he went and greeting gardeners and laborers as he passed...

"He addressed each person just as he had addressed them in the past. Ike Hoover, who had been head usher at the White House for forty years, said with tears in his eyes, 'It is the only happy day we had in nearly two years, and not one of us would exchange it for a hundred-dollar bill.'"

The same concern for the seemingly unimportant people helped sales representative Edward M. Sykes, Jr., of Chatham, New Jersey, retain an account. "Many years ago," he reported, "I called on customers for Johnson and Johnson in the Massachusetts area. One account was a drug store in Hingham. Whenever I went into this store I would always talk to the soda clerk and sales clerk for a few minutes before talking to the owner to obtain his order. One day I went up to the owner of the store, and he told me to leave as he was not interested in buying J&J products anymore because he felt they were concentrating their activities on food and discount stores to the detriment of the small drugstore. I left with my tail between my legs and drove around the town for several hours. Finally, I decided to go back and try at least to explain our position to the owner of the store.

"When I returned I walked in and as usual said hello to the soda clerk and sales clerk. When I walked up to the owner, he smiled at me and welcomed me back. He then gave me double the usual order. I looked at him with surprise and asked him what had happened since my visit only a few hours earlier. He pointed to the young man at the soda fountain and said that after I had left, the boy had come over and said that I was one of the few salespeople who called on the store who even bothered to say hello to him and to the others in the store. He told the owner that if any salesperson deserved his business, it was I. The owner agreed and remained a loyal customer. I never forgot that to be genuinely interested in other people is a most important quality for a salesperson to possess—for any person, for that matter."

I have discovered from personal experience that one can win the attention and time and cooperation of even the most sought-after people by becoming genuinely interested in them. Let me illustrate.

Years ago I conducted a course in fiction writing at the Brooklyn Institute of Arts and Sciences, and we wanted such distinguished and busy authors as Kathleen Norris, Fannie Hurst, Ida Tarbell, Albert Payson Terhune, and Rupert Hughes to come to Brooklyn and give us the benefit of their experience. So we wrote them, saying we admired their work and were deeply interested in getting their advice and learning the secrets of their success.

Each of these letters was signed by about 150 students. We said we realized that these authors were busy—too busy to prepare a lecture. So we enclosed a list of questions for them to answer about themselves and their methods of work. They liked that. Who wouldn't like it? So they left their homes and traveled to Brooklyn to give us a helping hand.

By using the same method, I persuaded Leslie M. Shaw, secretary of the treasury in Theodore Roosevelt's cabinet; George W. Wickersham, attorney general in Taft's cabinet; William Jennings Bryan; Franklin D. Roosevelt; and many other prominent men to come to talk to the students of my courses in public speaking.

All of us, be we workers in a factory, clerks in an office, or even a king upon his throne—all of us like people who admire us. Take the German kaiser, for example. At the close of World War I, he was probably the most savagely and universally despised man on this earth. Even his own nation turned against him when he fled over into Holland to save his neck. The hatred against him was so intense that millions of people would have loved to tear him limb from limb or burn him at the stake. In the midst of all this forest fire of fury, one little boy wrote the kaiser a simple, sincere letter glowing with kindliness and admiration. This little boy said that no matter what the others thought, he would always love Wilhelm as his emperor. The kaiser was deeply touched by his letter and invited the little boy to come see him. The boy came, so did his mother—and the kaiser married her. That little boy didn't need to read a book on how to win friends and influence people. He knew how instinctively.

If we want to make friends, let's put ourselves out to do things for other people—things that require time, energy, unselfishness, and thoughtfulness. When the Duke of Windsor was Prince of Wales, he was scheduled to tour South America, and before he started out on that tour he spent months studying Spanish so that he could make public talks in the language of the country; and the South Americans loved him for it.

For years I made it a point to find out the birthdays of my friends. How? Although I haven't the foggiest bit of faith in astrology, I began by asking the other party whether he believed the date of one's birth has anything to do with character and disposition. I then asked him or her to tell me the month and day of birth. If he or she said November 24, for example, I kept repeating to myself,

"November 24, November 24." The minute my friend's back was turned, I wrote down the name and birthday and later would transfer it to a birthday book. At the beginning of each year, I had these birthday dates scheduled in my calendar pad so that they came to my attention automatically. When the natal day arrived, there was my letter or telegram. What a hit it made! I was frequently the only person on earth who remembered.

If we want to make friends, let's greet people with animation and enthusiasm. When somebody calls you on the telephone use the same psychology. Say "Hello" in tones that bespeak how pleased you are to have the person call. Many companies train their telephone operators to greet all callers in a tone that radiates interest and enthusiasm. The callers feel the company is concerned about them. Let's remember that when we answer the telephone tomorrow.

Showing a genuine interest in others not only wins friends for you, but may develop in its customers a loyalty to your company. In an issue of the publication of the National Bank of North America of New York, the followng letter from Madeline Rosedale, a depositor, was published:

"I would like you to know how much I appreciate your staff. Everyone is so courteous, polite, and helpful. What a pleasure it is, after waiting in a long line, to have the teller greet you pleasantly.

"Last year my mother was hospitalized for five months. Frequently I went to Marie Petrucello, a teller. She was concerned about my mother and inquired about her progress."

Is there any doubt that Mrs. Rosedale will continue to use this bank?

Charles R. Walters, of one of the large banks in New York City, was assigned to prepare a confidential report on a certain corporation. He knew of only one person who possessed the facts he needed so urgently. As Mr. Walters was ushered into the president's office, a young woman stuck her head through a door and told the president that she didn't have any stamps for him that day.

"I am collecting stamps for my twelve-year-old son," the president explained to Mr. Walters.

Mr. Walters stated his mission and began asking questions. The president was vague, general, nebulous. He didn't want to talk, and apparently nothing could persuade him to talk. The interview was brief and barren.

"Frankly, I didn't know what to do," Mr. Walters said as he related the story to the class. "Then I remembered what his secretary had said to him—stamps, twelve-year-old son... And I also recalled that the foreign department of our bank collected stamps—stamps taken from letters pouring in from every continent washed by the seven seas.

"The next afternoon I called on this man and sent in word that I had some stamps for his boy. Was I ushered in with enthusiasm? Yes sir. He couldn't have shaken my hand with more enthusiasm if he had been running for Congress. He radiated smiles and good will. 'My George will love this one,' he kept saying as he fondled the stamps.

'And look at this! This is a treasure.'

"We spent half an hour talking stamps and looking at a picture of his boy, and he then devoted more than an hour of his time to giving me every bit of information I wanted—without my even suggesting that he do it. He told me all he knew, and then called in his subordinates and questioned them. He telephoned some of his associates. He loaded me down with facts, figures, reports, and correspondence. In the parlance of newspaper reporters, I had a scoop."

Here is another illustration:

C. M. Knaphle, Jr., of Philadelphia, had tried for years to sell fuel to a large chain-store organization. But the chain-store company continued to purchase its fuel from an out-of-town dealer and haul it right past the door of Knaphle's office. Mr. Knaphle made a speech one night before one of my classes, pouring out his hot wrath upon chain stores, branding them as a curse on the nation.

And still he wondered why he couldn't sell them.

I suggested that he try different tactics. To put it briefly, this is what happened. We staged a debate between members of the course on whether the spread of the chain store is doing the country more harm than good.

Knaphle, at my suggestion, took the negative side; he agreed to defend the chain stores, and then went straight to an executive of the chain-store organization that he despised and said: "I am not here to try to sell fuel. I have come to ask you to do me a favor." He then told about his debate and said, "I have come to you for help because I can't think of anyone else who would be more capable of giving me the facts I want. I'm anxious to win this debate, and I'll deeply appreciate whatever help you can give me."

Here is the rest of the story in Mr. Knaphle's own words:

"I had asked this man for precisely one minute of his time. It was with this understanding that he consented to see me. After I had stated my case, he motioned me to a chair and talked to me for exactly one hour and forty-seven minutes. He called in another executive who had written a book about chain stores. He wrote to the National Chain Store Association and secured for me a copy of a debate on the subject. He feels that the chain store is rendering a real service to humanity. He is proud of what he is doing for hundreds of communities. His eyes fairly glowed as he talked, and I must confess that he opened my eyes to things I had never dreamed of. He changed my whole mental attitude.

"As I was leaving, he walked with me to the door, put his arm around my shoulder, wished me well in my debate, and asked me to stop in and see him again and let him know how I made out. The last words he said to me were: 'Please see me again later in the spring. I should like to place an order with you for fuel.'

"To me that was almost a miracle. Here he was offering to buy fuel without my even suggesting it. I had made more headway in two hours by becoming genuinely interested in him and his problems than I could have made in ten years trying to get him interested in me and my product."

You didn't discover a new truth, Mr. Knaphle, for a long time ago, a hundred years before Christ was born, a Roman poet, Publilius Syrus, remarked: "We are interested in others when they are interested in us."

A show of interest, as with every other principle of human relations, must be sincere. It must pay off not only for the person showing the interest, but for the person receiving the attention. It is a two-way street— both parties benefit.

Martin Ginsberg, who took our course in Long Island, New York, reported how the special interest a nurse took in him profoundly affected his life:

"It was Thanksgiving Day and I was ten years old. I was in a welfare ward of a city hospital and was scheduled to undergo major orthopedic surgery the next day. I knew that I could only look forward to months of confinement, convalescence, and pain. My father was dead; my mother and I lived alone in a small apartment and we were on welfare. My mother was unable to visit me that day.

"As the day went on, I became overwhelmed with the feeling of loneliness, despair, and fear. I knew my mother was home alone worrying about me, not having anyone to be with, not having anyone to eat with, and not even having enough money to afford a Thanksgiving Day dinner.

"The tears welled up in my eyes, and I stuck my head

under the pillow and pulled the covers over it. I cried silently, but oh so bitterly, so much that my body racked with pain.

"A young student nurse heard my sobbing and came over to me. She took the covers off my face and started wiping my tears. She told me how lonely she was, having to work that day and not being able to be with her family. She asked me whether I would have dinner with her. She brought two trays of food: sliced turkey, mashed potatoes, cranberry sauce, and ice cream for dessert. She talked to me and tried to calm my fears. Even though she was scheduled to go off duty at 4:00 p.m., she stayed on her own time until almost 11:00 p.m. She played games with me, talked to me, and stayed with me until I finally fell asleep.

"Many Thanksgivings have come and gone since I was ten, but one never passes without my remembering that particular one and my feelings of frustration, fear, loneliness, and the warmth and tenderness of the stranger who somehow made it all bearable."

If you want others to like you, if you want to develop real friendships, if you want to help others at the same time as you help yourself, keep this principle in mind:

If We Want to Make Friends, Let's Greet People with Animation and Enthusiasm

Keep on raging – to stop the aging.

—Dale Carnegie

3

HOW TO DEAL WITH PEOPLE

There is only one way under high heaven to get anybody to do anything. Did you ever stop to think of that? Yes, just one way. And that is by making the other person want to do it.

Remember, there is no other way.

Of course, you can make someone want to give you his watch by sticking a revolver in his ribs. You can make your employees give you cooperation—until your back is turned—by threatening to fire them. You can make a child do what you want it to do by a whip or a threat. But these crude methods have sharply undesirable repercussions.

The only way I can get you to do anything is by giving you what you want.

What do you want?

Sigmund Freud said that everything you and 1 do springs from two motives: the sex urge and the desire to be great.

John Dewey, one of America's most profound philosophers, phrased it a bit differently. Dr. Dewey said that the deepest urge in human nature is "the desire to be important." Remember that phrase: "the desire to be important." It is significant. You are going to hear a lot about it in this book.

What do you want? Not many things, but the few things that you do wish, you crave with an insistence that will not be denied. Some of the things most people want include:

1. Health and the preservation of life
2. Food
3. Sleep
4. Money and the things money will buy
5. Life in the hereafter
6. Sexual gratification
7. The well-being of our children
8. A feeling of importance

Almost all these wants are usually gratified—all except one. But there is one longing—almost as deep, almost as imperious, as the desire for food or sleep—that is seldom gratified. It is what Freud calls "the desire to be great." It is what Dewey calls "the desire to be important."

Lincoln once began a letter saying: "Everybody likes a compliment." William James said: "The deepest principle in human nature is the craving to be appreciated." He didn't speak, mind you, of the "wish" or the "desire" or the "longing" to be appreciated. He said the "craving" to be appreciated.

Here is a gnawing and unfaltering human hunger, and the rare individual who honestly satisfies this heart hunger will hold people in the palm of his or her hand and "even the undertaker will be sorry when he dies."

The desire for a feeling of importance is one of the chief distinguishing differences between mankind and the animals. To illustrate: When I was a farm boy out in

Missouri, my father bred fine Duroc-Jersey hogs and pedigreed white-faced cattle. We used to exhibit our hogs and white-faced cattle at the country fairs and livestock shows throughout the Middle West. We won first prizes by the score. My father pinned his blue ribbons on a sheet of white muslin, and when friends or visitors came to the house, he would get out the long sheet of muslin. He would hold one end and I would hold the other while he exhibited the blue ribbons.

The hogs didn't care about the ribbons they had won. But Father did. These prizes gave him a feeling of importance.

If our ancestors hadn't had this flaming urge for a feeling of importance, civilization would have been impossible. Without it, we should have been just about like animals.

It was this desire for a feeling of importance that inspired Dickens to write his immortal novels. This desire inspired Sir Christopher Wren to design his symphonies in stone. This desire made Rockefeller amass millions that he never spent! And this same desire made the richest family in your town build a house far too large for its requirements.

This desire makes you want to wear the latest styles, drive the latest cars, and talk about your brilliant children.

It is this desire that lures many boys and girls into joining gangs and engaging in criminal activities. The average young criminal, according to E. P. Mulrooney, one-time police commissioner of New York, is filled with ego, and his first request after arrest is for those lurid newspapers that make him out a hero. The disagreeable prospect of serving time seems remote so long as he can gloat over his likeness sharing space with pictures of sports figures, movie and television stars, and politicians.

If you tell me how you get your feeling of importance, I'll tell you what you are. That determines your character. That is the most significant thing about you. For example, John D. Rockefeller got his feeling of importance by giving money to erect a modern hospital in Peking, China, to care for millions of poor people whom he had never seen and never would see. Dillinger, on the other hand, got his feeling of importance by being a bandit, a bank robber and killer. When the FBI agents were hunting him, he dashed into a farmhouse up in Minnesota and said, "I'm Dillinger!" He was proud of the fact that he was Public Enemy Number One. "I'm not going to hurt you, but I'm Dillinger!" he said.

Yes, the one significant difference between Dillinger and Rockefeller is how they got their feeling of importance.

History sparkles with amusing examples of famous people struggling for a feeling of importance. Even George Washington wanted to be called "His Mightiness, the President of the United States"; and Columbus pleaded for the title "Admiral of the Ocean and Viceroy of India." Catherine the Great refused to open letters that were not addressed to "Her Imperial Majesty"; and Mrs. Lincoln, in the White House, turned upon Mrs. Grant like a tigress and shouted, "How dare you be seated in my presence until I invite you!"

Our millionaires helped finance Admiral Byrd's expedition to the Antarctic in 1928 with the understanding that ranges of icy mountains would be named after them; and Victor Hugo aspired to have nothing less than the city of Paris renamed in his honor. Even Shakespeare, mightiest of the mighty, tried to add luster to his name by procuring a coat of arms for his family.

People sometimes become invalids in order to win sympathy and attention, and get a feeling of importance. For example, take Mrs. McKinley. She got a feeling of importance by forcing her husband, the President of the United States, to neglect important affairs of state while he reclined on the bed beside her for hours at a time, his arm about her, soothing her to sleep. She fed her gnawing desire for attention by insisting that he remain with her while she was having her teeth fixed, and once created a stormy scene when he had to leave her alone with the dentist while he kept an appointment with John Hay, his secretary of state.

The writer Mary Roberts Rinehart once told me of a bright, vigorous young woman who became an invalid in order to get a feeling of importance. "One day," said Mrs. Rinehart, "this woman had been obliged to face something, her age perhaps. The lonely years were stretching ahead and there was little left for her to anticipate.

"She took to her bed; and for ten years her old mother traveled to the third floor and back, carrying trays, nursing her. Then one day the old mother, weary with service, lay down and died. For some weeks, the invalid languished; then she got up, put on her clothing, and resumed living again."

Some authorities declare that people may actually go insane in order to find, in the dreamland of insanity, the feeling of importance that has been denied them in the harsh world of reality. There are more patients suffering from mental diseases in the United States than from all other diseases combined.

What is the cause of insanity?

Nobody can answer such a sweeping question, but we know that certain diseases, such as syphilis, break down and destroy the brain cells and result in insanity. In fact, about one-half of all mental diseases can be attributed to such physical causes as brain lesions, alcohol, toxins, and injuries. But the other half—and this is the appalling part of the story—the other half of the people who go insane apparently have nothing organically wrong with their brain cells. In post-mortem examinations, when their brain tissues are studied under the highest-powered microscopes, these tissues are found to be apparently just as healthy as yours and mine.

Why do these people go insane?

I put that question to the head physician of one of our most important psychiatric hospitals. This doctor, who has received the highest honors and the most coveted awards for his knowledge of this subject, told me frankly that he didn't know why people went insane. Nobody knows for sure. But he did say that many people who go insane find in insanity a feeling of importance that they were unable to achieve in the world of reality. Then he told me this story:

"I have a patient right now whose marriage proved to

be a tragedy. She wanted love, sexual gratification, children, and social prestige, but life blasted all her hopes. Her husband didn't love her. He refused even to eat with her and forced her to serve his meals in his room upstairs. She had no children, no social standing. She went insane; and, in her imagination, she divorced her husband and resumed her maiden name. She now believes she has married into English aristocracy, and she insists on being called Lady Smith.

"And as for children, she imagines now that she has had a new child every night. Each time I call on her she says: 'Doctor, I had a baby last night.'"

Life once wrecked all her dream ships on the sharp rocks of reality; but in the sunny, fantasy isles of insanity, all her barkentines race into port with canvas billowing and winds singing through the sails.

Tragic? Oh, I don't know. Her physician said to me: "If I could stretch out my hand and restore her sanity, I wouldn't do it. She's much happier as she is."

If some people are so hungry for a feeling of importance that they actually go insane to get it, imagine what miracle you and I can achieve by giving people honest appreciation this side of insanity.

One of the first people in American business to be paid a salary of over a million dollars a year (when there was no income tax and a person earning fifty dollars a week was considered well off) was Charles Schwab. He had been picked by Andrew Carnegie to become the first president of the newly formed United States Steel Company in 1921, when Schwab was only thirty-eight years old.

(Schwab later left U.S. Steel to take over the then-troubled Bethlehem Steel Company, and he rebuilt it into one of the most profitable companies in America.)

Why did Andrew Carnegie pay a million dollars a year, or more than three thousand dollars a day, to Charles Schwab? Why? Because Schwab was a genius? No. Because he knew more about the manufacture of steel than other people? Nonsense. Charles Schwab told me himself that he had many men working for him who knew more about the manufacture of steel than he did.

Schwab says that he was paid this salary largely because of his ability to deal with people. I asked him how he did it. Here is his secret set down in his own words—words that ought to be cast in eternal bronze and hung in every home and school, every shop and office in the land; words that children ought to memorize instead of wasting their time memorizing the conjugation of Latin verbs or the amount of the annual rainfall in Brazil; words that will all but transform your life and mine if we will only live them:

"I consider my ability to arouse enthusiasm among my people," said Schwab, "the greatest asset I possess, and the way to develop the best that is in a person is by appreciation and encouragement.

"There is nothing else that so kills the ambitions of a person as criticisms from superiors. I never criticize anyone. I believe in giving a person incentive to work. So I am anxious to praise but loath to fault. If I like anything, I am hearty in my approbation and lavish in my praise."

That is what Schwab did. But what do average people do? The exact opposite. If they don't like a thing, they bawl out their subordinates; if they do like it, they say nothing. As the old couplet says: "Once I did bad and that I heard ever/Twice I did good, but that I heard never."

"In my wide association in life, meeting with many and great people in various parts of the world," Schwab declared, "I have yet to find the person, however great and exalted his station, who did not do better work and put forth greater effort under a spirit of approval than he would ever do under a spirit of criticism."

That, he said frankly, was one of the outstanding reasons for the phenomenal success of Andrew Carnegie. Carnegie praised his associates publicly as well as privately.

Carnegie wanted to praise his assistants even on his tombstone. He wrote an epitaph for himself that read: "Here lies one who knew how to get around him men who were cleverer than himself."

Sincere appreciation was one of the secrets of the first John D. Rockefeller's success in handling men. For example, when one of his partners, Edward T. Bedford, lost a million dollars for the firm by a bad buy in South America, John D. might have criticized; but he knew Bedford had done his best—and the incident was closed. So Rockefeller found something to praise; he congratulated Bedford because he had been able to save sixty percent of the money he had invested. "That's splendid," said Rockefeller. "We don't always do as well as that upstairs."

I have among my clippings a story that I know never

376 • THE DALE CARNEGIE OMNIBUS: VOLUME 2

happened, but it illustrates a truth, so I'll repeat it:

According to this silly story, a farm woman, at the end of a heavy day's work, set before her menfolks a heaping pile of hay. And when they indignantly demanded whether she had gone crazy, she replied: "Why, how did I know you'd notice? I've been cooking for you men for the last twenty years and in all that time I ain't heard no word to let me know you wasn't just eating hay."

When a study was made a few years ago on runaway wives, what do you think was discovered to be the main reasons wives ran away? It was "lack of appreciation." And I'd bet that a similar study made of runaway husbands would come out the same way. We often take our spouses so much for granted that we never let them know we appreciate them.

Florenz Ziegfeld, the most spectacular producer who ever dazzled Broadway, gained his reputation by his subtle ability to "glorify the American girl." Time after time, he took drab litle creatures that no one ever looked at twice and transformed them on the stage into glamorous visions of mystery and seduction. Knowing the value of appreciation and confidence, he made women feel beautiful by the sheer power of his gallantry and consideration. He was practical: he raised the salary of chorus girls from $30 a week to as high as $175. And he was also chivalrous; on opening night at the Follies, he sent telegrams to the stars in the cast, and he deluged every chorus girl in the show with American Beauty roses.

I once succumbed to the fad of fasting and went for six days and nights without eating. It wasn't difficult. I was less hungry at the end of the sixth day than I was at the end of the second. Yet I know, as you know, people who would think they had committed a crime if they let their families or employees go for six days without food; but they will let them go for six days, and six weeks, and sometimes sixty years without giving them the hearty appreciation that they crave almost as much as they crave food.

When Alfred Lunt, one of the great actors of his time, played the leading role in *Reunion in Vienna*, he said, "There is nothing I need so much as nourishment for my self-esteem."

We nourish the bodies of our children and friends and employees, but how often do we nourish their self-esteem? We provide them with roast beef and potatoes to build energy, but we neglect to give them kind words of appreciation that would sing in their memories for years like the music of the morning stars.

Paul Harvey, in one of his radio broadcasts, "The Rest of the Story," told how showing sincere appreciation can change a person's life. He reported that years ago a teacher in Detroit asked Stevie Morris to help her find a mouse that was lost in the classroom. You see, she appreciated the fact that nature had given Stevie something no one else in the room had. Nature had given Stevie a remarkable pair of ears to compensate for his blind eyes. But this was really the first time Stevie had been shown appreciation for those talented ears. Now, years later, he says that this act of appreciation was the beginning of a new life. You see, from that time on he developed his gift of hearing and went on to become, under the stage name of Stevie

Wonder, one of *the* great pop singers and songwriters of the seventies.

Some readers are saying right now as they read these lines; "Oh, phooey! Flattery! Bear oil! I've tried that stuff. It doesn't work—not with intelligent people."

Of course, flattery seldom works with discerning people. It is shallow, selfish, and insincere. It ought to fail and it usually does. True, some people are so hungry, so thirsty, for appreciation that they will swallow anything, just as a starving man will eat grass and fishworms.

Even Queen Victoria was susceptible to flattery. Prime Minister Benjamin Disraeli confessed that he laid it on thick in dealing with the queen. To use his exact words, he said he "spread it on with a trowel." But Disraeli was one of the most polished, deft, and adroit men who ever ruled the far-flung British Empire. He was a genius in his line. What would work for him wouldn't necessarily work for you and me. In the long run, flattery will do you more harm than good. Flattery is counterfeit, and like counterfeit money, it will eventually get you into trouble if you pass it to someone else.

The difference between appreciation and flattery? That is simple. One is sincere and the other insincere. One comes from the heart out; the other from the teeth out. One is unselfish; the other selfish. One is universally admired; the other universally condemned.

I recently saw a bust of the Mexican hero General Álvaro Obregón in the Chapultepec palace in Mexico City. Below the bust are carved these wise words from General Obregón's philosophy: "Don't be afraid of enemies who attack you. Be afraid of friends who flatter you."

No! No! No! I am not suggesting flattery? Far from it. I'm talking about a new way of life. Let me repeat. *I am talking about a new way of life.*

King George V had a set of six maxims displayed on the walls of his study at Buckingham Palace. One of these maxims said: "Teach me neither to proffer nor receive cheap praise." That's all flattery is—cheap praise. I once read a definition of flattery that may be worth repeating: "Flattery is telling the other person precisely what he thinks about himself."

"Use what language you will," said Ralph Waldo Emerson, "you can never say anything but what you are."

If all we had to do was flatter, everybody would catch on and we should all be experts in human relations.

When we are not engaged in thinking about some definite problem, we usually spend about ninety-five percent of our time thinking about ourselves. Now, if we stop thinking about ourselves for a while and begin to think of the other person's good points, we won't have to resort to flattery so cheap and false that it can be spotted almost before it is out of the mouth.

One of the most neglected virtues of our daily existence is appreciation. Somehow, we neglect to praise our son or daughter when he or she brings home a good report card, and we fail to encourage our children when they first succeed in baking a cake or building a birdhouse. Nothing pleases children more than this kind of parental interest and approval.

The next time you enjoy filet mignon at the club, send

word to the chef that it was excellently prepared, and when a tired salesperson shows you unusual courtesy, please mention it.

Every minister, lecturer, and public speaker knows the discouragement of pouring himself or herself out to an audience and not receiving a single ripple of appreciative comment. What applies to professionals applies doubly to workers in offices, shops, and factories, and to our families and friends. In our interpersonal relations we should never forget that all our associates are human beings and hunger for appreciation. It is the legal tender that all souls enjoy.

Try leaving a friendly trail of little sparks of gratitude on your daily trips. You will be surprised how they will set small flames of friendship that will be rose beacons on your next visit.

Pamela Dunham of New Fairfield, Connecticut, had among her responsibilities on her job the supervision of a janitor who was doing a very poor job. The other employees would jeer at him and litter the hallways to show him what a bad job he was doing. It was so bad, productive time was being lost in the shop.

Without success, Pam tried various ways to motivate this person. She noticed that occasionally he did a particularly good piece of work. She made a point to praise him for it in front of the other people. Each day the job he did all around got better, and pretty soon he started doing all his work efficiently. Now he does an excellent job and other people give him appreciation and recognition. Honest appreciation got results where criticism and ridicule failed.

Hurting people not only does not change them, it is never called for. There is an old saying that I have cut out and pasted on my mirror, where I cannot help but see it every day:

> I shall pass this way but once; any good, therefore, that I can do or any kindness that I can show to any human being, let me do it now. Let me not defer nor neglect it, for I shall not pass this way again.

Emerson said: "Every man I meet is my superior in some way. In that, I learn of him."

If that was true of Emerson, isn't it likely to be a thousand times more true of you and me? Let's cease thinking of our accomplishments, our wants. Let's try to figure out the other person's good points. Then forget flattery. Give honest, sincere appreciation. Be "hearty in your approbation and lavish in your praise," and people will cherish your words and treasure them and repeat them over a lifetime—repeat them years after you have forgotten them.

One of the Most Neglected Virtues of Our Daily Existence is Appreciation.

4

"HE WHO CAN DO THIS HAS THE WHOLE WORLD WITH HIM. HE WHO CANNOT WALKS A LONELY WAY"

I often went fishing up in Maine during the summer. Personally I am very fond of strawberries and cream, but I have found that for some strange reason, fish prefer worms. So when I went fishing, I didn't think about what I wanted. I thought about what they wanted. I didn't bait the hook with strawberries and cream. Rather, I dangled a worm or a grasshopper in front of the fish and said: "Wouldn't you like to have that?"

Why not use the same common sense when fishing for people?

That is what Lloyd George, Great Britain's prime minister during World War I, did. When someone asked him how he managed to stay in power after the other wartime leaders—Wilson, Orlando, and Clemenceau—had been forgotten, he replied that if his staying on top might be attributed to any one thing, it would be to his having learned that it was necessary to bait the hook to suit the fish.

Why talk about what we want? That is childish. Absurd. Of course, you are interested in what you want. You are eternally interested in it. But no one else is. The rest of us are just like you: we are interested in what we want.

So the only way on earth to influence other people is to

talk about what *they* want and show them how to get it.

Remember that tomorrow when you are trying to get somebody to do something. If, for example, you don't want your children to smoke, don't preach at them, and don't talk about what you want; but show them that cigarettes may keep them from making the basketball team or winning the hundred-yard dash.

This is a good thing to remember regardless of whether you are dealing with children or calves or chimpanzees. For example: One day Ralph Waldo Emerson and his son tried to get a calf into a barn. But they made the common mistake of thinking only of what they wanted. Emerson pushed and his son pulled. But the calf was doing just what they were doing: he was thinking only of what he wanted; so he stiffened his legs and stubbornly refused to leave the pasture. The Irish housemaid saw their predicament. She couldn't write essays and books; but, on this occasion at least, she had more horse sense, or calf sense, than Emerson had. She thought of what the calf wanted; so she put her maternal finger in the calf's mouth and let the calf suck her finger as she gently led him into the barn.

Every act you have performed since the day you were born was performed because you wanted something. How about the time you gave a large contribution to the Red Cross? Yes, that is no exception to the rule. You gave the Red Cross the donation because you wanted to lend a helping hand: you wanted to do a beautiful, unselfish, divine act. "Inasmuch as ye have done it unto the least of these my brethren, ye have done it unto me."

If you hadn't wanted that feeling more than you wanted

your money, you would not have made the contribution. Of course, you might have made the contribution because you were ashamed to refuse or because a customer asked you to do it. But one thing is certain. You made the contribution because you wanted something.

Harry A. Overstreet in his illuminating book *Influencing Human Behavior* said: "Action springs out of what we fundamentally desire ...and the best piece of advice which can be given to would-be persuaders, whether in business, in the home, in the school, in politics, is: First, arouse in the other person an eager want. He who can do this has the whole world with him. He who cannot walks a lonely way."

Andrew Carnegie, the poverty-stricken Scotch lad who started to work at two cents an hour and finally gave away $365 million, learned early in life that the only way to influence people is to talk in terms of what the other person wants. He attended school only four years; yet he learned how to handle people.

An example of persuading comes from Stan Novak of Cleveland, Ohio, a participant in our course. Stan came home from work one evening to find his youngest son, Tim, kicking and screaming on the living room floor. He was to start kindergarten the next day and was protesting that he would not go. Stan's normal reaction would have been to banish the child to his room and tell him he'd just better make up his mind to go. He had no choice. But tonight, recognizing that this would not really help Tim start kindergarten in the best frame of mind, Stan sat down and thought, "If I were Tim, why would I be excited about going to kindergarten?" He and his wife made a list of all the fun things Tim would do such as finger-painting, singing songs, making new friends. Then they put them into action. "We all started finger-painting on the kitchen table—my wife, Lil, my other son, Bob, and myself, all having fun. Soon Tim was peeping around the corner. Next he was begging to participate. 'Oh, no! You have to go to kindergarten first to learn how to finger-paint.' With all the enthusiasm I could muster I went through the list talking in terms he could understand—telling him all the fun he would have in kindergarten. The next morning, I thought I was the first one up. I went downstairs and found Tim sitting sound asleep in the living room chair. 'What are you doing here?' I asked. 'I'm waiting to go to kindergarten. I don't want to be late.' The enthusiasm of our entire family had aroused in Tim an eager want that no amount of discussion or threat could have possibly accomplished."

Tomorrow you may want to persuade somebody to do something. Before you speak, pause and ask yourself: "How can I make this person want to do it?"

That question will stop us from rushing into a situation heedlessly, with futile chatter about our desires.

At one time I rented the grand ballroom of a certain New York hotel for twenty nights in each season in order to hold a series of lectures.

At the beginning of one season, I was suddenly informed that I should have to pay almost three times as much rent as formerly. This news reached me after the tickets had been printed and distributed and all announcements had been made.

Naturally, I didn't want to pay the increase, but what was the use of talking to the hotel about what I wanted? They were interested only in what they wanted. So a couple of days later I went to see the manager.

"I was a bit shocked when I got your letter," I said, "but I don't blame you at all. If I had been in your position, I should probably have written a similar letter myself. Your duty as the manager of the hotel is to make all the profit possible. If you don't do that, you will be fired and you ought to be fired. Now, let's take a piece of paper and write down the advantages and the disadvantages that will accrue to you, if you insist on this increase in rent."

Then I took a letterhead and ran a line through the center and headed one column "Advantages" and the other column "Disadvantages."

I wrote down under the head "Advantages" these words: "Ballroom free." Then I went on to say: "You will have the advantages of having the ballroom free to rent for dances and conventions. That is a big advantage, for affairs like that will pay you much more than you can get for a series of lectures. If I tie your ballroom up for twenty nights during the course of the season, it is sure to mean a loss of some very profitable business to you.

"Now, let's consider the disadvantages. First, instead of increasing your income from me, you are going to decrease it. In fact, you are going to wipe it out because I cannot pay the rent you are asking. I shall be forced to hold these lectures at some other place.

"There's another disadvantage to you also. These

lectures attract crowds of educated and cultured people to your hotel. That is good advertising for you, isn't it? In fact, if you spent five thousand dollars advertising in the newspapers, you couldn't bring as many people to look at your hotel as I can bring by these lectures. That is worth a lot to a hotel, isn't it?"

As I talked, I wrote these two "disadvantages" under the proper heading, and handed the sheet of paper to the manager, saying: "I wish you would carefully consider both the advantages and the disadvantages that are going to accrue to you and then give me your final decision."

I received a letter the next day, informing me that my rent would be increased only fifty percent instead of three hundred percent.

Mind you, I got this reduction without saying a word about what I wanted. I talked all the time about what the other person wanted and how he could get it.

Suppose I had done the human, natural thing; suppose I had stormed into his office and said, "What do you mean by raising my rent three hundred percent when you know the tickets have been printed and the announcements made? Three hundred percent! Ridiculous! Absurd! I won't pay it!"

What would have happened then? An argument would have begun to steam and boil and sputter—and you know how arguments end. Even if I had convinced him that he was wrong, his pride would have made it difficult for him to back down and give in.

Here is one of the best bits of advice ever given about the fine art of human relationships. "If there is any one secret of success," said Henry Ford, "it lies in the ability to get the other person's point of view and see things from that person's angle as well as from your own."

That is so good, I want to repeat it: "If there is any one secret of success, it lies in the ability to get the other person's point of view and see things from that person's angle as well as from your own."

That is so simple, so obvious, that anyone ought to see the truth of it at a glance; yet ninety percent of the people on this earth ignore it ninety percent of the time.

An example? Look at the letters that come across your desk tomorrow morning, and you will find that most of them violate this important canon of common sense. Take this one, a letter written by the head of the radio department of an advertising agency with offices scattered across the continent. This letter was sent to the managers of local radio stations throughout the country. (I have set down, in brackets, my reactions to each paragraph.)

Mr. John Blank,
Blankville,
Indiana

Dear Mr. Blank:

The company desires to retain its position in advertising agency leadership in the radio field.

[Who cares what your company desires? I am worried about my own problems. The bank is foreclosing the mortgage on my house, the bugs are destroying the hollyhocks, the stock market tumbled yesterday. I missed the eight-fifteen this morning, I wasn't invited to the Joneses' dance last night, the doctor tells me I have high blood pressure and neuritis and dandruff. And then what happens? I come down to the office this morning worried, open my mail, and here is some little whippersnapper off in New York yapping about what his company wants. Bah! If he only realized what sort of impression his letter makes, he would get out of the advertising business and start manufacturing sheep dip.]

This agency's national advertising accounts were the bulwark of the network. Our subsequent clearances of station time have kept us at the top of agencies year after year.

[You are big and rich and right at the top, aren't you? So what? I don't give two whoops in Hades if you are as big as General Motors and General Electric and the General Staff of the U.S. Army all combined. If you had as much sense as a half-witted hummingbird, you would realize that I am interested in how big I am—not how big you are. All this talk about your enormous success makes me feel small and unimportant.]

We desire to service our accounts with the last word on radio station information.

[You desire! You desire. You unmitigated ass. I'm not interested in what you desire or what the President of the United States desires. Let me tell you once and for all that I am interested in what I desire—and you haven't said a word about that yet in this absurd letter of yours.]

Will you, therefore, put the—company on your preferred list for weekly station information—every single detail that will be useful to an agency in intelligently booking time.

["Preferred list." You have your nerve! You make me feel insignificant by your big talk about your company—and then you ask me to put you on a "preferred" list, and you don't even say "please" when you ask it.]

A prompt acknowledgment of this letter, giving us your latest "doings," will be mutually helpful.

[You fool! You mail me a cheap form letter, a letter scattered far and wide like the autumn leaves, and you have the gall to ask me, when I am worried about the mortgage and the hollyhocks and my blood pressure, to sit down and dictate a personal note acknowledging your form letter—and you ask me to do it "promptly." What do you mean, "promptly"? Don't you know I am just as busy as you are—or, at least, I like to think I am. And while we are on the subject, who gave you the lordly right to order me around? You say it will be "mutually helpful." At last, at last, you have begun to see my viewpoint. But you are vague about how it will be to my advantage.]

Very truly yours,
John Doe
Manager, Radio Department

P.S. The enclosed reprint from the Blankville *Journal* will be of interest to you, and you may want to broadcast it over your station.

[Finally, down here in the postscript, you mention something that may help me solve one of my problems. Why didn't you begin your letter with—but what's the use? Any advertising man who is guilty of perpetrating such drivel as you have sent me has something wrong with his medulla oblongata. You don't need a letter giving our latest doings. What you need is a quart of iodine in your thyroid gland.]

Now, if people who devote their lives to advertising and who pose as experts in the art of influencing people to buy—if they write a letter like that, what can we expect from the butcher and baker or the auto mechanic?

Here is another letter, written by the superintendent of a large freight terminal to a student of this course, Edward Vermylen. What effect did this letter have on the man to whom it was addressed? Read it and then I'll tell you.

A. Zerega's Sons, Inc.
28 Front Street
Brooklyn, N.Y. 11201
Attention: Mr. Edward Vermylen

Gentlemen:

The operations at our outbound-rail-receiving station are handicapped because a material percentage of the total business is delivered us in the late afternoon. This condition results in congestion, overtime on the part of our forces, delays to trucks, and in some cases delays to freight. On November

10, we received from your company a lot of 510 pieces, which reached here at 4:20 p.m.

We solicit your cooperation toward overcoming the undesirable effects arising from late receipt of freight. May we ask that, on days on which you ship the volume which was received on the above date, effort be made either to get the truck here earlier or to deliver us part of the freight during the morning?

The advantage that would accrue to you under such an arrangement would be that of more expeditious discharge of your trucks and the assurance that your business would go forward on the date of its receipt.

Very truly yours,
J— B—, Supt.

After reading this letter, Mr. Vermylen, sales manager for A. Zerega's Sons, Inc., sent it to me with the following comment:

This letter had the reverse effect from that which was intended. The letter begins by describing the Terminal's difficulties, in which we are not interested, generally speaking. Our cooperation is then requested without any thought as to whether it would inconvenience us, and then, finally, in the last paragraph, the fact is mentioned that if we do cooperate it will mean more expeditious discharge of our trucks with the assurance that our freight will go forward on the date of its receipt.

In other words, that in which we are most interested is mentioned last and the whole effect is one of raising a spirit of antagonism rather than of cooperation.

Let's see if we can't rewrite and improve this letter. Let's not waste any time talking about our problems. As Henry Ford admonishes, let's "get the other person's point of view and see things from his or her angle, as well as from our own."

Here is one way of revising the letter. It may not be the best way, but isn't it an improvement?

Mr. Edward Vermylen
c/o A. Zerega's Sons, Inc.
28 Front St.
Brooklyn, N.Y. 11201

Dear Mr. Vermylen:

Your company has been one of our good customers for fourteen years. Naturally, we are very grateful for your patronage and are eager to give you the speedy, efficient service you deserve. However, we regret to say that it isn't possible for us to do that when your trucks bring us a large shipment late in the afternoon, as they did on November 10. Why? Because many other customers make late-afternoon deliveries also. Naturally, that causes congestion. That means your trucks are held up unavoidably at the pier and sometimes even your freight is delayed.

That's bad, but it can be avoided. If you make your deliveries at the pier in the morning when possible, your trucks will be able to keep moving, your freight will get immediate attention, and our workers will get home early at night to enjoy a dinner of the delicious macaroni and noodles that you manufacture.

Regardless of when your shipments arrive, we shall always cheerfully do all in our power to serve you promptly.

You are busy. Please don't trouble to answer this note.

Very truly yours,
J— B—, Supt.

Barbara Anderson, who worked in a bank in New York, desired to move to Phoenix, Arizona, because of the health of her son. Using the principles she had learned in our course, she wrote the following letter to twelve banks in Phoenix:

Dear Sir:

My ten years of bank experience should be of interest to a rapidly growing bank like yours.

In various capacities in bank operations with the Bankers Trust Company in New York, leading to my present assignment as branch manager, I have acquired skills in all phases of banking, including depositor relations, credits, loans, and administration.

I will be relocating to Phoenix in May and I am sure I can contribute to your growth and profit. I will be in Phoenix the week of April 3 and would appreciate the opportunity to show you how I can help your bank meet its goals.

Sincerely,
Barbara L. Anderson

Do you think Mrs. Anderson received any response from that letter? Eleven of the twelve banks invited her to be interviewed, and she had a choice of which bank's offer to accept. Why? Mrs. Anderson did not state what *she* wanted, but wrote in the letter how she could help them, and focused on *their* wants, not her own.

Thousands of salespeople are pounding the pavements today, tired, discouraged, and underpaid. Why? Because they are always thinking only of what they want. They don't realize that neither you nor I want to buy anything. If we did, we would go out and buy it. But both of us are eternally interested in solving our problems. And if salespeople can show us how their services or merchandise will help us solve our problems, they won't need to sell us. We'll buy. And customers like to feel that they are buying—not being sold.

Yet many salespeople spend a lifetime in selling without seeing things from the customer's angle. For example, for many years I lived in Forest Hills, a little community of private homes in the center of Greater New York. One day as I was rushing to the station, I chanced to meet a real-estate operator who had bought and sold property in that area for many years. He knew Forest Hills well, so I hurriedly asked him whether or not my stucco house was built with metal lath or hollow tile. He said he didn't know and told me what I already knew—that I could find out by calling the Forest Hills Garden Association. The following morning, I received a letter from him. Did he give me the information I wanted? He could have gotten it in sixty seconds by a telephone call. But he didn't. He told me again that I could get it by telephoning, and then asked me to let him handle my insurance.

He was not interested in helping me. He was interested only in helping himself.

J. Howard Lucas of Birmingham, Alabama, tells how two salespeople from the same company handled the same type of situation. He reported:

"Several years ago I was on the management team of a small company. Headquartered near us was the district office of a large insurance company. Their agents were assigned territories, and our company was assigned to two agents, who I shall refer to as Carl and John.

"One morning, Carl dropped by our office and casually mentioned that his company had just introduced a new life insurance policy for executives and thought we might be interested later on and he would get back to us when he had more information on it.

"The same day, John saw us on the sidewalk while returning from a coffee break, and he shouted: 'Hey, Luke, hold up, I have some great news for you fellows.'

He hurried up and very excitedly told us about an executive life insurance policy his company had introduced that very day. (It was the same policy that Carl had casually mentioned.) He wanted us to have one of the first issued. He gave us a few important facts about the coverage and ended saying, 'The policy is so new, I'm going to have someone from the home office come out tomorrow and explain it. Now, in the meantime, let's get the applications signed and on the way so he can have more information to work with.' His enthusiasm aroused in us an eager want for this policy even though we still did not have details. When they were made available to us, they confirmed John's initial understanding of the policy, and he not only sold each of us a policy, but later doubled our coverage.

"Carl could have had those sales, but he made no effort to arouse in us any desire for the policies."

The world is full of people who are grabbing and self-seeking. So the rare individual who unselfishly tries to serve others has an enormous advantage. He has little competition. Owen D. Young, a noted lawyer and one of America's great business leaders, once said: "People who can put themselves in the place of other people, who can understand the workings of their minds, need never worry about what the future has in store for them."

If out of reading this book you get just one thing—an increased tendency to think always in terms of other people's point of view, and see things from their angle—if you get that one thing out of this book, it may easily prove to be one of the building blocks of your career.

Looking at the other person's point of view and arousing an eager want for something is not to be construed as manipulating that person to do something that is only for your benefit and his or her detriment. Each party should gain from the negotiation. In the letters to Mr. Vermylen, both the sender and the receiver of the correspondence gained by implementing what was suggested. Both the bank and Mrs. Anderson won by her letter in that the bank obtained a valuable employee and Mrs. Anderson a suitable job. And in the example of John's sale of insurance to Mr. Lucas, both gained through the transaction.

Another example in which everybody gains through this principle of arousing an eager want comes from Michael E. Whidden of Warwick, Rhode Island, who is a territory salesman for the Shell Oil Company. Mike wanted to become the number-one salesperson in his district, but one service station was holding back. It was run by an older man who could not be motivated to clean up his station. It was in such poor shape that sales were declining significantly.

The manager would not listen to any of Mike's pleas to upgrade the station. After many exhortations and heart-to-heart talks—all of which had no impact—Mike decided to invite the manager to visit the newest Shell station in his territory.

The manager was so impressed by the facilities at the new station that when Mike visited him the next time, his station was cleaned up and had recorded a sales increase. This enabled Mike to reach the number-one spot in his district. All his talking and discussion hadn't helped, but by arousing an eager want in the manager, by showing him the modern station, he had accomplished his goal, and both the manager and Mike benefited.

Most people go through college and learn to read Virgil and master the mysteries of calculus without ever discovering how their own minds function. For instance: I once gave a course in Effective Speaking for the young college graduates who were entering the employ of the Carrier Corporation, the large air-conditioner manufacturer. One of the participants wanted to persuade the others to play basketball in their free time, and this is about what he said: "I want you to come out and play basketball. I like to play basketball, but the last few times I've been to the gymnasium there haven't been enough people to get up a game. Two or three of us got to throwing the ball around the other night—and I got a black eye. I wish all of you would come down tomorrow night. I want to play basketball."

Did he talk about anything you want? You don't want to go to a gymnasium that no one else goes to, do you? You don't care about what he wants. You don't want to get a black eye.

Could he have shown you how to get the things you want by using the gymnasium? Surely. More pep. Keener edge to the appetite. Clearer brain. Fun. Games. Basketball.

To repeat Professor Overstreet's wise advice: First, arouse in the other person an eager want. He who can do this has the whole world with him. He who cannot walks a lonely way.

One of the students in the training course was worried about his little boy. The child was underweight and refused to eat properly. They scolded and nagged. "Mother wants you to eat this and that." "Father wants you to grow up to be a big man."

Did the boy pay any attention to these pleas? Just about as much as you would pay to one fleck of sand on a sandy beach.

No one with a trace of horse sense would expect a child three years old to react to the viewpoint of a father thirty years old. Yet that was precisely what that father had expected. It was absurd. He finally saw that. So he said to himself: "What does that boy want? How can I tie up what I want to what he wants?"

It was easy for the father when he started thinking about it. His boy had a tricycle that he loved to ride up and down the sidewalk in front of the house in Brooklyn. A few doors down the street lived a bully—a bigger boy who would pull the little boy off his tricycle and ride it himself.

Naturally, the little boy would run screaming to his mother, and she would have to come out and take the bully off the tricycle and put her little boy on again. This happened almost every day.

What did the little boy want? It didn't take a Sherlock Holmes to answer that one. His pride, his anger, his desire for a feeling of importance—all the strongest emotions in his makeup—goaded him to get revenge, to smash the bully in the nose. And when his father explained that the boy would be able to wallop the daylights out of the bigger kid someday if he would only eat the things his mother wanted him to eat—when his father promised him that—there was no longer any problem of dietetics. That boy would have eaten spinach, sauerkraut, salt mackerel—anything in order to be big enough to whip the bully who had humiliated him so often.

After solving that problem, the parents tackled another: the boy had the unholy habit of wetting the bed.

He slept with his grandmother. In the morning, his grandmother would wake up and feel the sheet and say: "Look, Johnny, what you did again last night."

He would say: "No, I didn't do it. You did it."

Scolding, spanking, shaming him, reiterating that the parents didn't want him to do it—none of these things kept the bed dry. So the parents asked: "How can we make this boy want to stop wetting his bed?".

What were his wants? First, he wanted to wear pajamas like Daddy instead of wearing a nightgown like Grandmother. Grandmother was getting fed up with his nocturnal iniquities, so she gladly offered to buy him a pair of pajamas if he would reform. Second, he wanted a bed of his own. Grandma did object.

His mother took him to a department store in Brooklyn, winked at the salesgirl, and said: "Here is a little gentleman who would like to do some shopping."

The salesgirl made him feel important by saying: "Young man, what can I show you?"

He stood a couple of inches taller and said: "I want to buy a bed for myself."

When he was shown the one his mother wanted him to buy, she winked at the salesgirl and the boy was persuaded to buy it.

The bed was delivered the next day; and that night, when Father came home, the little boy ran to the door shouting: "Daddy! Daddy! Come upstairs and see my bed that I bought!"

The father, looking at the bed, obeyed Charles Schwab's injunction: he was "hearty in his approbation and lavish in his praise."

"You are not going to wet this bed, are you?" the father said.

"Oh, no, no! I am not going to wet this bed." The boy kept his promise, for his pride was involved. That was his bed. He and he alone had bought it. And he was wearing pajamas now like a little man. He wanted to act like a man. And he did.

Another father, K. T. Dutschmann, a telephone engineer, a student of the training course, couldn't get his three-year-old daughter to eat breakfast food. The usual scolding, pleading, coaxing methods had all ended in futility. So the parents asked themselves: "How can we make her want to do it?"

The little girl loved to imitate her mother, to feel big and grown up; so one morning they put her on a chair and let her make the breakfast food. At just the psychological moment, Father drifted into the kitchen while she was stirring the cereal and she said: "Oh, look, Daddy, I am making the cereal this morning."

She ate two helpings of the cereal without any coaxing, because she was interested in it. She had achieved a feeling of importance; she had found in making the cereal an avenue of self-expression.

William Winter once remarked that "self-expression is the dominant necessity of human nature." Why can't we adapt this same psychology to business dealings? When we have a brilliant idea, instead of making others think it is ours, why not let them cook and stir the idea themselves? They will then regard it as their own; they will like it and maybe eat a couple of helpings of it.

Remember: "First, arouse in the other person an eager want. He who can do this has the whole world with him. He who cannot walks a lonely way."

Look at Things from the Other Person's Vantage as Well as Your Own

Instead of worrying about what people say of you, why not spend time trying to accomplish something they will admire.

—Dale Carnegie

5

"IF YOU WANT TO GATHER HONEY, DON'T KICK OVER THE BEEHIVE"

On May 7, 1931, the most sensational manhunt New York City had ever known had come to its climax. After weeks of search, "Two Gun" Crowley—the killer, the gunman who didn't smoke or drink—was at bay, trapped in his sweetheart's apartment on West End Avenue.

One hundred and fifty policemen and detectives laid siege to his top-floor hideaway. They chopped holes in the roof; they tried to smoke out Crowley, the "cop killer," with teargas. Then they mounted their machine guns on surrounding buildings, and for more than an hour one of New York's fine residential areas reverberated with the crack of pistol fire and the rat-tat-tat of machine guns. Crowley, crouching behind an overstuffed chair, fired incessantly at the police. Ten thousand excited people watched the battle. Nothing like it had ever been seen before on the sidewalks of New York.

When Crowley was captured, Police Commissioner E. P. Mulrooney declared that the two-gun desperado was one of the most dangerous criminals ever encountered in the history of New York. "He will kill," said the commissioner, "at the drop of a feather."

But how did "Two Gun" Crowley regard himself? We know, because while the police were firing into the apartment, he wrote a letter addressed "To whom it may concern." And, as he wrote, the blood flowing from his wounds left a crimson trail on the paper. In this letter Crowley said: "Under my coat is a weary heart, but a kind one—one that would do nobody any harm."

A short time before this, Crowley had been having a necking party with his girlfriend on a country road out on Long Island. Suddenly a policeman walked up to the car and said: "Let me see your license."

Without saying a word, Crowley drew his gun and cut the policeman down with a shower of lead. As the dying officer fell, Crowley leaped out of the car, grabbed the officer's revolver, and fired another bullet into the prostrate body. And that was the killer who said: "Under my coat is a weary heart, but a kind one—one that would do nobody any harm."

Crowley was sentenced to the electric chair. When he arrived at the death house in Sing Sing, did he say, "This is what I get for killing people?" No, he said: "This is what I get for defending myself."

The point of the story is this: "Two Gun" Crowley didn't blame himself for anything.

Is that an unusual attitude among criminals? If you think so, listen to this:

"I have spent the best years of my life giving people the lighter pleasures, helping them have a good time, and all I get is abuse, the existence of a hunted man."

That's Al Capone speaking. Yes, America's most notorious Public Enemy—the most sinister gang leader who ever shot up Chicago. Capone didn't condemn himself. He actually regarded himself as a public benefactor—an unappreciated and misunderstood public benefactor.

And so did Dutch Schultz before he crumpled up under gangster bullets in Newark. Dutch Schultz, one of New York's most notorious rats, said in a newspaper interview that he was a public benefactor. And he believed it.

I have had some interesting correspondence with Lewis Lawes, who was warden of New York's infamous Sing Sing prison for many years, on this subject, and he declared that "few of the criminals in Sing Sing regard themselves as bad men. They are just as human as you and I. So they rationalize, they explain. They can tell you why they had to crack a safe or be quick on the trigger finger. Most of them attempt by a form of reasoning, fallacious or logical, to justify their antisocial acts even to themselves, consequently stoutly maintaining that they should never have been imprisoned at all."

If Al Capone, "Two Gun" Crowley, Dutch Schultz and the desperate men and women behind prison walls don't blame themselves for anything—what about the people with whom you and I come in contact?

John Wanamaker, founder of the stores that bear his name, once confessed: "I learned thirty years ago that it is foolish to scold. I have enough trouble overcoming my own limitations without fretting over the fact that God has not seen fit to distribute evenly the gift of intelligence."

Wanamaker learned this lesson early, but I personally had to blunder through this old world for a third of a century before it even began to dawn upon me that ninety-nine times out of a hundred, people don't criticize themselves for anything, no matter how wrong it may be.

Criticism is futile because it puts a person on the defensive and usually makes him strive to justify himself. Criticism is dangerous, because it wounds a person's precious pride, hurts his sense of importance, and arouses resentment.

B. F. Skinner, the world-famous psychologist, proved through his experiments that an animal rewarded for good behavior will learn much more rapidly and retain what it learns far more effectively than an animal punished for bad behavior. Later studies have shown that the same applies to humans. By criticizing, we do not make lasting changes and often incur resentment.

Hans Selye, another great psychologist, said, "As much as we thirst for approval, we dread condemnation."

The resentment that criticism engenders can demoralize employees, family members, and friends, and still not correct the situation that has been condemned.

George B. Johnston of Enid, Oklahoma, is the safety coordinator for an engineering company. One of his responsibilities is to see that employees wear their hard hats whenever they are on the job in the field. He reported that whenever he came across workers who were not wearing hard hats, he would tell them with a lot of authority of the regulation and that they must comply. As a result he would get sullen acceptance, and often after he left, the workers would remove the hats.

He decided to try a different approach. The next time he found some of the workers not wearing their hard hats, he asked if the hats were uncomfortable or did not fit properly. Then he reminded the men in a pleasant tone of voice that the hat was designed to protect them from injury and suggested that it always be worn on the job. The result was increased compliance with the regulation with no resentment or emotional upset.

You will find examples of the futility of criticism bristling on a thousand pages of history. Take, for example, the famous quarrel between Theodore Roosevelt and President Taft—a quarrel that split the Republican party, put Woodrow Wilson in the White House, and wrote bold, luminous lines across the First World War and altered the flow of history. Let's review the facts quickly. When Theodore Roosevelt stepped out of the White House in 1908, he supported Taft, who was elected president. Then Theodore Roosevelt went off to Africa to shoot lions. When he returned, he exploded. He denounced Taft for his conservatism, tried to secure the nomination for a third term himself, formed the Bull Moose party, and all but demolished the GOP. In the election that followed, William Howard Taft and the Republican party carried only two states, Vermont and Utah—the most disastrous defeat the party had ever known.

Theodore Roosevelt blamed Taft, but did President Taft blame himself? Of course not. With tears in his eyes, Taft said: "I don't see how I could have done any differently from what I have."

Who was to blame? Roosevelt or Taft? Frankly, I don't know, and I don't care. The point I am trying to make is that all of Theodore Roosevelt's criticism didn't persuade Taft that he was wrong. It merely made Taft strive to justify himself and to reiterate with tears in his eyes: "I don't see how I could have done any differently from what I have."

Or, take the Teapot Dome oil scandal. It kept the newspapers ringing with indignation in the early 1920s. It rocked the nation! Within the memory of living men, nothing like it had ever happened before in American public life. Here are the bare facts of the scandal: Albert B. Fall, secretary of the interior in Harding's cabinet, was entrusted with the leasing of government oil reserves at Elk Hill and Teapot Dome—oil reserves that had been set aside for the future use of the Navy. Did Secretary Fall permit competitive bidding? No sir. He handed the fat, juicy contract outright to his friend Edward L. Doheny. And what did Doheny do? He gave Secretary Fall what he was pleased to call a "loan" of one hundred thousand dollars. Then in a high-handed manner, Secretary Fall ordered United States Marines into the district to drive off competitors whose adjacent wells were sapping oil out of the Elk Hill reserves. These competitors, driven off their ground at the ends of guns and bayonets, rushed into court—and blew the lid off the Teapot Dome scandal. A stench arose so vile that it ruined the Harding administration, nauseated an entire nation, threatened to wreck the Republican party, and put Albert B. Fall behind prison bars.

Fall was condemned viciously—condemned as few men in public life have ever been. Did he repent? Never!

Years later Herbert Hoover intimated in a public speech that President Harding's death had been due to mental anxiety and worry because a friend had betrayed him. When Mrs. Fall heard that, she sprang from her chair, she wept, she shook her fists at fate and screamed: "What? Harding betrayed by Fall? No! My husband never betrayed anyone. This whole house full of gold would not tempt my husband to do wrong. He is the one who has been betrayed and led to the slaughter and crucified."

There you are; human nature in action, wrongdoers, blaming everybody but themselves. We are all like that. So when you and I are tempted to criticize someone tomorrow, let's remember Al Capone, "Two Gun" Crowley, and Albert Fall. Let's realize that criticisms are like homing pigeons. They always return home. Let's realize that the person we are going to correct and condemn will probably justify himself or herself, and condemn us in return; or, like the gentle Taft, will say: "I don't see how I could have done any differently from what I have."

On the morning of April 15, 1865, Abraham Lincoln lay dying in a hall bedroom of a cheap lodging house directly across the street from Ford's Theater, where John Wilkes Booth had shot him. Lincoln's long body lay stretched diagonally across a sagging bed that was too short for him. A cheap reproduction of Rosa Bonheur's famous painting *The Horse Fair* hung above the bed, and a dismal gas jet flickered yellow light.

As Lincoln lay dying, Secretary of War Stanton said, "There lies the most perfect ruler of men that the world has ever seen."

What was the secret of Lincoln's success in dealing with people? I studied the life of Abraham Lincoln for ten years and devoted all of three years to writing and rewriting a book entitled *Lincoln the Unknown*. I believe I have made as detailed and exhaustive a study of Lincoln's personality and home life as it is possible for any being to make. I made a special study of Lincoln's method of dealing with people. Did he indulge in criticism? Oh, yes. As a young man in the Pigeon Creek Valley of Indiana, he not only criticized but also wrote letters and poems ridiculing people and dropped these letters on the country roads where they were sure to be found. One of these letters aroused resentments that burned for a lifetime.

Even after Lincoln had become a practising lawyer in Springfield, Illinois, he attacked his opponents openly in letters published in the newspapers. But he did this just once too often.

In the autumn of 1842 he ridiculed a vain, pugnacious politician by the name of James Shields. Lincoln lampooned him through an anonymous letter published in the Springfield *Journal*. The town roared with laughter. Shields, sensitive and proud, boiled with indignation. He found out who wrote the letter, leaped on his horse, started after Lincoln, and challenged him to fight a duel. Lincoln didn't want to fight. He was opposed to dueling, but he couldn't get out of it and save his honor. He was given the choice of weapons. Since he had very long arms, he chose cavalry broadswords and took lessons in sword fighting from a West Point graduate. On the appointed day, he and Shields met on a sandbar in the Mississippi

River, prepared to fight to the death, but at the last minute, their seconds interrupted and stopped the duel.

That was the most lurid personal incident in Lincoln's life. It taught him an invaluable lesson in the art of dealing with people. Never again did he write an insulting letter. Never again did he ridicule anyone. And from that time on, he almost never criticized anybody for anything.

Time after time, during the Civil War, Lincoln put a new general at the head of the Army of the Potomac, and each one in turn—McClellan, Pope, Burnside, Hooker, Meade—blundered tragically and drove Lincoln to pacing the floor in despair. Half the nation savagely condemned these incompetent generals, but Lincoln, "with malice toward none, with charity for all," held his peace. One of his favorite quotations was "Judge not, that ye be not judged."

And when Mrs. Lincoln and others spoke harshly of the southern people, Lincoln replied: "Don't criticize them; they are just what we would be under similar circumstances."

Yet if any man ever had occasion to criticize, surely it was Lincoln. Let's take just one illustration:

The Battle of Gettysburg was fought during the first three days of July 1863. During the night of July 4, Lee began to retreat southward while storm clouds deluged the country with rain. When Lee reached the Potomac with his defeated army, he found a swollen, impassible river in front of him, and a victorious Union Army behind him. Lee was in a trap. He couldn't escape. Lincoln saw that. Here was a golden, heaven-sent opportunity—the opportunity to capture Lee's army and end the war immediately. So, with a surge of high hope, Lincoln ordered Meade not to call a council of war but to attack Lee immediately. Lincoln telegraphed his orders and then sent a special messenger to Meade demanding immediate action.

And what did General Meade do? He did the very opposite of what he was told to do. He called a council of war in direct violation of Lincoln's orders. He hesitated. He procrastinated. He telegraphed all manner of excuses. He refused point-blank to attack Lee. Finally the waters receded and Lee escaped over the Potomac with his forces.

Lincoln was furious. "What does this mean?" Lincoln cried to his son Robert. "Great God! What does this mean? We had them within our grasp, and had only to stretch forth our hands and they were ours; yet nothing I could say or do could make the army move. Under the circumstances, almost any general could have defeated Lee. If I had gone up there, I could have whipped him myself."

In bitter disappointment, Lincoln sat down and wrote Meade this letter. And remember, at this period of his life Lincoln was extremely conservative and restrained in his phraseology. So this letter coming from Lincoln in 1863 was tantamount to the severest rebuke.

My dear General,

I do not believe you appreciate the magnitude of the misfortune involved in Lee's escape. He was within our easy grasp, and to have closed upon him would, in connection with our other late successes, have ended the war. As it is, the war will be prolonged indefinitely. If you could not safely attack Lee last Monday, how can you possibly do so south of the river, when you can take with you very few—no more than two-thirds of the force you then had in hand? It would be unreasonable to expect and I do not expect that you can now effect much. Your golden opportunity is gone, and I am distressed immeasurably because of it.

What do you suppose Meade did when he read the letter?

Meade never saw that letter. Lincoln never mailed it. It was found among his papers after his death.

My guess is—and this is only a guess—that after writing that letter, Lincoln looked out of the window and said to himself, "Just a minute. Maybe I ought not to be so hasty. It is easy enough for me to sit here in the quiet of the White House and order Meade to attack; but if I had been up at Gettysburg, and if I had seen as much blood as Meade has seen during the last week, and if my ears had been pierced with the screams and shrieks of the wounded and dying, maybe I wouldn't be so anxious to attack either. If I had Meade's timid temperament, perhaps I would have done just what he had done. Anyhow, it is water under the bridge now. If I send this letter, it will relieve my feelings, but it will make Meade try to justify himself. It will make him condemn me. It will arouse hard feelings, impair all his further usefulness as a commander, and perhaps force him to resign from the army."

So, as I have already said, Lincoln put the letter aside, for he had learned by bitter experience that sharp criticisms and rebukes almost invariably end in futility.

Theodore Roosevelt said that when he, as president, was confronted with a perplexing problem, he used to lean back and look up at a large painting of Lincoln that hung above his desk in the White House and ask himself, "What would Lincoln do if he were in my shoes? How would he solve this problem?"

The next time we are tempted to admonish somebody, let's pull a five-dollar bill out of our pocket, look at Lincoln's picture on the bill, and ask, "How would Lincoln handle this problem if he had it?"

Mark Twain lost his temper occasionally and wrote letters that turned the paper brown. For example, he once wrote to a man who had aroused his ire: "The thing for you is a burial permit. You have only to speak and I will see that you get it." On another occasion he wrote to an editor about a proofreader's attempts to "improve my spelling and punctuation." He ordered: "Set the matter according to my copy hereafter and see that the proofreader retains his suggestions in the mush of his decayed brain."

The writing of these stinging letters made Mark Twain feel better. They allowed him to blow off steam, and the letters didn't do any real harm, because Mark's wife secretly lifted them out of the mail. They were never sent.

Do you know someone you would like to change and regulate and improve? Good! This is fine. I am all in favor

416 · THE DALE CARNEGIE OMNIBUS: VOLUME 2

of it. But why not begin on yourself? From a purely selfish standpoint, that is a lot more profitable than trying to improve others—yes, and a lot less dangerous. "Don't complain about the snow on your neighbor's roof," said Confucius, "when your own doorstep is unclean."

When I was still young and trying hard to impress people, I wrote a foolish letter to Richard Harding Davis, an author who once loomed large on the literary horizon of America. I was preparing a magazine article about authors, and I asked Davis to tell me about his method of work. A few weeks earlier, I had received a letter from someone with this notation at the bottom: "Dictated but not read." I was quite impressed. I felt that the writer must be very big and busy and important. I wasn't the slightest bit busy, but I was eager to make an impression on Richard Harding Davis, so I ended my short note with the words: "Dictated but not read."

He never troubled to answer the letter. He simply returned it to me with this scribbled across the bottom: "Your bad manners are exceeded only by your bad manners." True, I had blundered, and perhaps I deserved this rebuke. But, being human, I resented it. I resented it so sharply that when I read of the death of Richard Harding Davis ten years later, the one thought that still persisted in my mind—I am ashamed to admit—was the hurt he had given me.

If you and I want to stir up a resentment tomorrow that may rankle across the decades and endure until death, just let us indulge in a little stinging criticism.

When dealing with people, let us remember we are not

dealing with creatures of logic. We are dealing with creatures of emotion, creatures bristling with prejudices and motivated by pride and vanity.

Bitter criticism caused the sensitive Thomas Hardy, one of the finest novelists ever to enrich English literature, to give up forever the writing of fiction. Criticism drove Thomas Chatterton, the English poet, to suicide.

Benjamin Franklin, tactless in his youth, became so diplomatic, so adroit at handling people, that he was made American ambassador to France. The secret of his success? "I will speak ill of no man," he said, "...and speak all the good I know of everybody."

Any fool can criticize, condemn, and complain—and most fools do.

But it takes character and self-control to be understanding and forgiving.

"A great man shows his greatness," said Carlyle, "by the way he treats little men."

Bob Hoover, a famous test pilot and frequent performer at air shows, was returning to his home in Los Angeles from an air show in San Diego. As described in the magazine *Flight Operations,* at three hundred feet in the air, both engines suddenly stopped. By deft maneuvering he managed to land the plane, but it was badly damaged although nobody was hurt.

Hoover's first act after the emergency landing was to inspect the airplane's fuel. Just as he suspected, the World War II propeller plane he had been flying had been fueled with jet fuel rather than gasoline.

Upon returning to the airport, he asked to see the mechanic who had serviced his airplane. The young man was sick with the agony of his mistake. Tears streamed down his face as Hoover approached. He had just caused the loss of a very expensive plane and could have caused the loss of three lives as well.

You can imagine Hoover's anger. One could anticipate the tongue-lashing that this proud and precise pilot would unleash for that carelessness. But Hoover didn't scold the mechanic; he didn't even criticize him. Instead, he put his big arm around the man's shoulder and said, "To show you I'm sure that you'll never do this again, I want you to service my F-51 tomorrow."

Often parents are tempted to criticize their children. You would expect me to say "Don't." But I will not. I am merely going to say, "Before you criticize them, read one of the classics of American journalism, 'Father Forgets.'" It originally appeared as an editorial in the *People's Home Journal*. We are reprinting it here with the author's permission, as condensed in the *Reader's Digest*.

"Father Forgets" is one of those little pieces that—dashed off in a moment of sincere feeling—strikes an echoing chord in so many readers as to become a perennial reprint favorite. Since its first appearance, "Father Forgets" has been reproduced, writes the author, W. Livingston Larned, "in hundreds of magazines and house organs, and in newspapers the country over. It has been reprinted almost as extensively in many foreign languages. I have given personal permission to thousands who wished to read it from school, church, and lecture platforms. It has been 'on the air' on countless occasions and programs. Oddly enough, college periodicals have used it, and high-school magazines. Sometimes a little piece seems mysteriously to 'click.' This one certainly did."

FATHER FORGETS
W. Livingston Larned

Listen, son: I am saying this as you lie asleep, one little paw crumpled under your cheek and the blond curls stickily wet on your damp forehead. I have stolen into your room alone. Just a few minutes ago, as I sat reading my paper in the library, a stifling wave of remorse swept over me. Guiltily I came to your bedside.

There are the things I was thinking, son: I had been cross to you. I scolded you as you were dressing for school because you gave your face merely a dab with a towel. I took you to task for not cleaning your shoes. I called out angrily when you threw some of your things on the floor.

At breakfast I found fault, too. You spilled things. You gulped down your food. You put your elbows on the table. You spread butter too thick on your bread. And as you started off to play and I made for my train, you turned and waved a hand and called, "Goodbye, Daddy!" and I frowned, and said in reply, "Hold your shoulders back!"

Then it began all over again in the late afternoon. As I came up the road I spied you, down on your knees, playing marbles. There were holes in your stockings. I humiliated you before your boyfriends by marching you ahead of me to the house. Stockings were expensive—and if you had to buy them you would be more careful! Imagine that, son, from a father!

Do you remember, later, when I was reading in the library, how you came in timidly, with a sort of hurt look in your eyes? When I glanced up over my paper, impatient at the interruption, you hesitated at the door. "What is it you want?" I snapped.

You said nothing, but ran across in one tempestuous plunge, and threw your arms around my neck and kissed me, and your small arms tightened with an affection that God had set blooming in your heart and which even neglect could not wither. And then you were gone, pattering up the stairs.

Well, son, it was shortly afterwards that my paper slipped from my hands and a terrible sickening fear came over me. What has habit been doing to me? The habit of finding fault, of reprimanding—this was my reward to you for being a boy. It was not that I did not love you; it was that I expected too much of youth. I was measuring you by the yardstick of my own years.

And there was so much that was good and fine and true in your character. The little heart of you was as big as the dawn itself over the wide hills. This was shown by your spontaneous impulse to rush in and kiss me good night. Nothing else matters tonight, son. I have come to your bedside in the darkness, and I have knelt there, ashamed!

It is a feeble atonement; I know you would not

understand these things if I told them to you during your waking hours. But tomorrow I will be a real daddy! I will chum with you, and suffer when you suffer, and laugh when you laugh. I will bite my tongue when impatient words come. I will keep saying as if it were a ritual: "He is nothing but a boy—a little boy!"

I am afraid I have visualized you as a man. Yet as I see you now, son, crumpled and weary in your cot, I see that you are still a baby. Yesterday you were in your mother's arms, your head on her shoulder. I have asked too much, too much.

Instead of condemning people, let's try to understand them. Let's try to figure out why they do what they do. That's a lot more profitable and intriguing than criticism; and it breeds sympathy, tolerance, and kindness. "To know all is to forgive all."

As Dr. Johnson said: "God himself, sir, does not propose to judge man until the end of his days."

Why should you and I?

Instead of Condemning People, Try to Understand Them

6

THE HIGH ROAD TO REASON

If your temper is aroused and you tell 'em a thing or two, you will have a fine time unloading your feelings. But what about the other person? Will he share your pleasure? Will your belligerent tones, your hostile attitude, make it easy for him to agree with you?

"If you come at me with your fists doubled," said Woodrow Wilson, "I think I can promise you that mine will double as fast as yours; but if you come to me and say, 'Let us sit down and take counsel together, and, if we differ from each other, understand why it is that we differ, just what the points at issue are,' we will presently find that we are not so far apart after all, that the points on which we differ are few and the points on which we agree are many, and that if we only have the patience and the candor and the desire to get together, we will get together."

Nobody appreciated the truth of Woodrow Wilson's statement more than John D. Rockefeller, Jr. Back in 1915, Rockefeller was the most fiercely despised man in Colorado. One of the bloodiest strikes in the history of American industry had been shocking the state for two terrible years. Irate, belligerent miners were demanding higher wages from the Colorado Fuel and Iron Company; Rockefeller controlled that company. Property had been destroyed, troops had been called out. Blood had been shed. Strikers had been shot, their bodies riddled with bullets.

At a time like that, with the air seething with hatred, Rockefeller wanted to win the strikers to his way of thinking. And he did it. How? Here's the story. After weeks spent in making friends, Rockefeller addressed the representatives of the strikers. This speech, in its entirety, is a masterpiece. It produced astonishing results. It calmed the tempestuous waves of hate that threatened to engulf Rockefeller. It won him a host of admirers. It presented facts in such a friendly manner that the strikers went back to work without saying another word about the increase in wages for which they had fought so violently.

The opening of that remarkable speech follows. Note how it fairly glows with friendliness. Rockefeller, remember, was talking to men who, a few days previously, had wanted to hang him by the neck to a sour apple tree; yet he couldn't have been more gracious, more friendly if he had addressed a group of medical missionaries. His speech was radiant with such phrases as I am proud to be here, having visited in your homes, met many of your wives and children, we meet here not as strangers, but as friends…spirit of mutual friendship, our common interests, it is only by your courtesy that I am here.

"This is a red-letter day in my life," Rockefeller began. "It is the first time I have ever had the good fortune to meet the representatives of the employees of this great company, its officers and superintendents, together, and I can assure you that I am proud to be here, and that I shall remember this gathering as long as I live. Had this meeting been held two weeks ago, I should have stood here a stranger to most of you, recognizing a few faces.

Having had the opportunity last week of visiting all the camps in the southern coal field and of talking individually with practically all of the representatives, except those who were away; having visited in your homes, met many of your wives and children, we meet here not as strangers, but as friends, and it is in that spirit of mutual friendship that I am glad to have this opportunity to discuss with you our common interests.

"Since this is a meeting of the officers of the company and the representatives of the employees, it is only by your courtesy that I am here, for I am not so fortunate as to be either one or the other; and yet I feel that I am intimately associated with you men, for, in a sense, I represent both the stockholders and the directors."

Isn't that a superb example of the fine art of making friends out of enemies?

Suppose Rockefeller had taken a different tack. Suppose he had argued with these miners and hurled devastating facts in their faces. Suppose he had told them by his tone and insinuations that they were wrong. Suppose that, by all the rules of logic, he had proved that they were wrong. What would have happened? More anger would have been stirred up, more hatred, more revolt.

If a man's heart is rankling with discord and ill feeling toward you, you can't win him to your way of thinking with all the logic in Christendom. Scolding parents and domineering bosses and husbands and nagging wives ought to realize that people don't want to change their minds. They can't be forced or driven to agree with you or me. But they may possibly be led to, if we are gentle and friendly, ever so gentle and ever so friendly.

Lincoln said that, in effect, over a hundred years ago. Here are his words:

It is an old and true maxim that "a drop of honey catches more flies than a gallon of gall." So with men, if you would win a man to your cause, first convince him that you are his sincere friend. Therein is a drop of honey that catches his heart; which, say what you will, is the great high road to his reason.

Business executives have learned that it pays to be friendly to strikers. For example, when twenty-five hundred employees in the White Motor Company's plant struck for higher wages and a union shop, Robert F. Black, then president of the company, didn't lose his temper and condemn and threaten and talk of tyranny and communists. He actually praised the strikers. He published an advertisement in the Cleveland papers, complimenting them on "the peaceful way in which they laid down their tools." Finding the strike pickets idle, he bought them a couple of dozen baseball bats and gloves and invited them to play ball on vacant lots. For those who preferred bowling, he rented a bowling alley.

This friendliness on Mr. Black's part did what friendliness always does: it begot friendliness. So the strikers borrowed brooms, shovels, and rubbish carts, and began picking up matches, papers, cigarette stubs, and cigar butts around the factory. Imagine it! Imagine strikers tidying up the factory grounds while battling for higher wages and recognition of the union. Such an event had

426 • THE DALE CARNEGIE OMNIBUS: VOLUME 2

never been heard of before in the long, tempestuous history of American labor wars. That strike ended with a compromise settlement within a week—ended without any ill feeling or rancor.

Daniel Webster, who looked like a god and talked like Jehovah, was one of the most successful advocates who ever pleaded a case; yet he ushered in his most powerful arguments with such friendly remarks as: "It will be for the jury to consider," "This may, perhaps, be worth thinking of," "Here are some facts that I trust you will not lose sight of," or "You, with your knowledge of human nature, will easily see the significance of these facts." No bulldozing. No high-pressure methods. No attempt to force his opinions on others. Webster used the soft-spoken, quiet, friendly approach, and it helped to make him famous.

You may never be called upon to settle a strike or address a jury, but you may want to get your rent reduced. Will the friendly approach help you then? Let's see.

O. L. Straub, an engineer, wanted to get his rent reduced. And he knew his landlord was hard-boiled. "I wrote him," Mr. Straub said in a speech before the class, "notifying him that I was vacating my apartment as soon as my lease expired. The truth was, I didn't want to move. I wanted to stay if I could get my rent reduced. But the situation seemed hopeless. Other tenants had tried—and failed. Everyone told me that the landlord was extremely difficult to deal with. But I said to myself, 'I am studying a course in how to deal with people, so I'll try it on him— and see how it works.'

"He and his secretary came to see me as soon as he got my letter. I met him at the door with a friendly greeting. I fairly bubbled with good will and enthusiasm. I didn't begin talking about how high the rent was. I began talking about how much I liked his apartment house. Believe me, I was 'hearty in my approbation and lavish in my praise.' I complimented him on the way he ran the building and told him I should like so much to stay for another year but I couldn't afford it.

"He had evidently never had such a reception from a tenant. He hardly knew what to make of it.

"Then he started to tell me his troubles. Complaining tenants. One had written him fourteen letters, some of them positively insulting. Another threatened to break his lease unless the landlord kept the man on the floor above from snoring. 'What a relief it is,' he said, 'to have a satisfied tenant like you.' And then, without my even asking him to do it, he offered to reduce my rent a little. I wanted more, so I named the figure I could afford to pay, and he accepted without a word.

"As he was leaving, he turned to me and asked, 'What decorating can I do for you?'

"If I had tried to get the rent reduced by the methods the other tenants were using, I am positive I should have met the same failure they encountered. It was the friendly, sympathetic, appreciative approach that won."

Dean Woodcock of Pittsburgh, Pennsylvania, is the superintendent of a department of the local electric company. His staff was called upon to repair some equipment on top of a pole. This type of work had formerly been performed by a different department and had only recently been transferred to Woodcock's section. Although his people had been trained in the work, this was the first time they had ever actually been called upon to do it. Everybody in the organization was interested in seeing if and how they could handle it. Mr. Woodcock, several of his subordinate managers, and members of other departments of the utility went to see the operation. Many cars and trucks were there, and a number of people were standing around watching the two lone men on top of the pole.

Glancing around, Woodcock noticed a man up the street getting out of his car with a camera. He began taking pictures of the scene. Utility people are extremely conscious of public relations, and suddenly Woodcock realized what this setup looked like to the man with the camera—overkill, dozens of people being called out to do a two-person job. He strolled up the street to the photographer.

"I see you're interested in our operation."

"Yes, and my mother will be more than interested. She owns stock in your company. This will be an eye-opener for her. She may even decide her investment was unwise. I've been telling her for years there's a lot of waste motion in companies like yours. This proves it. The newspapers might like these pictures, too."

"It does look like it, doesn't it? I'd think the same thing in your position. But this is a unique situation, …" and Dean Woodcock went on to explain how this was the first job of this type for his department and how everyone from executives down was interested. He assured the man that under normal conditions two people could handle the job. The photographer put away his camera, shook Woodcock's hand, and thanked him for taking the time to explain the situation to him.

Dean Woodcock's friendly approach saved his company much embarrassment and bad publicity.

Another member of one of our classes, Gerald H. Winn of Littleton, New Hampshire, reported how, by using a friendly approach, he obtained a very satisfactory settlement on a damage claim.

"Early in the spring," he reported, "before the ground had thawed from winter freezing, there was an unusually heavy rainstorm and the water, which normally would have run off to nearby ditches and storm drains along the road, took a new course onto a building lot where I had just built a new home.

"Not being able to run off, the water pressure built up around the foundation of the house. The water forced itself under the concrete basement floor, causing it to explode, and the basement filled with water. This ruined the furnace and the hot-water heater. The cost to repair this damage was in excess of two thousand dollars. I had no insurance to cover this type of damage.

"However, I soon found out that the owner of the subdivision had neglected to put in a storm drain near the house which could have prevented this problem. I made an appointment to see him. During the twenty-five-minute trip to his office, I carefully reviewed the situation and, remembering the principles I learned in this course,

I decided that showing my anger would not serve any worthwhile purpose. When I arrived, I kept very calm and started by talking about his recent vacation to the West Indies; then, when I felt the timing was right, I mentioned the 'little' problem of water damage. He quickly agreed to do his share in helping to correct the problem.

"A few days later he called and said he would pay for the damage and also put in a storm drain to prevent the same thing from happening in the future.

"Even though it was the fault of the owner of the subdivision, if I had not begun in a friendly way, there would have been a great deal of difficulty in getting him to agree to the total liability."

Years ago, when I was a barefoot boy walking through the woods to a country school out in northwest Missouri, I read a fable by Aesop about the sun and the wind. They quarreled about which was the stronger, and the wind said, "I'll prove I am. See the old man down there with a coat? I bet I can get his coat off him quicker than you can."

So the sun went behind a cloud, and the wind blew until it was almost a tornado, but the harder it blew, the tighter the old man clutched his coat to him.

Finally, the wind calmed down and gave up, and then the sun came out from behind the clouds and smiled kindly on the old man. Presently, he mopped his brow and pulled off his coat. The sun then told the wind that gentleness and friendliness were always stronger than fury and force.

The use of gentleness and friendliness is demonstrated

day after day by people who have learned that a drop of honey catches more flies than a gallon of gall. F. Gale Connor of Lutherville, Maryland, proved this when he had to take his four-month-old car to the service department of the car dealer for the third time. He told our class: "It was apparent that talking to, reasoning with, or shouting at the service manager was not going to lead to a satisfactory resolution of my problems.

"I walked over to the showroom and asked to see the agency owner, Mr. White. After a short wait, I was ushered into Mr. White's office. I introduced myself and explained to him that I had bought my car from his dealership because of the recommendations of friends who had had previous dealings with him. I was told that his prices were very competitive and his service was outstanding. He smiled with satisfaction as he listened to me. I then explained the problem I was having with the service department. 'I thought you might want to be aware of any situation that might tarnish your fine reputation,' I added. He thanked me for calling this to his attention and assured me that my problem would be taken care of. Not only did he personally get involved, but he also lent me his car to use while mine was being repaired."

Aesop was a Greek slave who lived at the court of Croesus and spun immortal fables six hundred years before Christ. Yet the truths he taught about human nature are just as true in Boston and Birmingham now as they were twenty-six centuries ago in Athens. The sun can make you take off your coat more quickly than the wind;

and kindliness, the friendly approach, and appreciation can make people change their minds more readily than all the bluster and storming in the world.

Remember what Lincoln said: "A drop of honey catches more flies than a gallon of gall."

Be Friendly

It isn't what you have, or who you are, or where you are, or what you are doing that makes you happy or unhappy. It is what you think about.

—Dale Carnegie

7

HOW TO GET COOPERATION

Don't you have much more faith in ideas that you discover for yourself than in ideas that are handed to you on a silver platter? If so, isn't it bad judgment to try to ram your opinions down the throats of other people? Isn't it wiser to make suggestions—and let the other person think out the conclusion?

Adolph Seltz of Philadelphia, sales manager in an automobile showroom and a student in one of my courses, suddenly found himself confronted with the necessity of injecting enthusiasm into a discouraged and disorganized group of automobile salespeople. Calling a sales meeting, he urged his people to tell him exactly what they expected from him. As they talked, he wrote their ideas on the blackboard. He then said: "I'll give you all these qualities you expect from me. Now I want you to tell me what I have a right to expect from you." The replies came quick and fast: loyalty, honesty, initiative, optimism, teamwork, eight hours a day of enthusiastic work. The meeting ended with a new courage, a new inspiration—one salesperson volunteered to work fourteen hours a day—and Mr. Seltz reported to me that the increase of sales was phenomenal.

"The people had made a sort of moral bargain with me," said Mr. Seltz, "and as long as I lived up to my part in it, they were determined to live up to theirs. Consulting them about their wishes and desires was just the shot in the arm they needed."

No one likes to feel that he or she is being sold something or told to do a thing. We much prefer to feel that we are buying of our own accord or acting on our own ideas. We like to be consulted about our wishes, our wants, our thoughts.

Take the case of Eugene Wesson. He lost countless thousands of dollars in commissions before he learned this truth. Mr. Wesson sold sketches for a studio that created designs for stylists and textile manufacturers. Mr. Wesson had called on one of the leading stylists in New York once a week, every week for three years. "He never refused to see me," said Mr. Wesson, "but he never bought. He always looked over my sketches very carefully and then said: 'No, Wesson, I guess we don't get together today.'"

After 150 failures, Wesson realized he must be in a mental rut, so he resolved to devote one evening a week to the study of influencing human behavior, to help him develop new ideas and generate new enthusiasm.

He decided on this new approach. With half a dozen unfinished artists' sketches under his arm, he rushed over to the buyer's office. "I want you to do me a little favor, if you will," he said. "Here are some uncompleted sketches. Won't you please tell me how we could finish them up in such a way that you could use them?"

The buyer looked at the sketches for a while without uttering a word. Finally he said: "Leave these with me for a few days, Wesson, and then come back and see me."

Wesson returned three days later, got his suggestions, took the sketches back to the studio, and had them finished according to the buyer's ideas. The result? All accepted.

After that, this buyer ordered scores of other sketches from Wesson, all drawn according to the buyer's ideas. "I realized why I had failed for years to sell him," said Mr. Wesson. "I had urged him to buy what I thought he ought to have. Then I changed my approach completely. I urged him to give me his ideas. This made him feel that he was creating the designs. And he was. I didn't have to sell him. He bought."

Letting the other person feel that the idea is his or hers not only works in business and politics, it works in family life as well. Paul M. Davis of Tulsa, Oklahoma, told his class how he applied this principle:

"My family and I enjoyed one of the most interesting sightseeing vacation trips we have ever taken. I had long dreamed of visiting such historic sites as the Civil War battlefield in Gettysburg, Independence Hall in Philadelphia, and our nation's capital. Valley Forge, Jamestown, and the restored colonial village of Williamsburg were high on the list of things I wanted to see.

"In March my wife, Nancy, mentioned that she had ideas for our summer vacation which included a tour of the western states, visiting points of interest in New Mexico, Arizona, California, and Nevada. She had wanted to make this trip for several years. But we couldn't, obviously, make both trips.

"Our daughter, Anne, had just completed a course in U.S. history in junior high school and had become very interested in the events that shaped our country's growth. I asked her how she would like to visit the places she had learned about on our next vacation. She said she would love to.

"Two evenings later as we sat around the dinner table, Nancy announced that if we all agreed, the summer's vacation would be to the eastern states, that it would be a great trip for Anne and thrilling for all of us. We all concurred."

This same psychology was used by an X-ray manufacturer to sell his equipment to one of the largest hospitals in Brooklyn. This hospital was building an addition and preparing to equip it with the finest X-ray department in America. Dr. L—, who was in charge of the X-ray department, was overwhelmed with sales representatives, each caroling the praises of his own company's equipment.

One manufacturer, however, was more skillful. He knew far more about handling human nature than the others did. He wrote a letter something like this:

Our factory has recently completed a new line of X-ray equipment. The first shipment of these machines has just arrived at our office. They are not perfect. We know that, and we want to improve them. So we should be deeply obligated to you if you could find time to look them over and give us your ideas about how they can be made more serviceable to your profession. Knowing how occupied you are, I shall be glad to send my car for you at any hour you specify.

"I was surprised to get that letter," Dr. L—said as he related the incident before the class. "I was both surprised and complimented. I had never had an X-ray manufacturer seeking my advice before. It made me feel important. I was busy every night that week, but I canceled a dinner appointment in order to look over the equipment. The more I studied it, the more I discovered for myself how much I liked it.

"Nobody had tried to sell it to me. I felt that the idea of buying that equipment for the hospital was my own. I sold myself on its superior qualities and ordered it installed."

Ralph Waldo Emerson in his essay "Self-Reliance" stated: "In every work of genius we recognize our own rejected thoughts; they come back to us with a certain alienated majesty."

Colonel Edward M. House wielded an enormous influence in national and international affairs while Woodrow Wilson occupied the White House. Wilson leaned upon Colonel House for secret counsel and advice more than he did upon even members of his own cabinet.

What method did the colonel use in influencing the President? Fortunately, we know, for House himself revealed it to Arthur D. Howden Smith, and Smith quoted House in an article in *The Saturday Evening Post*.

"'After I got to know the President,' House said, 'I

learned the best way to convert him to an idea was to plant it in his mind casually, but so as to interest him in it—so as to get him thinking about it on his own account. The first time this worked it was an accident. I had been visiting him at the White House and urged a policy on him which he appeared to disapprove. But several days later, at the dinner table, I was amazed to hear him trot out my suggestion as his own.'"

Did House interrupt him and say, "That's not your idea. That's mine"? Oh, no. Not House. He was too adroit for that. He didn't care about credit. He wanted results. So he let Wilson continue to feel that the idea was his. House did even more than that. He gave Wilson public credit for these ideas.

Let's remember that everyone we come in contact with is just as human as Woodrow Wilson. So let's use Colonel House's technique.

A man up in the beautiful Canadian province of New Brunswick used this technique on me and won my patronage. I was planning at the time to do some fishing and canoeing in New Brunswick. So I wrote the tourist bureau for information. Evidently my name and address were put on a mailing list, for I was immediately overwhelmed with scores of letters and booklets and printed testimonials from camps and guides. I was bewildered. I didn't know which to choose. Then one camp owner did a clever thing. He sent me the names and telephone numbers of several New York people who had stayed at his camp and he invited me to telephone them and discover for myself what he had to offer.

I found to my surprise that I knew one of the men on

his list. I telephoned him, found out what his experience had been, and then wired the camp the date of my arrival.

The others had been trying to sell me their service, but one let me sell myself. That organization won.

Twenty-five centuries ago, Lao-tse, a Chinese sage, said some things that readers of this book might use today:

"The reason why rivers and seas receive the homage of a hundred mountain streams is that they keep below them. Thus they are able to reign over all the mountain streams. So the sage, wishing to be above men, putteth himself below them; wishing to be before them, he putteth himself behind them. Thus, though his place be above men, they do not feel his weight; though his place be before them, they do not count it an injury."

Let the Other Person Feel that the Idea is His or Hers

Men of age object too much, consult too long, adventure too little, repent too soon, and seldom drive business home to the full period, but content themselves with a mediocrity of success.

—Dale Carnegie

8

AN APPEAL THAT EVERYBODY LIKES

I was reared on the edge of the Jesse James country out in Missouri, and I visited the James farm at Kearney, Missouri, where the son of Jesse James was then living.

His wife told me stories of how Jesse robbed trains and held up banks and then gave money to the neighboring farmers to pay off their mortgages.

Jesse James probably regarded himself as an idealist at heart, just as Dutch Schultz, "Two Gun" Crowley, Al Capone, and many other organized crime "godfathers" did generations later. The fact is that all people you meet have a high regard for themselves and like to be fine and unselfish in their own estimation.

J. Pierpont Morgan observed, in one of his analytical interludes, that a person usually has two good reasons for doing a thing: one that sounds good and a real one. The person himself will think of the real reason. You don't need to emphasize that. But all of us, being idealists at heart, like to think of motives that sound good. So, in order to change people, appeal to the nobler motives.

Is that too idealistic to work in business? Let's see. Let's take the case of Hamilton J. Farrell of the Farrell-Mitchell Company of Glenolden, Pennsylvania. Mr. Farrell had a disgruntled tenant who threatened to move. The tenant's lease still had four months to run; nevertheless, he served notice that he was vacating immediately, regardless of lease.

"These people had lived in my house all winter—the most expensive part of the year," Mr. Farrell said as he told the story to the class, "and I knew it would be difficult to rent the apartment again before fall. I could see all that rent income going over the hill and believe me, I saw red.

"Now, ordinarily, I would have waded into that tenant and advised him to read his lease again. I would have pointed out that if he moved, the full balance of his rent would fall due at once—and that I could, *and would*, take steps to collect.

"However, instead of flying off the handle and making a scene, I decided to try other tactics. So I started like this: 'Mr. Doe,' I said, 'I have listened to your story, and I still don't believe you intend to move. Years in the renting business have taught me something about human nature, and I sized you up in the first place as being a man of your word. In fact, I'm so sure of it that I'm willing to take a gamble.

"'Now, here's my proposition. Lay your decision on the table for a few days and think it over. If you come back to me between now and the first of the month, when the rent is due, and tell me you still intend to move, I give you my word I will accept your decision as final. I will give you the privilege of moving and admit to myself I've been wrong in my judgment. But I still believe you're a man of your word and will live up to your contract. For after all, we are either men or monkeys—and the choice usually lies with ourselves!'

"Well, when the new month came around, this gentleman came to see me and paid his rent in person. He and his wife had talked it over, he said—and decided to stay. They had concluded that the only honorable thing to do was to live up to their lease."

When the late Lord Northcliffe found a newspaper using a picture of him which he didn't want published, he wrote the editor a letter. But did he say, "Please do not publish that picture of me anymore; I don't like it"? No, he appealed to a nobler motive. He appealed to the respect and love that all of us have for motherhood. He wrote, "Please do not publish that picture of me anymore. My mother doesn't like it."

When John D. Rockefeller, Jr., wished to stop newspaper photographers from snapping pictures of his children, he, too, appealed to the nobler motives. He didn't say: "I don't want the pictures published." No, he appealed to the desire, deep in all of us, to refrain from harming children. He said: "You know how it is, boys. You've got children yourselves, some of you. And you know it's not good for youngsters to get too much publicity."

When Cyrus H. K. Curtis, a poor boy from Maine, was starting on the meteoric career which was destined to make him millions as owner of *The Saturday Evening Post* and the *Ladies Home Journal*, he couldn't afford to pay his contributors the prices that other magazines paid. He couldn't afford to hire first-class authors to write for money alone. So he appealed to their nobler motives. For example, he persuaded even Louisa May Alcott, the immortal author of *Little Women*, to write for him when she was at the flood tide of her fame; and he did it by offering to send a check for a hundred dollars, not to her, but to her favorite charity.

Right here the skeptic may say: "Oh, that stuff is all right for Northcliffe and Rockefeller or a sentimental novelist. But I'd like to see you make it work with the tough babies I have to collect bills from!"

You may be right. Nothing will work in all cases—and nothing will work with all people. If you are satisfied with the results you are getting, why change? If you are not satisfied, why not experiment?

At any rate, I think you will enjoy reading this true story told by James L. Thomas, a former student of mine:

Six customers of a certain automobile company refused to pay their bills for servicing. None of the customers protested the entire bill, but each claimed that some one charge was wrong. In each case, the customer had signed for the work done, so the company knew it was right—and said so. That was the first mistake.

Here are the steps the credit department took to collect these overdue bills. Do you suppose they succeeded?

They called on the customers and told them bluntly that they had come to collect a bill that was long past due.

They made it very plain that the company was absolutely and unconditionally right; therefore, the customer was absolutely and unconditionally wrong.

They intimated that they, the company, knew more about automobiles than the customer could ever hope to know. So what was the argument about?

Result: They argued.

Did any of these methods reconcile the customer and

settle the account? You can answer that one yourself.

At this stage of affairs, the credit manager was about to open fire with a battery of legal talent, when fortunately the matter came to the attention of the general manager. The manager investigated these defaulting clients and discovered that they all had the reputation of paying their bills promptly. Something was wrong here—something was drastically wrong about the method of collection. So he called in James L. Thomas and told him to collect these "uncollectible" accounts.

Here, in his words, are the steps Mr. Thomas took:

"My visit to each customer was likewise to collect a bill long past due—a bill that we knew was absolutely right. But I didn't say a word about that. I explained I had called to find out what it was the company had done, or failed to do.

"I made it clear that, until I heard the customer's story, I had no opinion to offer. I told him the company made no claims to being infallible.

"I told him I was interested only in his car, and that he knew more about his car than anyone else in the world; that he was the authority on the subject.

"I let him talk, and I listened to him with all the interest and sympathy that he wanted—and expected.

"Finally, when the customer was in a reasonable mood, I put the whole thing up to his sense of fair play. I appealed to the nobler motives. 'First,' I said, 'I want you to know I also feel this matter has been badly mishandled. You've been inconvenienced and annoyed and irritated by one of our representatives. That should never have happened.

I'm sorry and, as a representative of the company, I apologize. As I sat here and listened to your side of the story, I could not help being impressed by your fairness and patience. And now, because you are fair-minded and patient, I am going to ask you do to something for me. It's something that you can do better than anyone else, something you know more about than anyone else. Here is your bill; I know it is safe for me to adjust it, just as you would do if you were the president of my company. I am going to leave it all up to you. Whatever you say goes.'

"Did he adjust the bill? He certainly did, and got quite a kick out of it. The bills ranged from $150 to $400—but did the customer give himself the best of it? Yes, one of them did! One of them refused to pay a penny of the disputed charge; but the other five all gave the company the best of it! And here's the cream of the whole thing: we delivered new cars to all six of these customers within the next two years!"

"Experience has taught me," says Mr. Thomas, "that when no information can be secured about the customer the only sound basis on which to proceed is to assume that he or she is sincere, honest, truthful, and willing and anxious to pay the charges, once convinced they are correct. To put it differently and perhaps more clearly, people are honest and want to discharge their obligations. The exceptions to that rule are comparatively few, and I am convinced that the individuals who are inclined to chisel will in most cases react favorably if you make them feel that you consider them honest, upright, and fair."

446 • THE DALE CARNEGIE OMNIBUS: VOLUME 2

THE DALE CARNEGIE OMNIBUS: VOLUME 2

In Order to Change People, Appeal to the Nobler Motives

Most of the important things in the world have been accomplished by people who have kept on trying when there seemed to be no hope at all.

—Dale Carnegie

9

A SURE WAY OF MAKING
ENEMIES AND HOW TO AVOID IT

When Theodore Roosevelt was in the White House, he confessed that if he could be right seventy-five percent of the time, he would reach the highest measure of his expectation.

If that was the highest rating that one of the most distinguished men of the twentieth century could hope to obtain, what about you and me?

If you can be sure of being right only fifty-five percent of the time, you can go down to Wall Street and make a million dollars a day. If you can't be sure of being right even fifty-five percent of the time, why should you tell other people they are wrong?

You can tell people they are wrong by a look or an intonation or a gesture just as eloquently as you can in words—and if you tell them they are wrong, do you make them want to agree with you? Never! For you have struck a direct blow at their intelligence, judgment, pride, and self-respect. That will make them want to strike back. But it will never make them want to change their minds. You may then hurl at them all the logic of a Plato or an Immanuel Kant, but you will not alter their opinions, for you have hurt their feelings.

Never begin by announcing, "I am going to prove so-and-so to you." That's bad. That's tantamount to saying:

"I'm smarter than you are. I'm going to tell you a thing or two and make you change your mind."

That is a challenge. It arouses opposition and makes the listener want to battle with you before you even start. It is difficult, under even the most benign conditions, to change people's minds. So why make it harder? Why handicap yourself?

Well, I can't hope to be any smarter than Socrates, so I have quit telling people they are wrong. And I find that it pays.

If a person makes a statement that you think is wrong—yes, even that you know is wrong—isn't it better to begin by saying: "Well, now, look. I thought otherwise, but I may be wrong. I frequently am. And if I am wrong, I want to be put right. Let's examine the facts."

There's magic, positive magic, in such phrases as: "I may be wrong. I frequently am. Let's examine the facts."

Nobody in the heavens above or on the earth will ever object to your saying: "I may be wrong. Let's examine the facts."

One of our class members who used this approach in dealing with customers was Harold Reinke, a Dodge dealer in Billings, Montana. He reported that because of the pressures of the automobile business, he was often hard-boiled and callous when dealing with customers complaints. This caused flared tempers, loss of business, and general unpleasantness.

He told his class: "Recognizing that this was getting me nowhere fast, I tried a new tack. I would say something like this: 'Our dealership has made so many mistakes that

I am frequently ashamed. We have erred in your case. Tell me about it.'

"This approach becomes quite disarming, and by the time the customer releases his feelings, he is usually much more reasonable when it comes to settling the matter. In fact, several customers have thanked me for having such an understanding attitude. And two of them have even brought in friends to buy new cars. In this highly competitive market, we need more of this type of customer, and I believe that showing respect for all customers opinions and treating them diplomatically and courteously will help beat the competition."

You will never get into trouble by admitting that you may be wrong. That will stop all argument and inspire your opponent to be just as fair and open and broad-minded as you are. It will make him want to admit that he, too, may be wrong.

If you know positively that a person is wrong, and you bluntly tell him or her so, what happens? Let me illustrate. Mr. S, a young New York attorney, once argued a rather important case before the United States Supreme Court (Lustgarten v. Fleet Corporation 280 U.S. 320). The case involved a considerable sum of money and an important question of law. During the argument, one of the Supreme Court justices said to him: "The statute of limitations is six years, is it not?"

Mr. S stopped, stared at the justice for a moment, and then said bluntly, "Your Honor, there is no statute of limitations in admiralty."

"A hush fell on the court," said Mr. S, as he related his

experience to one of the author's classes, "and the temperature in the room seemed to drop to zero. I was right. Justice was wrong. And I had told him so. But did that make him friendly? No. I still believe that I had the law on my side. And I know that I spoke better than I ever spoke before. But I didn't persuade. I made the enormous blunder of telling a very learned and famous man that he was wrong."

Few people are logical. Most of us are prejudiced and biased. Most of us are blighted with preconceived notions, with jealousy, suspicion, fear, envy, and pride. And most citizens don't want to change their minds about their religion or their haircut or communism or their favorite movie star.

Carl Rogers, the eminent psychologist, wrote in his book *On Becoming a Person*:

> I have found it of enormous value when I can permit myself to understand the other person. The way in which I have worded this statement may seem strange to you. Is it necessary to permit oneself to understand another? I think it is. Our first reaction to most of the statements [which we hear from other people] is an evaluation or judgment, rather than an understanding of it. When someone expresses some feeling, attitude or belief, our tendency is almost immediately to feel "that's right," or "that's stupid," "that's abnormal," "that's unreasonable," "that's incorrect," "that's not nice." Very rarely do we permit ourselves to *understand* precisely what the meaning

of the statement is to the other person.

I once employed an interior decorator to make some draperies for my home. When the bill arrived, I was dismayed.

A few days later, a friend dropped in and looked at the draperies. The price was mentioned, and she exclaimed with a note of triumph: "What? That's awful. I am afraid he put one over on you."

True? Yes, she had told the truth, but few people like to listen to truths that reflect on their judgment. So, being human, I tried to defend myself. I pointed out that the best is eventually the cheapest, that one can't expect to get quality and artistic taste at bargain-basement prices, and so on and on.

The next day another friend dropped in, admired the draperies, bubbled over with enthusiasm, and expressed a wish that she could afford such exquisite creations for her home. My reaction was totally different. "Well, to tell the truth," I said, "I can't afford them myself. I paid too much. I'm sorry I ordered them."

When we are wrong, we may admit it to ourselves. And if we are handled gently and tactfully, we may admit it to others and even take pride in our frankness and broad-mindedness. But not if someone else is trying to ram the unpalatable fact down our esophagus.

Horace Greeley, the most famous editor in America during the time of the Civil War, disagreed violently with Lincoln's policies. He believed that he could drive Lincoln into agreeing with him by a campaign of argument, ridicule, and abuse. He waged this bitter campaign month after month, year after year. In fact, he wrote a brutal, bitter, sarcastic, and personal attack on President Lincoln the night Booth shot him.

But did all this bitterness make Lincoln agree with Greeley? Not at all. Ridicule and abuse never do.

If you want some excellent suggestions about dealing with people and managing yourself and improving your personality, read Benjamin Franklin's autobiography—one of the most fascinating life stories ever written, one of the classics of American literature. Ben Franklin tells how he conquered the iniquitous habit of argument and transformed himself into one of the most able, suave, and diplomatic men in American history.

One day, when Ben Franklin was a blundering youth, an old Quaker friend took him aside and lashed him with a few stinging truths, something like this:

> Ben, you are impossible. Your opinions have a slap in them for everyone who differs with you. They have become so offensive that nobody cares for them. Your friends find they enjoy themselves better when you are not around. You know so much that no man can tell you anything. Indeed, no man is going to try, for the effort would lead only to discomfort and hard work. So you are not likely ever to know any more than you do now, which is very little.

One of the finest things I know about Ben Franklin is

the way he accepted that smarting rebuke. He was big enough and wise enough to realize that it was true, to sense that he was headed for failure and social disaster. So he made a right-about-face. He began immediately to change his insolent, opinionated ways.

"I made it a rule," said Franklin, "to forbear all direct contradiction to the sentiment of others, and all positive assertion of my own. I even forbade myself the use of every word or expression in the language that imported a fix'd opinion, such as 'certainly,' 'undoubtedly,' etc., and I adopted, instead of them, 'I conceive,' 'I apprehend,' or 'I imagine' a thing to be so or so, or 'it so appears to me at present.' When another asserted something that I thought an error, I deny'd myself the pleasure of contradicting him abruptly, and of showing immediately some absurdity in his proposition: and in answering I began by observing that in certain cases or instances his opinion would be right, but in the present case there appear'd or seem'd to me some difference, etc. I soon found the advantage of this change in my manner; the conversations I engag'd in went on more pleasantly. The modest way in which I propos'd my opinions procur'd them a readier reception and less contradiction; I had less mortification when I was found to be in the wrong, and I more easily prevail'd with others to give up their mistakes and join with me when I happened to be in the right.

"And this mode, which I at first put on with some violence to natural inclination, became at length so easy, and so habitual to me, that perhaps for these fifty years past no one has ever heard a dogmatical expression escape me. And to this habit (after my character of integrity) I think it principally owing that I had earned so much weight with my fellow citizens when I proposed new institutions, or alterations in the old, and so much influence in public councils when I became a member; for I was but a bad speaker, never eloquent, subject to much hesitation in my choice of words, hardly correct in language, and yet I generally carried my points."

How do Ben Franklin's methods work in business? Let's take two examples.

Katherine A. Allred of Kings Mountain, North Carolina, is an industrial engineering supervisor for a yarn-processing plant. She told one of our classes how she handled a sensitive problem before and after taking our training:

"Part of my responsibility," she reported, "deals with setting up and maintaining incentive systems and standards for our operators so they can make more money by producing more yarn. The system we were using had worked fine when we had only two or three different types of yarn, but recently we had expanded our inventory and capabilities to enable us to run more than twelve different varieties. The present system was no longer adequate to pay the operators fairly for the work being performed and give them an incentive to increase production. I had worked up a new system which would enable us to pay the operator by the class of yarn she was running at any one particular time. With my new system in hand, I entered the meeting determined to prove to the management that my system was the right approach. I told them in detail how they were wrong and showed where they were being unfair and how I had all the answers they needed. To say the least, I failed miserably! I had become so busy defending my position on the new system that I had left them no opening to graciously admit their problems on the old one. The issue was dead.

"After several sessions of this course, I realized all too well where I had made my mistakes. I called another meeting and this time I asked where they felt their problems were. We discussed each point, and I asked them their opinions on which was the best way to proceed. With a few low-keyed suggestions, at proper intervals, I let them develop my system themselves. At the end of the meeting when I actually presented my system, they enthusiastically accepted it.

"I am convinced now that nothing good is accomplished and a lot of damage can be done if you tell a person straight out that he or she is wrong. You only succeed in stripping that person of self-dignity and making yourself an unwelcome part of any discussion."

Let's take another example—and remember these cases I am citing are typical of the experiences of thousands of other people. R. V. Crowley was a salesman for a lumber company in New York. Crowley admitted that he had been telling hard-boiled lumber inspectors for years that they were wrong. And he had won the arguments too. But it hadn't done any good. "For these lumber inspectors," said Mr. Crowley, "are like baseball umpires. Once they make a decision, they never change it."

Mr. Crowley saw that his firm was losing thousands of dollars through the arguments he won. So while taking my course, he resolved to change tactics and abandon arguments. With what results? Here is the story as he told it to the fellow members of his class:

"One morning the phone rang in my office. A hot and bothered person at the other end proceeded to inform me that a car of lumber we had shipped into his plant was entirely unsatisfactory. His firm had stopped unloading and requested that we make immediate arrangements to remove the stock from their yard. After about one-fourth of the car had been unloaded, their lumber inspector reported that the lumber was running fifty-five percent below grade. Under the circumstances, they refused to accept it.

"I immediately started for his plant and on the way turned over in my mind the best way to handle the situation. Ordinarily, under such circumstances, I should have quoted grading rules and tried, as a result of my own experience and knowledge as a lumber inspector, to convince the other inspector that the lumber was actually up to grade, and that he was misinterpreting the rules in his inspection. However, I thought I would apply the principles learned in this training.

"When I arrived at the plant, I found the purchasing agent and the lumber inspector in a wicked humor, both set for an argument and a fight. We walked out to the car that was being unloaded, and I requested that they continue to unload so that I could see how things were going. I asked the inspector to go right ahead and lay out the rejects, as he had been doing, and to put the good pieces in another pile.

"After watching him for a while it began to dawn on me that his inspection actually was much too strict and that he was misinterpreting the rules. This particular lumber was white pine, and I knew the inspector was thoroughly schooled in hard woods but not a competent, experienced inspector on white pine. White pine happened to be my own strong suit, but did I offer any objection to the way he was grading the lumber? None whatever. I kept on watching and gradually began to ask questions as to why certain pieces were not satisfactory. I didn't for one instant insinuate that the inspector was wrong. I emphasized that my only reason for asking was in order that we could give his firm exactly what they wanted in future shipments.

"By asking questions in a very friendly, cooperative spirit, and insisting continually that they were right in laying out boards not satisfactory to their purpose, I got him warmed up, and the strained relations between us began to thaw and melt away. An occasional carefully put remark on my part gave birth to the idea in his mind that possibly some of these rejected pieces were actually within the grade that they had bought, and that their requirements demanded a more expensive grade. I was very careful, however, not to let him think I was making an issue of this point.

"Gradually his whole attitude changed. He finally admitted to me that he was not experienced on white pine and began to ask me questions about each piece as it came out of the car. I would explain why such a piece came within the grade specified, but kept on insisting that we did not want him to take it if it was unsuitable for their purpose. He finally got to the point where he felt guilty every time he put a piece in the rejected pile. And at last he saw that the mistake was on their part for not having specified as good a grade as they needed.

"The ultimate outcome was that he went through the entire carload again after I left, accepted the whole lot, and we received a check in full.

"In that one instance alone, a little tact, and the determination to refrain from telling the other man he was wrong, saved my company a substantial amount of cash, and it would be hard to place a money value on the good will that was saved."

Martin Luther King, Jr., was asked how, as a pacifist, he could be an admirer of Air Force General Daniel "Chappie" James, then the nation's highest-ranking black officer. Dr. King replied, "I judge people by their own principles—not by my own."

In a similar way, General Robert E. Lee once spoke to the president of the Confederacy, Jefferson Davis in the most glowing terms about a certain officer under his command. Another officer was astonished. "General," he said, "do you not know that the man of whom you speak so highly is one of your bitterest enemies who misses no opportunity to malign you?" "Yes," replied General Lee, "but the president asked my opinion of him; he did not ask for his opinion of me."

By the way, I am not revealing anything new in this

chapter. Two thousand years ago, Jesus said: "Agree with thine adversary quickly."

And twenty-two hundred years before Christ was born, Pharaoh Akhtoi of Egypt gave his son some shrewd advice—advice that is sorely needed today. "Be diplomatic," counseled the pharaoh. "It will help you gain your point."

In other words, don't argue with your customer or your spouse or your adversary. Don't tell them they are wrong, don't get them stirred up. Use a little diplomacy.

Be Diplomatic

Most of us have far more courage than we ever dreamed possible.

—Dale Carnegie

10

HOW TO CRITICIZE
AND NOT BE HATED FOR IT

Charles Schwab was passing through one of his steel mills one day at noon when he came across some of his employees smoking. Immediately above their heads was a sign that said No Smoking. Did Schwab point to the sign and say, "Can't you read?" Oh, no, not Schwab. He walked over to the men, handed each one a cigar, and said, "I'll appreciate it, boys, if you will smoke these on the outside." They knew that he knew that they had broken a rule—and they admired him because he said nothing about it and gave them a little present and made them feel important. Couldn't keep from loving a man like that, could you?

John Wanamaker used the same technique. Wanamaker used to make a tour of his great store in Philadelphia every day. Once he saw a customer waiting at a counter. No one was paying the slightest attention to her. The salespeople? Oh, they were in a huddle at the far end of the counter laughing and talking among themselves. Wanamaker didn't say a word. Quietly slipping behind the counter, he waited on the woman himself and then handed the purchase to the salespeople to be wrapped as he went on his way.

Public officials are often criticized for not being accessible to their constituents. They are busy people, and the fault sometimes lies in overprotective assistants who don't want to overburden their bosses with too many visitors. Carl Langford, who had been mayor of Orlando, Florida, the home of Disney World, for many years, frequently admonished his staff to allow people to see him. He claimed he had an "open-door" policy; yet the citizens of his community were blocked by secretaries and administrators when they called.

Finally the mayor found the solution. He removed the door from his office! His aides got the message, and the mayor had a truly open administration from the day his door was symbolically thrown away.

Simply changing one three-letter word can often spell the difference between failure and success in changing people without giving offense or arousing resentment.

Many people begin their criticism with sincere praise followed by the word "but" and ending with a critical statement. For example, in trying to change a child's careless attitude toward studies, we might say, "We're really proud of you, Johnnie, for raising your grades this term. *But* if you had worked harder on your algebra, the results would have been better."

In this case, Johnnie might feel encouraged until he heard the word "but." He might then question the sincerity of the original praise. To him, the praise might seem only to be a contrived lead-in to a critical inference of failure. Credibility would be strained, and we probably would not achieve our objective of changing Johnnie's attitude toward his studies.

This could be easily overcome by changing the word

"but" to "and." "We're really proud of you, Johnnie, for raising your grades this term, *and* if you continue the same conscientious efforts next term, your algebra grade can be up with all the others."

Now, Johnnie would accept the praise because there was no follow-up of an inference of failure. We have called his attention to the behavior we wished to change indirectly, and the chances are he will try to live up to our expectations.

Calling attention indirectly to someone's mistakes works wonders with sensitive people who may resent bitterly any direct criticism. Marge Jacob of Woonsocket, Rhode Island, told one of our classes how she convinced some sloppy construction workers to clean up after themselves when they were building additions to her house.

For the first few days of the work, when Mrs. Jacob returned from her job, she noticed that the yard was strewn with the cut ends of lumber. She didn't want to antagonize the builders, because they did excellent work. So after the workers had gone home, she and her children picked up and neatly piled all the lumber debris in a corner. The following morning she called the foreman to one side and said, "I'm really pleased with the way the front lawn was left last night; it is nice and clean and does not offend the neighbors." From that day forward the workers picked up and piled the debris to one side, and the foreman came in each day seeking approval of the condition the lawn was left in after a day's work.

One of the major areas of controversy between

members of the army reserves and their regular army trainers is haircuts. The reservists consider themselves civilians (which they are most of the time) and resent having to cut their hair short.

Master Sergeant Harley Kaiser of the 542nd USAR School addressed himself to this problem when he was working with a group of reserve noncommissioned officers. As an old-time regular-army master sergeant, he might have been expected to yell at his troops and threaten them. Instead he chose to make his point indirectly.

"Gentlemen," he started, "you are leaders. You will be most effective when you lead by example. You must be the example for your men to follow. You know what the army regulations say about haircuts. I am going to get my hair cut today, although it is still much shorter than some of yours. You look at yourself in the mirror, and if you feel you need a haircut to be a good example, we'll arrange time for you to visit the post barbershop."

The result was predictable. Several of the candidates did look in the mirror and went to the barbershop that afternoon and received "regulation" haircuts. Sergeant Kaiser commented the next morning that he already could see the development of leadership qualities in some of the members of the squad.

On March 8, 1887, the eloquent Henry Ward Beecher died. The following Sunday, Lyman Abbott was invited to speak in the pulpit left silent by Beecher's passing. Eager to do his best, he wrote, rewrote, and polished his sermon with the meticulous care of a Flaubert. Then he read it to his wife. It was poor—as most written speeches are. She might have said, if she had had less judgment, "Lyman, that is terrible. That'll never do. You'll put people to sleep. It reads like an encyclopedia. You ought to know better than that after all the years you have been preaching. For heaven's sake, why don't you talk like a human being? Why don't you act natural? You'll disgrace yourself if you ever read that stuff."

That's what she *might* have said. And, if she had, you know what would have happened. And she knew too. So, she merely remarked that it would make an excellent article for the *North American Review.* In other words, she praised it and at the same time subtly suggested that it wouldn't do as a speech. Lyman Abbott saw the point, tore up his carefully prepared manuscript, and preached without even using notes.

Don't Call Attention to People's Mistakes Directly

Most of us have far more courage than we ever dreamed we possessed.

—Dale Carnegie

11

NO ONE LIKES TO TAKE ORDERS

I once had the pleasure of dining with Mrs. Ida Tarbell, the dean of American biographers. When I told her I was writing this book, we began discussing this all-important subject of getting along with people, and she told me that while she was writing her biography of Owen D. Young, she interviewed a man who had sat for three years in the same office with Mr. Young. This man declared that during all that time he had never heard Owen D. Young give a direct order to anyone. He always gave suggestions, not orders. Owen D. Young never said, for example, "Do this or do that," or "Don't do this or don't do that." He would say, "You might consider this," or "Do you think that would work?" Frequently he would say, after he had dictated a letter, "What do you think of this?" In looking over a letter of one of his assistants, he would say, "Maybe if we were to phrase it this way it would be better." He always gave people the opportunity to do things themselves; he never told his assistants to do things; he let them do them, let them learn from their mistakes.

A technique like that makes it easy for a person to correct errors. A technique like that saves a person's pride and gives him or her a feeling of importance. It encourages cooperation instead of rebellion.

Resentment caused by a brash order may last a long time—even if the order was given to correct an obviously bad situation. Dan Santarelli, a teacher at a vocational school in Wyoming, Pennsylvania, told one of our classes how one of his students had blocked the entraceway to one of the school's shops by illegally parking his car in it. One of the other instructors stormed into the classroom and asked in an arrogant tone, "Whose car is blocking the driveway?" When the student who owned the car responded, the instructor screamed: "Move that car and move it right now, or I'll wrap a chain around it and drag it out of there."

Now that student was wrong. The car should not have been parked there. But from that day on, not only did that student resent the instructor's action, but all the students in the class did everything they could to give the instructor a hard time and make his job unpleasant.

How could he have handled it differently? If he had asked in a friendly way, "Whose car is in the driveway?" and then suggested that if it were moved, other cars could get in and out, the student would have gladly moved it and neither he nor his classmates would have been upset and resentful.

Asking questions not only makes an order more palatable; it often stimulates the creativity of the persons whom you ask. People are more likely to accept an order if they have had a part in the decision that caused the order to be issued.

When Ian Macdonald of Johannesburg, South Africa, the general manager of a small manufacturing plant specializing in precision machine parts, had the opportunity to accept a very large order, he was convinced that he would not meet the promised delivery date. The work already scheduled in the shop and the short completion time needed for this order made it seem impossible for him to accept the order.

Instead of pushing his people to accelerate their work and rush the order through, he called everybody together, explained the situation to them, and told them how much it would mean to the company and to them if they could make it possible to produce the order on time. Then he started asking questions:

"Is there anything we can do to handle this order?"

"Can anyone think of different ways to process it through the shop that will make it possible to take the order?"

"Is there any way to adjust our hours or personnel assignments that would help?"

The employees came up with many ideas and insisted that he take the order. They approached it with a "We can do it" attitude, and the order was accepted, produced, and delivered on time.

An effective leader will…

Make People Part of the Decision

An old man was asked what had robbed him of joy in his life. His reply was, "Things that never happened."

—Dale Carnegie

12
LET THE OTHER PERSON SAVE FACE

Years ago the General Electric Company was faced with the delicate task of removing Charles Steinmetz from the head of a department. Steinmetz, a genius of the first magnitude when it came to electricity, was a failure as the head of the calculating department. Yet the company didn't dare offend the man. He was indispensable—and highly sensitive. So they gave him a new title. They made him consulting engineer of the General Electric Company—a new title for work he was already doing—and let someone else head the department.

Steinmetz was happy.

So were the officers of G.E. They had gently maneuvered their most temperamental star, and they had done it without a storm—by letting him save face.

Letting someone save face! How important, how vitally important, that is! And how few of us ever stop to think of it! We ride roughshod over the feelings of others, getting our own way, finding fault, issuing threats, criticizing a child or an employee in front of others, without even considering the hurt to the other person's pride. Whereas a few minutes' thought, a considerate word or two, a genuine understanding of the other person's attitude, would go so far toward alleviating the sting!

Let's remember this the next time we are faced with the

distasteful necessity of discharging or reprimanding an employee.

"Firing employees is not much fun. Getting fired is even less fun." (I'm quoting now from a letter written me by Marshall A. Granger, a certified public accountant.) "Our business is mostly seasonal. Therefore we have to let a lot of people go when the income tax rush is over.

"It's a byword in our profession that no one enjoys wielding the ax. Consequently, the custom has developed of getting it over as soon as possible, and usually in the following way: 'Sit down, Mr. Smith. The season's over, and we don't seem to see any more assignments for you. Of course, you understand you were employed only for the busy season anyhow, etc., etc.'

"The effect on these people is one of disappointment and a feeling of being 'let down.' Most of them are in the accounting field for life, and they retain no particular love for the firm that drops them so casually.

"I recently decided to let our seasonal personnel go with a little more tact and consideration. So I call each one in only after carefully thinking over his or her work during the winter. And I've said something like this: 'Mr. Smith, you've done a fine job (if he has). That time we sent you to Newark, you had a tough assignment. You were on the spot, but you came through with flying colors, and we want you to know the firm is proud of you. You've got the stuff—you're going a long way, wherever you're working. This firm believes in you, and is rooting for you, and we don't want you to forget it.'

"Effect? The people go away feeling a lot better about

being fired. They don't feel 'let down'. They know that if we had work for them, we'd keep them on. And when we need them again, they come to us with a keen personal affection."

At one session of our course, two class members discussed the negative effects of faultfinding versus the positive effects of letting the other person save face.

Fred Clark of Harrisburg, Pennsylvania, told of an incident that occurred in his company: "At one of our production meetings, a vice-president was asking very pointed questions of one of our production supervisors regarding a production process. His tone of voice was aggressive and aimed at pointing out faulty performance on the part of the supervisor. Not wanting to be embarrassed in front of his peers, the supervisor was evasive in his responses. This caused the vice-president to lose his temper, berate the supervisor, and accuse him of lying.

"Any working relationship that might have existed prior to this encounter was destroyed in a few brief moments. This supervisor, who was basically a good worker, was useless to our company from that time on. A few months later he left our firm and went to work for a competitor, where I understand he is doing a fine job."

Another class member, Anna Mazzone, related how a similar incident had occurred at her job—but what a difference in approach and results! Ms. Mazzone, a marketing specialist for a food packer, was given her first major assignment—the test marketing of a new product. She told the class: "When the results of the test came in, I was devastated. I had made a serious error in my planning, and the entire test had to be done all over again. To make this worse, I had no time to discuss it with my boss before the meeting in which I was to make my report on the project.

"When I was called on to give the report, I was shaking with fright. I had all I could do to keep from breaking down, but I resolved I would not cry and have all those men make remarks about women not being able to handle an assignment because they are too emotional. I made my report briefly and stated that due to an error I would repeat the study before the next meeting. I sat down, expecting my boss to blow up.

"Instead, he thanked me for my work and remarked that it was not unusual for a person to make an error on a new project and that he had confidence that the repeat survey would be accurate and meaningful to the company. He assured me, in front of my colleagues, that he had faith in me and knew I had done my best, and that my lack of experience, not my lack of ability, was the reason for the failure.

"I left that meeting with my head up in the air and with the determination that I would never let that boss of mine down again."

Even if we are right and the other person is definitely wrong, we only destroy ego by causing someone to lose face. The legendary French aviation pioneer and author Antoine de Saint-Exupéry wrote: "I have no right to say or do anything that diminishes a man in his own eyes. What matters is not what I think of him, but what he thinks of himself. Hurting a man in his dignity is a crime."

Let People Save Face

13

TALK ABOUT YOUR OWN MISTAKES FIRST

My niece, Josephine Carnegie, had come to New York to be my secretary. She was nineteen, had graduated from high school three years previously, and her business experience was a trifle more than zero. She became one of the most proficient secretaries west of Suez, but in the beginning, she was—well, susceptible to improvement. One day when I started to criticize her, I said to myself: "Just a minute, Dale Carnegie; just a minute. You are twice as old as Josephine. You have ten thousand times as much business experience. How can you possibly expect her to have your viewpoint, your judgment, your initiative—mediocre though they may be? And just a minute, Dale, what were you doing at nineteen? Remember the asinine mistakes and blunders you made? Remember the time you did this …and that…?"

After thinking the matter over, honestly and impartially, I concluded that Josephine's batting average at nineteen was better than mine had been—and that, I'm sorry to confess, isn't paying Josephine much of a compliment.

So after that, when I wanted to call Josephine's attention to a mistake, I used to begin by saying, "You have made a mistake, Josephine, but the Lord knows, it's no worse than many I have made. You were not born with judgment. That comes only with experience, and you are better than I was at your age. I have been guilty of so many stupid, silly things myself, I have very little inclination to criticize you or anyone. But don't you think it would have been wiser if you had done so and so?"

It isn't nearly so difficult to listen to a recital of your faults if the person criticizing begins by humbly admitting that he, too, is far from impeccable.

E. G. Dillistone, an engineer in Brandon, Manitoba, Canada, was having problems with his new secretary. Letters he dictated were coming to his desk for signature with two or three spelling mistakes per page. Mr. Dillistone reported how he handled this:

"Like many engineers, I have not been noted for my excellent English or spelling. For years I have kept a little black thumb-index book for words I had trouble spelling. When it became apparent that merely pointing out the errors was not going to cause my secretary to do more proofreading and dictionary work, I resolved to take another approach. When the next letter came to my attention that had errors in it, I sat down with the typist and said:

"'Somehow this word doesn't look right. It's one of the words I always have had trouble with. That's the reason I started this spelling book of mine. (I opened the book to the appropriate page.) Yes, here it is. I'm very conscious of the spelling now because people do judge us by our letters, and misspellings make us look less professional.'

"I don't know whether she copied my system or not, but since that conversation, her frequency of spelling errors has been significantly reduced."

The polished Prince Bernhard von Bülow learned the sharp necessity of doing this back in 1909. Von Bülow was then the imperial chancellor of Germany, and on the throne sat Wilhelm II—Wilhelm, the haughty; Wilhelm, the arrogant; Wilhelm, the last of the German kaisers, building an army and navy that he boasted could whip their weight in wildcats.

Then an astonishing thing happened. The kaiser said things, incredible things, things that rocked the continent and started a series of explosions heard around the world. To make matters worse, the kaiser made silly, egotistical, absurd announcements in public. He made them while he was a guest in England, and he gave his royal permission to have them printed in the *Daily Telegraph*. For example, he declared that he was the only German who felt friendly toward the English; that he was constructing a navy against the menace of Japan; that he, and he alone, had saved England from being humbled in the dust by Russia and France; that it had been *his* campaign plan that enabled England's Lord Roberts to defeat the Boers in South Africa; and so on and on.

No other such amazing words had ever fallen from the lips of a European king in peacetime within a hundred years. The entire continent buzzed with the fury of a hornet's nest. England was incensed. German statesmen were aghast. And in the midst of all this consternation, the kaiser became panicky and suggested to Prince von Bülow, the imperial chancellor, that he take the blame. Yes, he wanted von Bülow to announce that it was all his responsibility, that he had advised his monarch to say these incredible things.

"But Your Majesty," von Bülow protested, "it seems to me utterly impossible that anybody either in Germany or England could suppose me capable of having advised Your Majesty to say any such thing."

The moment those words were out of von Bülow's mouth, he realized he had made a grave mistake. The Kaiser blew up.

"You consider me a donkey," he shouted, "capable of blunders you yourself could never have committed."

Von Bülow knew that he ought to have praised before he condemned; but since it was too late, he did the next best thing. He praised after he had criticized. And it worked a miracle.

"I'm far from suggesting that," he answered respectfully. "Your Majesty surpasses me in many respects; not only, of course, in naval and military knowledge, but above all, in natural science. I have often listened in admiration when Your Majesty explained the barometer, or wireless telegraphy, or the Roentgen rays. I am shamefully ignorant of all branches of natural science, have no notion of chemistry or physics, and am quite incapable of explaining the simplest of natural phenomena. But," von Bülow continued, "in compensation, I possess some historical knowledge and perhaps certain qualities useful in politics, especially in diplomacy."

The kaiser beamed. Von Bülow had praised him. Von Bülow had exalted him and humbled himself. The kaiser could forgive anything after that. "Haven't I always told you," he exclaimed with enthusiasm, "that we complete one another famously? We should stick together, and we will!"

He shook hands with von Bülow, not once, but several times. And later in the day he waxed so enthusiastic that he exclaimed with doubled fists, "If anyone says anything to me against Prince von Bülow, *I shall punch him in the nose.*"

Von Bülow saved himself in time—but, canny diplomat that he was, he nevertheless had made one error: he should have *begun* by talking about his own shortcomings and Wilhelm's superiority—not by intimating that the kaiser was a half-wit in need of a guardian.

If a few sentences humbling oneself and praising the other party can turn a haughty, insulted kaiser into a staunch friend, imagine what humility and praise can do for you and me in our daily contacts. Rightly used, they will work veritable miracles in human relations.

Admitting one's own mistakes—even when one hasn't corrected them—can help convince somebody to change his or her behavior. This was illustrated more recently by Clarence Zerhusen of Timonium, Maryland, when he discovered his fifteen-year-old son was experimenting with cigarettes.

"Naturally, I didn't want David to smoke," Mr. Zerhusen told us, "but his mother and I smoked cigarettes; we were giving him a bad example all the time. I explained to Dave how I started smoking at about his age and how the nicotine had gotten the best of me and now it was nearly impossible for me to stop. I reminded him how irritating my cough was and how he had been after me to give up cigarettes not many years before. I didn't exhort him to stop or make threats or warn him about their dangers. All I did was point out how I was hooked on cigarettes and what it had meant to me.

"He thought about it for a while and decided he wouldn't smoke until he had graduated from high school. As the years went by David never did start smoking and has no intention of ever doing so.

"As a result of that conversation I made the decision to stop smoking myself, and with the support of my family, I have succeeded."

Admit to Your Own Faults Before Pointing the Finger at Others

One of the most tragic things I know about human nature is that all of us tend to put off living. We are all dreaming of some magical rose garden over the horizon instead of enjoying the roses that are blooming outside our windows today.

—Dale Carnegie

PART II

STOP WORRYING

14

FOUR GOOD WORKING HABITS THAT WILL HELP PREVENT FATIGUE AND WORRY

GOOD WORKING HABIT NO. 1
Clear your desk of all papers except those relating to the immediate problem at hand.

Roland L. Williams, President of the Chicago and Northwestern Railway, once said, "A person with his desk piled high with papers on various matters will find his work much easier and more accurate if he clears that desk of all but the immediate problem on hand. I call this good housekeeping, and it is the number-one step toward efficiency."

If you visit the Library of Congress in Washington, D.C., you will find five words painted on the ceiling—five words written by the poet Pope:

"Order is Heaven's first law."

Order ought to be the first law of business, too. But is it? No, the average desk is cluttered up with papers that haven't been looked at for weeks. In fact, the publisher of a New Orleans newspaper once told me that his secretary cleared up one of his desks and found a typewriter that had been missing for two years!

The mere sight of a desk littered with unanswered mail and reports and memos is enough to breed confusion, tension, and worries. It is much worse than that. The constant reminder of "a million things to do and no time to do them" can worry you not only into tension and fatigue, but also into high blood pressure, heart trouble, and stomach ulcers.

Dr. John H. Stokes, professor, Graduate School of Medicine, University of Pennsylvania, read a paper before the National Convention of the American Medical Association—a paper entitled "Functional Neuroses as Complications of Organic Disease." In that paper, Dr. Stokes listed eleven conditions under the title: "What to Look for in the Patient's State of Mind." Here is the first item on that list:

> The sense of must or obligation; the unending stretch of things ahead that simply have to be done.

But how can such an elementary procedure as clearing your desk and making decisions help you avoid this high pressure, this sense of *must*, this sense of an "unending stretch of things ahead" that simply have to be done? Dr. William L. Sadler, the famous psychiatrist, told of a patient who, by using this simple device, avoided a nervous breakdown. The man was an executive in a big Chicago firm. When he came to Dr. Sadler's office, he was tense, nervous, worried. He knew he was heading for a tailspin, but he couldn't quit work. He had to have help.

"While this man was telling me his story," Dr. Sadler says, "my telephone rang. It was the hospital calling; and instead of deferring the matter, I took time right then to come to a decision. I always settle questions, if possible, right on the spot. I had no sooner hung up than the phone rang again. Again an urgent matter, which I took time to discuss. The third interruption came when a colleague of mine came to my office for advice on a patient who was critically ill. When I had finished with him, I turned to my caller and began to apologize for keeping him waiting. But he had brightened up. He had a completely different look on his face."

"Don't apologize, doctor!" this man said to Sadler. "In the last ten minutes, I think I've got a hunch as to what is wrong with me. I'm going back to my office and revise my working habits… But before I go, do you mind if I take a look in your desk?"

Dr. Sadler opened up the drawers of his desk. All empty—except for supplies. "Tell me," said the patient, "where do you keep your unfinished business?"

"Finished!" said Sadler.

"And where do you keep your unanswered mail?"

"Answered!" Sadler told him. "My rule is never to lay down a letter until I have answered it. I dictate the reply to my secretary at once."

Six weeks later, this same executive invited Dr. Sadler to come to his office. He was changed—and so was his desk. He opened the desk drawers to show there was no unfinished business inside of the desk. "Six weeks ago," this executive said, "I had three different desks in two different offices—and was snowed under by my work. I was never finished. After talking to you, I came back here and cleared out a wagonload of reports and old papers. Now I work at one desk, settle things as they come up, and don't have a mountain of unfinished business nagging at me and making me tense and worried. But the most astonishing thing is I've recovered completely. There is nothing wrong anymore with my health!"

Charles Evans Hughes, former Chief Justice of the United States Supreme Court, said: "Men do not die from overwork. They die from dissipation and worry." Yes, from dissipation of their energies—and worry because they never seem to get their work done.

GOOD WORKING HABIT NO. 2
Do things in the order of their importance.

Henry L. Doherty, founder of the nationwide Cities Service Company, said that regardless of how much salary he paid, there were two abilities he found it almost impossible to find.

Those two priceless abilities: first, the ability to think. Second, the ability to do things in the order of their importance.

Charles Luckman, the lad who started from scratch and climbed in twelve years to president of the Pepsodent Company, got a salary of a hundred thousand dollars a year, and made a million dollars besides—that lad declared that he owed much of his success to developing the two abilities that Henry L. Doherty said he found almost impossible to find. Charles Luckman said: "As far back as I can remember, I have gotten up at five o'clock in the morning because I can think better then than any other time—I can think better then and plan my day, plan to do things in the order of their importance."

Frank Bettger, one of America's most successful insurance salesmen, didn't wait until five o'clock in the morning to plan his day. He planned it the night before—set a goal for himself—a goal to sell a certain amount of insurance that day. If he failed, that amount was added to his next day—and so on.

I know from long experience that one is not always able to do things in the order of their importance, but I also know that some kind of plan to do first things first is infinitely better than extemporizing as you go along.

If George Bernard Shaw had not made it a rigid rule to do first things first, he would probably have failed as a writer and might have remained a bank cashier all his life. His plan called for writing five pages each day for nine heartbreaking years, even though he made a total of thirty dollars in those nine years—about a penny a day. Even Robinson Crusoe wrote out a schedule of what he would do each hour of the day.

GOOD WORKING HABIT NO. 3
When you face a problem, solve it then and there if you have the facts necessary to make a decision. Don't keep putting off decisions.

One of my former students, the late H. P. Howell, told me that when he was a member of the board of directors of U.S. Steel, the meetings of the board were often long-drawn-out affairs—many problems were discussed, few decisions were made. The result: each member of the board had to carry home bundles of reports to study.

Finally, Mr. Howell persuaded the board of directors to take up one problem at a time and come to a decision. No procrastination—no putting off. The decision might be to ask for additional facts; it might be to do something or to do nothing. But a decision was reached on each problem before passing on to the next. Mr. Howell told me that the results were striking and salutary: the docket was cleared. The calender was clean. No longer was it necessary for each member to carry home a bundle of reports. No longer was there a worried sense of unresolved problems.

A good rule, not only for the board of directors of U.S. Steel, but for you and me.

GOOD WORKING HABIT NO. 4
Learn to organize, deputize and supervise.

Many business persons are driving themselves to premature graves because they have never learned to delegate responsibility to others, insisting on doing everything themselves. Result: details and confusion overwhelm them. They are driven by a sense of hurry, worry, anxiety and tension. It is hard to learn to delegate responsibilities. I know. It was hard for me, awfully hard. I also know from experience the disasters that can be caused by delegating authority to the wrong people. But difficult as it is to delegate authority, executives must do it if they are to avoid worry, tension and fatigue.

Executives who build up big businesses and don't learn to organize, deputize and supervise usually pop off with heart trouble in their fifties or early sixties—heart trouble caused by tension and worries. Want a specific instance? Look at the death notices in your local paper.

Our fatigue is often caused not by work, but by worry, frustration and resentment.

—Dale Carnegie

Only the prepared speaker deserves to be confident.

—Dale Carnegie.

15

HOW TO BANISH THE BOREDOM THAT PRODUCES FATIGUE, WORRY AND RESENTMENT

One of the chief causes of fatigue is boredom. To illustrate, let's take the case of Alice, an executive who lives on your street. Alice came home one night utterly exhausted. She *acted* fatigued. She *was* fatigued. She had a headache. She had a backache. She was so exhausted she wanted to go to bed without waiting for dinner. Her mother pleaded… She sat down at the table. The telephone rang. The boy friend! An invitation to a dance! Her eyes sparkled. Her spirits soared. She rushed upstairs, put on her Alice-Blue gown, and danced until three o'clock in the morning; and when she finally did get home, she was not the slightest bit exhausted. She was, in fact, so exhilarated she couldn't fall asleep.

Was Alice really and honestly tired eight hours earlier, when she looked and acted exhausted? Sure she was. She was exhausted because she was bored with her work, perhaps bored with life. There are millions of Alices. You may be one of them.

It is a well-known fact that your emotional attitude usually has far more to do with producing fatigue than has physical exertion. A few years ago, Joseph E. Barmack, Ph.D., published in the *Archives of Psychology* a report of some of his experiments, showing how boredom produces fatigue. Dr. Barmack put a group of students through a series of tests in which, he knew, they could have little interest. The result? The students felt tired and sleepy, complained of headaches and eyestrain, felt irritable. In some cases, even their stomachs were upset. Was it all "imagination"? No. Metabolism tests were taken of these students. These tests showed that the blood pressure of the body and the consumption of oxygen actually decrease when a person is bored, and that the whole metabolism picks up immediately as soon as he begins to feel interest and pleasure in his work!

We rarely get tired when we are doing something interesting and exciting. For example, I recently took a vacation in the Canadian Rockies up around Lake Louise. I spent several days trout fishing along Corral Creek, fighting my way through brush higher than my head, stumbling over logs, struggling through fallen timber—yet after eight hours of this, I was not exhausted. Why? Because I was excited, exhilarated. I had a sense of high achievement: six cut-throat trout. But suppose I had been bored by fishing, then how do you think I would have felt? I would have been worn out by such strenuous work at an altitude of seven thousand feet.

Even in such exhausting activities as mountain climbing, boredom may tire you far more than the strenuous work involved. For example, Mr. S. H. Kingman, president of the Farmers and Mechanics Savings Bank of Minneapolis, told me of an incident that is a perfect illustration of that statement. In July, 1953, the Canadian government asked the Canadian Alpine Club to furnish guides to train the members of the Prince of Wales Rangers in mountain climbing. Mr. Kingman was one of the guides chosen to train these soldiers. He told me how he and the other guides—men ranging from forty-two to fifty-nine years of age—took these young army men on long hikes across glaciers and snow fields and up a sheer cliff of forty feet, where they had to climb with ropes and tiny footholds and precarious handholds. They climbed Michael's Peak, the Vice-President Peak, and other unnamed peaks in the Little Yoho Valley in the Canadian Rockies. After fifteen hours of mountain climbing, these young men, who were in the pink of condition (they had just finished a six-week course in tough Commando training), were utterly exhausted.

Was their fatigue caused by using muscles that had not been hardened by Commando training? Anyone who had ever been through Commando training would hoot at such a ridiculous question! No, they were utterly exhausted because they were bored by mountain climbing. They were so tired that many of them fell asleep without waiting to eat. But the guides—men who were two and three times as old as the soldiers—were they tired? Yes, but not exhausted. The guides ate dinner and stayed up for hours, talking about the day's experiences. They were not exhausted because they were interested.

When Dr. Edward Thorndike of Columbia was conducting experiments in fatigue, he kept young men awake for almost a week by keeping them constantly interested. After much investigation, Dr. Thorndike is reported to have said: "Boredom is the only real cause of diminution of work."

If you are a mental worker, it is seldom the amount of work you do that makes you tired. You may be tired by the amount of work you do *not* do. For example, remember the day last week when you were constantly interrupted. No letters answered. Appointments broken. Trouble here and there. Everything went wrong that day. You accomplished nothing whatever, yet you went home exhausted—and with a splitting head.

The next day everything clicked at the office. You accomplished forty times more than you did the previous day. Yet you went home fresh as a snowy-white gardenia. You have had that experience. So have I.

The lesson to be learned? Just this: our fatigue is often caused not by work, but by worry, frustration, and resentment.

While writing this chapter, I went to see a revival of Jerome Kern's delightful musical comedy *Show Boat*. Captain Andy, captain of the *Cotton Blossom*, says in one of his philosophical interludes: "The lucky folks are the ones that get to do things they enjoy doing." Such folk are lucky because they have more energy, more happiness, less worry and less fatigue. Where your interests are, there is your energy also. Walking ten blocks with a nagging wife or husband can be more fatiguing than walking ten miles with an adoring sweetheart.

And so what? What can you do about it? Well, here is what one stenographer did about it—a stenographer working for an oil company in Tulsa, Oklahoma. For several days each month, she had one of the dullest jobs imaginable: filling out printed forms for oil leases, inserting figures and statistics. This task was so boring that she resolved, in self-defense, to make it interesting. How? She had a daily contest with herself. She counted the number of forms she filled out each morning, and then tried to excel that record in the afternoon. She counted each day's total and tried to better it the next day. Result? She was soon able to fill out more of these dull printed forms than any other stenographer in her division. And what did all this get her? Praise? No... Thanks? No... Promotion? No... Increased pay? No... But it did help to prevent the fatigue that is spawned by boredom. It did give her a mental stimulant. Because she had done her best to make a dull job interesting, she had more energy, more zest, and got far more happiness out of her leisure hours.

I happen to know this story is true, because I married that girl.

Here is the story of another stenographer who found it paid to act *as if* her work were interesting. She used to fight her work. But no more. She is Miss Vallie G. Golden, of Elmhurst, Illinois. Here is her story, as she wrote it to me:

"There are four stenographers in my office and each of us is assigned to take letters from several men. Once in a while we get jammed up in these assignments. One day, when an assistant department head insisted that I do a long letter over, I started to rebel. I tried to point out to him that the letter could be corrected without being retyped—and he retorted that if I didn't do it over, he would find someone else who would! I was absolutely fuming! But as I started to retype this letter, it suddenly occurred to me that there were a lot of other people who would jump at the chance to do the work I was doing. Also, that I was being paid a salary to do just that work. I began to feel better. I suddenly made up my mind to do my work as if I actually enjoyed it—even though I despised it. Then I made this important discovery: if I do my work *as if* I really enjoy it, then I do enjoy it to some extent. I also found I can work faster when I enjoy my work. So there is seldom any need now for me to work overtime. This new attitude of mine gained me the reputation of being a good worker. And when one of the department superintendents needed a private secretary, he asked for me for the job—because, he said, I was willing to do extra work without being sulky! This matter of the power of a changed mental attitude," wrote Miss Golden, "has been a tremendously important discovery to me. It has worked wonders!"

Miss Golden used the wonder-working "as if" philosophy of Professor Hans Vaihinger. He taught us to act "as if" we were happy—and so on.

If you act "as if" you are interested in your job, that bit of acting will tend to make your interest real. It will also tend to decrease your fatigue, your tensions, and your worries.

A few years ago, Harlan A. Howard made a decision that completely altered his life. He resolved to make a dull job interesting—and he certainly had a dull one:

washing plates, scrubbing counters, and dishing out ice cream in the high-school lunchroom while the other boys were playing ball or kidding the girls. Harlan Howard despised his job—but since he had to stick to it, he resolved to study ice cream—how it was made, what ingredients were used, why some ice creams were better than others. He studied the chemistry of ice cream, and became a whiz in the high-school chemistry course. He was so interested now in food chemistry that he entered the Massachusetts State College and majored in the field of "food technology." When the New York Cocoa Exchange offered a hundred-dollar prize for the best paper on uses of cocoa and chocolate—a prize open to all college students—who do you suppose won it? ...That's right. Harlan Howard.

When he found it difficult to get a job, he opened a private laboratory in the basement of his home in Amherst, Massachusetts. Shortly after that, a new law was passed. The bacteria in milk had to be counted. Harlan A. Howard was soon counting bacteria for the fourteen milk companies in Amherst—and he had to hire two assistants.

Where will he be twenty-five years from now? Well, the men who are now running the business of food chemistry will be retired then, or dead; and their places will be taken by young lads who are now radiating initiative and enthusiasm. Twenty-five years from now, Harlan A. Howard will probably be one of the leaders in his profession, while some of his classmates to whom he used to sell ice cream over the counter will be sour, unemployed, cussing the government, and complaining that they never had a chance. Harlan A. Howard might never have had a chance, either, if he hadn't resolved to make a dull job interesting.

Years ago, there was another young man who was bored with his dull job of standing at a lathe, turning out bolts in a factory. His first name was Sam. Sam wanted to quit, but he was afraid he couldn't find another job. Since he had to do this dull work, Sam decided he would make it interesting. So he ran a race with the mechanic operating a machine beside him. One of them was to trim off the rough surfaces on his machine, and the other was to trim the bolts down to the proper diameter. They would switch machines occasionally and see who could turn out the most bolts. The foreman, impressed with Sam's speed and accuracy, soon gave him a better job. That was the start of a whole series of promotions. Thirty years later, Sam— Samuel Vauclain—was president of the Baldwin Locomotive Works. But he might have remained a mechanic all his life if he had not resolved to make a dull job interesting.

H. V. Kaltenborn—the famous radio news analyst— once told me how he made a dull job interesting. When he was twenty-two years old, he worked his way across the Atlantic on a cattle boat, feeding and watering the steers. After making a bicycle tour of England, he arrived in Paris, hungry and broke. Pawning his camera for five dollars, he put an ad in the Paris edition of *The New York Herald* and got a job selling stereopticon machines. I can remember those old-fashioned stereoscopes that we used to hold up before our eyes to look at two pictures exactly alike. As we looked, a miracle happened. The two lenses in the stereoscope transformed the two pictures into a single scene with the effect of a third dimension. We saw distance. We got an astounding sense of perspective.

Well, as I was saying, Kaltenborn started out selling these machines from door to door in Paris—and he couldn't speak French. But he earned five thousand dollars in commissions the first year, and made himself one of the highest-paid salesmen in France that year. H. V. Kaltenborn told me that this experience did as much to develop within him the qualities that make for success as did any single year of study at Harvard. Confidence? He told me himself that after that experience, he felt he could have sold *The Congressional Record* to French housewives.

That experience gave him an intimate understanding of French life that later proved invaluable in interpreting, on the radio, European events.

How did he manage to become an expert salesman when he couldn't speak French? Well, he had his employer write out his sales talk in perfect French, and he memorized it. He would ring a doorbell, a housewife would answer, and Kaltenborn would begin repeating his memorized sales talk with an accent so terrible it was funny. He would show the housewife his pictures, and when she asked a question, he would shrug his shoulders and say, "An American …an American." He would then take off his hat and point to a copy of the sales talk in perfect French that he had pasted in the top of his hat. The housewife would laugh, he would laugh—and show her more pictures. When H. V. Kaltenborn told me about this, he confessed that the job had been far from easy. He told me that there was only one quality that pulled him through: his determination to make the job interesting. Every morning before he started out, he looked into the mirror and gave himself a pep talk: *"Kaltenborn, you have to do this if you want to eat. Since you have to do it—why not have a good time doing it? Why not imagine every time you ring a doorbell that you are an actor before the footlights and that there's an audience out there looking at you? After all, what you are doing is just as funny as something on the stage. So why not put a lot of zest and enthusiasm into it?"*

Mr. Kaltenborn told me that these daily pep talks helped him transform a task that he had once hated and dreaded into an adventure that he liked and made highly profitable.

When I asked Mr. Kaltenborn if he had any advice to give to the young men of America who are eager to succeed, he said: "Yes, go to bat with yourself every morning. We talk a lot about the importance of physical exercise to wake us up out of the half-sleep in which so many of us walk around. But we need, even more, some spiritual and mental exercises every morning to stir us into action. Give yourself a pep talk every day."

Is giving yourself a pep talk every day silly, superficial, childish? No, on the contrary, it is the very essence of sound psychology. "Our life is what our thoughts make it." These words are just as true today as they were eighteen centuries ago when Marcus Aurelius first wrote them in his book on *Meditations*: "Our life is what our thoughts make it."

By talking to yourself every hour of the day, you can direct yourself to think thoughts of courage and happiness, thoughts of power and peace. By talking to yourself about the things you have to be grateful for, you can fill your mind with thoughts that soar and sing.

By thinking the right thoughts, you can make any job less distasteful. Your boss wants you to be interested in your job so that he or she will make more money. But let's forget about what the boss wants. Think only of what getting interested in your job will do for you. Remind yourself that it may double the amount of happiness you get out of life, for you spend about one half of your waking hours at your work, and if you don't find happiness in your work, you may never find it anywhere. Keep reminding yourself that getting interested in your job will take your mind off your worries, and, in the long run, will probably bring promotion and increased pay. Even if it doesn't do that, it will reduce fatigue to a minimum and help you enjoy your hours of leisure.

People rarely succeed unless they have fun in what they are doing.

—Dale Carnegie

Remember happiness doesn't depend upon who you are or what you have; it depends solely on what you think.

—Dale Carnegie

16

FIND YOURSELF AND BE YOURSELF

I have a letter from Mrs. Edith Allred, of Mount Airy, North Carolina: "As a child, I was extremely sensitive and shy," she says in her letter. "I was always overweight and my cheeks made me look even fatter than I was. I had an old-fashioned mother who thought it was foolish to make clothes look pretty. She always said: 'Wide will wear while narrow will tear'; and she dressed me accordingly. I never went parties; never had any fun; and when I went to school, I never joined the other children in outside activities, not even athletics. I was morbidly shy. I felt I was 'different' from everybody else and entirely undesirable.

"When I grew up, I married a man who was several years my senior. But I didn't change. My in-laws were a poised and self-confident family. They were everything I should have been but simply was not. I tried my best to be like them, but I couldn't. Every attempt they made to draw me out of myself only drove me further into my shell. I became nervous and irritable. I avoided all friends. I got so bad I even dreaded the sound of the doorbell ringing! I was a failure. I knew it; and I was afraid my husband would find it out. So, whenever we were in public, I tried to be gay, and overacted my part. I knew I overacted; and I would be miserable for days afterwards. At last I became so unhappy that I could see no point in prolonging my existence. I began to think of suicide."

What happened to change this unhappy woman's life? Just a chance remark!

"A chance remark," Mrs. Allred continued, "transformed my whole life. My mother-in-law was talking one day of how she brought her children up, and she said, 'No matter what happened, I always insisted on their being themselves.' ...'On being themselves.' ...That remark is what did it! In a flash, I realized I had brought all this misery on myself by trying to fit myself into a pattern to which I did not conform.

"I changed overnight! I started being myself. I tried to make a study of my own personality. Tried to find out *what I was*. I studied my strong points. I learned all I could about colors and styles, and dressed in a way that I felt was becoming to me. I reached out to make friends. I joined an organization—a small one at first—and was petrified with fright when they put me on a program. But each time I spoke, I gained a little courage. It took a long while—but today I have more happiness than I ever dreamed possible. In rearing my own children, I have always taught them the lesson I had to learn from such bitter experience: *No matter what happens, always be yourself!*"

This problem of being unwilling to be yourself is "as old as history," says Dr. James Gordon Gilkey, "and as universal as human life." This problem of being unwilling to be yourself is the hidden spring behind many neuroses and psychoses and complexes. Angelo Patri has written thirteen books and thousands of syndicated newspaper articles on the subject of child training, and he says: "Nobody is so miserable as he who longs to be somebody and something other than the person he is in body and mind."

This craving to be something you are not is especially rampant in Hollywood. Sam Wood, one of Hollywood's best-known directors, said the greatest headache he has with aspiring young actors is exactly this problem: to make them be themselves. They all want to be second-rate Lana Turners or third-rate Clark Gables. "The public has already had that flavor," Sam Wood keeps telling them; "now it wants something else."

Before he started directing such pictures as *Goodbye, Mr. Chips* and *For Whom the Bell Tolls*, Sam Wood spent years in the real-estate business, developing sales personalities. He declares that the same principles apply in the business world as in the world of moving pictures. You won't get anywhere playing the ape. You can't be a parrot. "Experience has taught me," says Sam Wood, "that it is safest to drop, as quickly as possible, people who pretend to be what they aren't."

I asked Paul Boynton, then employment director for a major oil company, what is the biggest mistake people make in applying for jobs. He ought to know: he has interviewed more than sixty thousand job seekers; and he has written a book entitled *6 Ways to Get a Job*. He replied: "The biggest mistake people make in applying for jobs is in not being themselves. Instead of taking their hair down and being completely frank, they often try to give you the answers they think you want." But it doesn't work, because nobody wants a phony. Nobody ever wants a counterfeit coin.

A certain daughter of a streetcar conductor had to learn that lesson the hard way. She longed to be a singer. But her face was her misfortune. She had a large mouth and protruding buck teeth. When she first sang in public—in a New Jersey night club—she tried to pull down her upper lip to cover her teeth. She tried to act "glamorous." The results? She made herself ridiculous. She was headed for failure.

However, there was a man in this night club who heard the girl sing and thought she had talent. "See here," he said bluntly, "I've been watching your performance and I know what it is you're trying to hide. You're ashamed of your teeth!" The girl was embarrassed, but the man continued, "What of it? Is there any particular crime in having buck teeth? Don't try to hide them! Open your mouth, and the audience will love you when they see you're not ashamed. Besides," he said shrewdly, "those teeth you're trying to hide may make your fortune!"

Cass Daley took his advice and forgot about her teeth. From that time on, she thought only about her audience. She opened her mouth wide and sang with such gusto and enjoyment that she became a top star in movies and radio. Other comedians tried to copy her!

The renowned William James was speaking of people who had never found themselves when he declared that the average person develops only ten percent of his or her latent mental abilities. "Compared to what we ought to be," he wrote, "we are only half awake. We are making use of only a small part of our physical and mental resources. Stating the thing broadly, human individuals thus far live within their limits. They possess powers of various sorts which they habitually fail to use."

You and I have such abilities, so let's not waste a second worrying because we are not like other people. You are something new in this world. Never before, since the beginning of time, has there ever been anybody exactly like you; and never again throughout all the ages to come will there ever be anybody exactly like you again. The science of genetics informs us that you are what you are largely as a result of twenty-four chromosomes contributed by your father and twenty-four chromosomes contributed by your mother. These forty-eight chromosomes comprise everything that determines what you inherit. In each chromosome there may be, says Amram Scheinfeld, "anywhere from scores to hundreds of genes—with a single gene, in some cases, able to change the whole life of an individual." Truly, we are "fearfully and wonderfully" made.

Even after your mother and father met and mated, there was only one chance in 300,000 billion that the person who is specifically you would be born! In other words, if you had 300,000 billion brothers and sisters, they might all have been different from you. Is all this guesswork? No. It is a scientific fact. If you would like to read more about it, consult *You and Heredity*, by Amram Scheinfeld.

I can talk with conviction about this subject of being yourself because I feel deeply about it. I know what I am talking about. I know from bitter and costly experience. To illustrate: when I first came to New York from the cornfields of Missouri, I enrolled in the American Academy of Dramatic Arts. I aspired to be an actor. I had what I thought was a brilliant idea, a shortcut to success, an idea so simple, so foolproof, that I couldn't understand why thousands of ambitious people hadn't already discovered it. It was this: I would study how the famous actors of that day—John Drew, Walter Hampden, and Otis Skinner—got their effects. Then I would imitate the best points of each one of them and make myself into a shining, triumphant combination of all of them. How silly! How absurd! I had to waste years of my life imitating other people before it penetrated through my thick Missouri skull that I had to be myself, and that I couldn't possibly be anyone else.

That distressing experience ought to have taught me a lasting lesson. But it didn't. Not me. I was too dumb. I had to learn it all over again. Several years later, I set out to write what I hoped would be the best book on public speaking for businessmen that had ever been written. I had the same foolish idea about writing this book that I had formerly had about acting: I was going to *borrow* the ideas of a lot of other writers and put them all in one book—a book that would have everything. So I got scores of books on public speaking and spent a year incorporating their ideas into my manuscript. But it finally dawned on me once again that I was playing the fool. This hodgepodge of other men's ideas that I had written was so synthetic, so dull, that no businessman would ever plod through it. So I tossed a year's work into the wastebasket and started all over again. This time I said to myself: "You've got to be Dale Carnegie, with all his faults and limitations. You can't possibly be anybody else." So I quit trying to be a combination of other men, and rolled up my sleeves and did what I should have done in the first place: I wrote a textbook on public speaking out of my own experiences, observations, and convictions as a speaker and a teacher of speaking. I learned—for all time, I hope—the lesson that Sir Walter Raleigh learned. (I am *not* talking about the Sir Walter who threw his coat in the mud for the queen to step on. I am talking about the Sir Walter Raleigh who was professor of English literature at Oxford back in 1904.) "I can't write a book commensurate with Shakespeare," he said, "but I can write a book by me."

Be yourself. Act on the sage advice that Irving Berlin gave the late George Gershwin. When Berlin and Gershwin first met, Berlin was famous but Gershwin was a struggling young composer working for thirty-five dollars a week in Tin Pan Alley. Berlin, impressed by Gershwin's ability, offered Gershwin a job as his musical secretary at almost three times the salary he was then getting. "But don't take the job," Berlin advised. "If you do, you may develop into a second-rate Berlin. But if you insist on being yourself, someday you'll become a first-rate Gershwin."

Gershwin heeded that warning and slowly transformed himself into one of the significant American composers of his generation.

Charlie Chaplin, Will Rogers, Mary Margaret McBride, Gene Autry, and millions of others had to learn the lesson I am trying to hammer home in this chapter. They had to learn the hard way—just as I did.

When Charlie Chaplin first started making films, the director of the picture insisted on Chaplin's imitating a popular German comedian of that day. Charlie Chaplin got nowhere until he acted himself. Bob Hope had a similar experience: spent years in a singing-and-dancing act—and got nowhere until he began to wisecrack and be himself. Will Rogers twirled a rope in vaudeville for years without saying a word. He got nowhere until he discovered his unique gift for humor and began to talk as he twirled his rope.

When Mary Margaret McBride first went on the air, she tried to be an Irish comedian and failed. When she tried to be just what she was—a plain country girl from Missouri—she became one of the most popular radio stars in New York.

When Gene Autry tried to get rid of his Texas accent and dressed like city boys and claimed he was from New York, people merely laughed behind his back. But when he started twanging his banjo and singing cowboy ballads, Gene Autry started out on a career that made him the world's most popular cowboy both in pictures and on the radio.

You are something new in this world. Be glad of it. Make the most of what nature gave you. In the last analysis, all art is autobiographical. You can sing only what you are. You can paint only what you are. You must be what your experiences, your environment, and your heredity have made you. For better or for worse, you must cultivate your own little garden. For better or for worse, you must play your own little instrument in the orchestra of life.

As Emerson said in his essay on "Self-Reliance": "There is a time in every man's education when he arrives at the conviction that envy is ignorance; that imitation is suicide; that he must take himself for better, for worse, as his portion; that though the wide universe is full of good, no kernel of nourishing corn can come to him but through his toil bestowed on that plot of ground which is given to him to till. The power which resides in him is new in nature, and none but he knows what that is which he can do, nor does he know until he has tried."

That is the way Emerson said it. But here is the way a poet—the late Douglas Malloch—said it:

> If you can't be a pine on the top of the
> hill
>   Be a scrub in the valley—but be
> The best little scrub by the side of the
> rill;
>   Be a bush, if you can't be a tree.
>
> If you can't be a bush, be a bit of the
> grass,
>   And some highway happier make;
> If you can't be a muskie, then just be a
> bass—
>   But the liveliest bass in the lake!

*We can't all be captains, we've got to
be crew,*
    There's something for all of us here.
*There's big work to do and there's lesser
to do*
    And the task we must do is the near.

*If you can't be a highway, then just be
a trail,*
    If you can't be the sun, be a star;
*It isn't by size that you win or you
fail—*
    Be the best of whatever you are!

*Speakers who talk about what life has taught them
never fail to keep the attention of their listeners.*

—Dale Carnegie

*Success is getting what you want. Happiness is
wanting what you get.*

—Dale Carnegie

17

HOW TO OVERCOME TIREDNESS

Here is an astounding and significant fact: Mental work alone can't make you tired. Sounds absurd. But a few years ago, scientists tried to find out how long the human brain could labor without reaching "a diminished capacity for work," the scientific definition of fatigue. To the amazement of these scientists, they discovered that blood passing through the brain, when it is active, shows no fatigue at all! If you took blood from the veins of a day laborer while he was working, you would find it full of "fatigue toxins" and fatigue products. But if you took a drop of blood from the brain of an Albert Einstein, it would show no fatigue toxins whatever at the end of the day.

So far as the brain is concerned, it can work "as well and as swiftly at the end of eight or even twelve hours of effort as at the beginning." The brain is utterly tireless… So what makes you tired?

Psychiatrists declare that most of our fatigue derives from our mental and emotional attitudes. One of England's most distinguished psychiatrists, J. A. Hadfield, says in his book *The Psychology of Power*: "The greater part of the fatigue from which we suffer is of mental origin; in fact exhaustion of purely physical origin is rare."

One of America's most distinguished psychiatrists, Dr.

A. A. Brill, goes even further. He declares, "One hundred percent of the fatigue of the sedentary worker in good health is due to psychological factors, by which we mean emotional factors."

What kinds of emotional factors tire the sedentary (or sitting) worker? Joy? Contentment? No! Never! Boredom, resentment, a feeling of not being appreciated, a feeling of futility, hurry, anxiety, worry—those are the emotional factors that exhaust the sitting worker, make him susceptible to colds, reduce his output, and send him home with a nervous headache. Yes, we get tired because our emotions produce nervous tensions in the body.

The Metropolitan Life Insurance Company pointed that out in a leaflet on fatigue: "Hard work by itself," said this great life insurance company, "seldom causes fatigue which cannot be cured by a good sleep or rest… Worry, tenseness, and emotional upsets are three of the biggest causes of fatigue. Often they are to blame when physical or mental work seems to be the cause… Remember that a tense muscle is a working muscle. Ease up! Save energy for important duties."

Stop now, right where you are, and give yourself a checkup. As you read these lines, are you scowling at the book? Do you feel a strain between the eyes? Are you sitting relaxed in your chair? Or are you hunching up your shoulders? Are the muscles of your face tense? Unless your entire body is as limp and relaxed as an old rag doll, you are at this very moment producing nervous tensions and muscular tensions. *You are producing nervous tensions and nervous fatigue!*

Why do we produce these unnecessary tensions in

doing mental work? Daniel W. Josselyn said, "I find that the chief obstacle …is the almost universal belief that hard work requires a feeling of effort, else it is not well done." So we scowl when we concentrate. We hunch up our shoulders. We call on our muscles to make the motion of *effort*, which in no way assists our brain in its work.

Here is an astonishing and tragic truth: millions of people who wouldn't dream of wasting dollars go right on wasting and squandering their energy with the recklessness of seven drunken sailors in Singapore.

What is the answer to this nervous fatigue? Relax! Relax! Relax! Learn to relax while you are doing your work!

Easy? No. You will probably have to reverse the habits of a lifetime. But it is worth the effort, for it may revolutionize your life! William James said, in his essay "The Gospel of Relaxation": "The American overtension and jerkiness and breathlessness and intensity and agony of expression …are *bad habits*, nothing more or less." Tension is a habit. Relaxing is a habit. And bad habits can be broken, good habits formed.

How do you relax? Do you start with your mind, or do you start with your nerves? You don't start with either. You always begin to relax with your muscles!

Let's give it a try. To show how it is done, suppose we start with your eyes. Read this paragraph through, and when you've reached the end, lean back, close your eyes, *and say to your eyes* silently, "Let go. Let go. Stop straining, stop frowning. Let go. Let go." Repeat that over and over very slowly for a minute….

Didn't you notice that after a few seconds the muscles of the eyes *began to obey*? Didn't you feel as though some hand had wiped away the tension? Well, incredible as it seems, you have sampled in that one minute the whole key and secret to the art of relaxing. You can do the same thing with the jaw, with the muscles of the face, with the neck, with the shoulders, the whole of the body. But the most important organ of all is the eye. Dr. Edmund Jacobson of the University of Chicago has gone so far as to say that if you can completely relax the muscles of the eyes, you can forget all your troubles! The reason the eyes are so important in relieving nervous tension is that they burn up one fourth of all the nervous energies consumed by the body. That is also why so many people with perfectly sound vision suffer from "eyestrain." They are tensing the eyes.

Vicki Baum, the famous novelist, said that when she was a child, she met an old man who taught her one of the most important lessons she ever learned. She had fallen down and cut her knees and hurt her wrist. The old man picked her up. He had once been a circus clown, and as he brushed her off, he said, "The reason you injured yourself was because you don't know how to relax. You have to pretend you are as limp as a sock, as an old crumpled sock. Come, I'll show you how to do it."

That old man taught Vicki Baum and the other children how to fall, how to do flip-flops, and how to turn somersaults. And always he insisted, "Think of yourself as an old crumpled sock. Then you've *got* to relax!

You can relax in odd moments, almost anywhere you are. Only don't make an effort to relax. *Relaxation is the absence of all tension and effort.* Think ease and relaxation. Begin by thinking relaxation of the muscles of your eyes and your face, saying over and over, "Let go ...let go ... let go and relax." Feel the energy flowing out of your facial muscles to the center of your body. Think of yourself as being as free from tension as a baby.

That is what Galli-Curci, the great soprano, used to do. Helen Jepson told me that she used to see Galli-Curci before a performance, sitting in a chair with all her muscles relaxed and her lower jaw so limp it actually sagged. An excellent practice—it kept her from becoming too nervous before her stage entrance; it prevented fatigue.

Here are four suggestions that will help you learn to relax:

1. Relax in odd moments. Let your body go limp like an old sock. I keep an old, maroon-colored sock on my desk as I work—keep it there as a reminder of how limp I ought to be. If you haven't got a sock, a cat will do. Did you ever pick up a kitten sleeping in the sunshine? If so, both ends sagged like a wet newspaper. Even the yogis in India say that if you want to master the art of relaxation, study the cat. I never saw a tired cat, a cat with a nervous breakdown, or a cat suffering from insomnia, worry, or stomach ulcers. You will probably avoid these disasters if you learn to relax as the cat does.

2. Work, as much as possible, in a comfortable

position. Remember that tensions on the body produce aching shoulders and nervous fatigue.

3. Check yourself four or five times a day, and say to yourself, "Am I making my work harder than it actually is? Am I using muscles that have nothing to do with the work I am doing?" This will help you form the *habit* of relaxing, and as Dr. David Harold Fink says, "Among those who know psychology best, it is habits two to one."

4. Test yourself again at the end of the day, by asking yourself, "Just how tired am I? If I am tired, it is not because of the mental work I have done, but the way I have done it." "I measure my accomplishments," said Daniel W. Josselyn, "not by how tired I am at the end of the day, or when irritability proves that my nerves are tired, I know beyond question that it has been an inefficient day both as to quantity and quality." If every businessperson in America would learn that same lesson, our death rate from "hypertension" diseases would drop overnight. And we would stop filling up our sanitariums and asylums with people who have been broken by fatigue and worry.

Take a chance! All life is a chance. The man who goes farthest is generally the one who is willing to do and dare.

—Dale Carnegie

18

DO THIS AND CRITICISM CAN'T HURT YOU

I once interviewed Major General Smedley Butler—old "Gimlet-Eye." Old "Hell-Devil" Butler! Remember him? One of the most colorful, swashbuckling generals who ever commanded the United States Marines.

He told me that when he was young, he was desperately eager to be popular, wanted to make a good impression on everyone. In those days the slightest criticism smarted and stung. But he confessed that thirty years in the Marines had toughened his hide. "I have been berated and insulted," he said, "and denounced as a yellow dog, a snake, and a skunk. I have been cursed by the experts. I have been called every possible combination of unprintable, cuss words in the English language. Bother me? Huh! When I hear somebody cussing me now, I never turn my head to see who is talking."

Maybe old "Gimlet-Eye" Butler was too indifferent to criticism, but one thing is sure: most of us take the little jibes and javelins that are hurled at us far too seriously. I remember the time, years ago, when a reporter from the New York *Sun* attended a demonstration meeting of my adult-education classes and lampooned me and my work. Was I burned up? I took it as a personal insult. I telephoned Gil Hodges, the chairman of the Executive Committee of the *Sun* and practically demanded that he print an article stating the facts—instead of ridicule. I was determined to make the punishment fit the crime.

I am ashamed now of the way I acted. I realize now that half the people who bought the paper never saw that article. Half of those who read it regarded it as a source of innocent merriment. Half of those who gloated over it forgot all about it in a few weeks.

I realize now that people are not thinking about you and me or caring what is said about us. They are thinking about themselves—before breakfast, after breakfast, and right on until ten minutes past midnight. They would be a thousand times more concerned about a slight headache of their own than they would about the news of your death or mine.

Even if you and I are lied about, ridiculed, double-crossed, knifed in the back, and sold down the river by one out of every six of our most intimate friends—let's not indulge in an orgy of self-pity. Instead, let's remind ourselves that that's precisely what happened to Jesus. One of His twelve most intimate friends turned traitor for a bribe that would amount, in our modern money, to about nineteen dollars. Another one of His twelve most intimate friends openly deserted Jesus the moment He got into trouble, and declared three times that he didn't even know Jesus—and swore as he said it. One out of six! That is what happened to Jesus. Why should you and I expect a better score?

I discovered years ago that although I couldn't keep people from criticizing me unjustly, I could do something infinitely more important: I could determine whether I would let the unjust condemnation disturb me.

Let's be clear about this: I am not advocating ignoring all criticism. Far from it. I am talking about *ignoring only unjust criticism*. I once asked Eleanor Roosevelt how she handled unjust criticism—and Allah knows she had a lot of it. She probably had more ardent friends and more violent enemies than any other woman who ever lived in the White House.

She told me that as a young girl she was almost morbidly shy, afraid of what people might say. She was so afraid of criticism that one day she asked her aunt, Theodore Roosevelt's sister, for advice. She said: "Auntie Bye, I want to do so-and-so. But I'm afraid of being criticized."

Teddy Roosevelt's sister looked her in the eye and said: "Never be bothered by what people say, as long as you know in your heart you are right." Eleanor Roosevelt told me that that bit of advice proved to be her Rock of Gibraltar years later, when she was in the White House. She told me that the only way we can avoid all criticism is to be like a Dresden-china figure and stay on a shelf. "Do what you feel in your heart to be right—for you'll be criticized, anyway. You'll be 'damned if you do, and damned if you don't.'" That is her advice.

When the late Matthew C. Brush was president of the American International Corporation, I asked him if he was ever sensitive to criticism, and he replied, "Yes, I was very sensitive to it in my early days. I was eager then to have all the employees in the organization think I was perfect. If they didn't, it worried me. I would try to please first one person who had been sounding off against me; but the very thing I did to patch it up with him would make someone else mad. Then when I tried to fix it up with this person, I would stir up a couple of other bumblebees. I finally discovered that the more I tried to pacify and to smooth over injured feelings in order to escape personal criticism, the more certain I was to increase my enemies. So finally I said to myself, 'If you get your head above the crowd, you're going to be criticized. So get used to the idea.' That helped me tremendously. From that time on I made it a rule to do the very best I could and then put up my old umbrella and let the rain of criticism drain off me instead of run down my neck."

Deems Taylor went a bit further: he let the rain of criticism run down his neck and had a good laugh over it—in public. When he was giving his comments during the intermission of the Sunday-afternoon radio concerts of the New York Philharmonic Symphony Orchestra, one woman wrote him a letter calling him "a liar, a traitor, a snake, and a moron." Mr. Taylor says in his book, *Of Men and Music*: "I have a suspicion that she didn't care for that talk." On the following week's broadcast, Mr. Taylor read this letter over the radio to millions of listeners—and received another letter from the same lady a few days later, "expressing her unaltered opinion," says Mr. Taylor, "that I was *still* a liar, a traitor, a snake, and a moron." We can't keep from admiring a man who takes criticism like that. We admire his serenity, his unshaken poise, and his sense of humor.

When Charles Schwab was addressing the student body at Princeton, he confessed that one of the most important lessons he had ever learned was taught to him by an old German who worked in Schwab's steel mill. This old German got involved in a hot wartime argument with the other steelworkers, and they tossed him into the river. "When he came into my office," Mr. Schwab said, "covered with mud and water, I asked him what he had said to the men who had thrown him into the river, and he replied, 'I just laughed.'"

Mr. Schwab declared that he had adopted that old German's words as his motto: "Just laugh."

That motto is especially good when you are the victim of unjust criticism. You can answer the man who answers you back, but what can you say to the man who "just laughs"?

Lincoln might have broken under the strain of the Civil War if he hadn't learned the folly of trying to answer all the vitriolic condemnations hurled at him. His description of how he handled his critics has become a literary gem—a classic. General MacArthur had a copy of it hanging above his headquarters desk during the war, and Winston Churchill had a framed copy of it on the wall of his study at Chartwell. It goes like this: "If I were to try to read, much less to answer, all the attacks made on me, this shop might as well be closed for any other business. I do the very best I know how—the very best I can; and I mean to keep on doing so until the end. If the end brings me out all right, then what is said against me won't matter; if the end brings me out wrong, then ten angels swearing I was right would make no difference."

If you want to gather honey, don't kick over the beehive.

—Dale Carnegie

19

WOULD YOU TAKE A MILLION DOLLARS
FOR WHAT YOU HAVE?

I have known Harold Abbott for years. He lived in Webb City, Missouri. He used to be my lecture manager. One day he and I met in Kansas City and he drove me down to my farm at Belton, Missouri. During that drive, I asked him how he kept from worrying, and he told me an inspiring story that I shall never forget.

"I used to worry a lot," he said, "but one spring day in 1934, I was walking down West Dougherty Street in Webb City when I saw a sight that banished all my worries. It all happened in ten seconds, but during those ten seconds I learned more about how to live than I had learned in the previous ten years. For two years I had been running a grocery store in Webb City." Harold Abbott said, as he told me the story, "I had not only lost all my savings, but I had incurred debts that took me seven years to pay back. My grocery store had been closed the previous Saturday; and now I was going to the Merchants and Miners Bank to borrow money so I could go to Kansas City to look for a job. I walked like a beaten man. I had lost all my fight and faith. Then suddenly I saw coming down the street a man who had no legs. He was sitting on a little wooden platform equipped with wheels from roller skates. He propelled himself along the street with a block of wood in each hand. I met him just after he had crossed the street and was starting to lift himself up a few inches over the curb to the sidewalk. As he tilted his little wooden platform to an angle, his eyes met mine. He greeted me with a grand smile. 'Good morning, sir. It is a fine morning, isn't it?' he said with spirit. As I stood looking at him, I realized how rich I was. I had two legs. I could walk. I felt ashamed of my self-pity. I said to myself, if he can be happy, cheerful, and confident without legs, I certainly can with legs. I could already feel my chest lifting. I had intended to ask the Merchants and Miners Bank for only one hundred dollars. But now I had courage to ask for *two* hundred. I had intended to say that I wanted to go to Kansas City to *try* to get a job. But now I announced confidently that I wanted to go to Kansas City to *get* a job. I got the loan; and I got the job.

I now have the following words pasted on my bathroom mirror, and I read them every morning as I shave:

> *I had the blues because I had no shoes,*
> *Until upon the street, I met a man who had no feet.*

I once asked Eddie Rickenbacker what was the biggest lesson he had learned from drifting about with his companions in life rafts for twenty-one days, hopelessly lost in the Pacific. "The biggest lesson I learned from that experience," he said, "was that if you have all the fresh water you want to drink and all the food you want to eat, you ought never to complain about anything."

Time ran an article about a sergeant who had been wounded on Guadalcanal. Hit in the throat by a shell fragment, this sergeant had had seven blood transfusions. Writing a note to his doctor, he asked: "Will I live?" The doctor replied: "Yes." He wrote another note, asking, "Will I be able to talk?" Again the answer was yes. He then wrote another note, saying: "Then what in the hell am I worrying about?"

Why don't you stop right now and ask yourself, "What in the hell am I worrying about?" You will probably find that it is comparatively unimportant and insignificant.

About ninety percent of the things in our lives are right and about ten percent are wrong. If we want to be happy, all we have to do is to concentrate on the ninety percent that are right and ignore the ten percent that are wrong. If we want to be worried and bitter and have stomach ulcers, all we have to do is to concentrate on the ten percent that are wrong and ignore the ninety percent that are glorious.

The words "Think and Thank" are inscribed in many of the Cromwellian churches of England. These words ought to be inscribed on our hearts, too: "Think and Thank." Think of all we have to be grateful for, and thank God for all our boons and bounties.

Jonathan Swift, author of *Gulliver's Travels*, was the most devastating pessimist in English literature. He was so sorry that he had been born that he wore black and fasted on his birthdays; yet, in his despair, this supreme pessimist of English literature praised the great health-giving powers of cheerfulness and happiness. "The best doctors in the world," he declared, "are Doctor Diet, Doctor Quiet, and Doctor Merryman."

You and I may have the services of "Doctor Merryman" free every day by keeping our attention fixed on all the incredible riches we possess—riches exceeding by far the fabled treasures of Ali Baba. Would you sell both your eyes for a billion dollars? What would you take for your two legs? Your hands? Your hearing? Your children? Your family? Add up your assets, and you will find that you won't sell what you have for all the gold ever amassed by the Rockefellers, the Fords, and the Morgans combined.

But do we appreciate all this? Ah, no. As Schopenhauer said: "We seldom think of what we have but always of what we lack." Yes, the tendency to "seldom think of what we have but always of what we lack" is the greatest tragedy on earth. It has probably caused more misery than all the wars and diseases in history.

It caused John Palmer to turn "from a regular guy into an old grouch," and almost wrecked his home. I know because he told me so.

Mr. Palmer lived in Paterson, New Jersey. "Shortly after I returned from the Army," he said, "I started in business for myself. I worked hard day and night. Things were going nicely. Then trouble started. I couldn't get parts and materials. I was afraid I would have to give up my business. I worried so much that I changed from a regular guy into an old grouch. I became so sour and cross that—well, I didn't know it then but I now realize that I came very near to losing my happy home. Then one day a young, disabled veteran who works for me said, 'Johnny, you ought to be ashamed of yourself. You take on as if you were the only person in the world with troubles. Suppose you do have to shut up shop for a while—so what? You can start up again when things get normal. You've got a lot to be thankful for. Yet you are always growling. Boy, how I wish I were in your shoes! Look at me. I've got only one arm, and half of my face is shot away, and yet I am not complaining. If you don't stop your growling and grumbling, you will lose not only your business, but also your health, your home, and your friends!'

"Those remarks stopped me dead in my tracks. They made me realize how well off I was. I resolved then and there that I would change and be my old self again—and I did."

A friend of mine, Lucile Blake, had to tremble on the edge of tragedy before she learned to be happy about what she had instead of worrying over what she lacked.

I met Lucile years ago, when we were both studying short-story writing in the Columbia University School of Journalism. Some years ago, she got the shock of her life. She was living then in Tucson, Arizona. She had—well, here is the story as she told it to me:

"I had been living in a whirl: studying the organ at the University of Arizona, conducting a speech clinic in town, and teaching a class in musical appreciation at the Desert Willow Ranch, where I was staying. I was going in for parties, dances, horseback rides under the stars. One morning I collapsed. My heart! 'You will have to lie in bed for a year of complete rest,' the doctor said. He didn't encourage me to believe I would ever be strong again.

"In bed for a year! To be an invalid—perhaps to die! I was terror-stricken! Why did all this have to happen to me? What had I done to deserve it? I wept and wailed. I was bitter and rebellious. But I did go to bed as the doctor advised. A neighbor of mine, Mr. Rudolf, an artist, said to me, 'You think now that spending a year in bed will be a tragedy. But it won't be. You will have time to think and get acquainted with yourself. You will make more spiritual growth in these next few months than you have made during all your previous life.' I became calmer, and tried to develop a new sense of values. I read books of inspiration. One day I heard a radio commentator say: 'You can express only what is in your own consciousness.' I had heard words like these many times before, but now they reached down inside me and took root. I resolved to think only the thoughts I wanted to live by: thoughts of joy, happiness, health. I forced myself each morning, as soon as I awoke, to go over all the things I had to be grateful for. No pain. A lovely young daughter. My eyesight. My hearing. Lovely music on the radio. Time to read. Good food. Good friends. I was so cheerful and had so many visitors that the doctor put up a sign saying that only one visitor at a time would be allowed in my cabin—and only at certain hours.

"Many years have passed since then, and I now lead a full, active life. I am deeply grateful now for that year I spent in bed. It was the most valuable and the happiest year I spent in Arizona. The habit I formed then of counting my blessings each morning still remains with me. It is one of my most precious possessions. I am ashamed to realize that I never really learned to live until I feared I was going to die."

My dear Lucile Blake, you may not realize it, but you learned the same lesson that Dr. Samuel Johnson learned two hundred years ago. "The habit of looking on the best side of every event," said Dr. Johnson, "is worth more than a thousand pounds a year."

Those words were uttered, mind you, not by a professional optimist, but by a man who had known anxiety, rags, and hunger for twenty years—and finally became one of the most eminent writers of his generation and the most celebrated conversationalist of all time.

Logan Pearsall Smith packed a lot of wisdom into a few words when he said: "There are two things to aim at in life: first, to get what you want; and, after that, to enjoy it. Only the wisest of mankind achieve the second."

Would you like to know how to make even dishwashing at the kitchen sink a thrilling experience? If so, read an inspiring book of incredible courage by Borghild Dahl. It is called *I Wanted to See*.

This book was written by a woman who was practically blind for half a century. "I had only one eye," she writes, "and it was so covered with dense scars that I had to do all my seeing through one small opening in the left of the eye. I could see a book only by holding it up close to my face and by straining my one eye as hard as I could to the left."

But she refused to be pitied, refused to be considered "different." As a child, she wanted to play hopscotch with other children, but she couldn't see the markings. So after the other children had gone home, she got down on the ground and crawled along with her eyes near the marks. She memorized every bit of the ground where she and her friends played and soon became an expert at running games. She did her reading at home, holding a book of large print so close to her eyes that her eyelashes brushed the pages. She earned two college degrees: a B.A. from the University of Minnesota and a Master of Arts from Columbia University.

She started teaching in the tiny village of Twin Valley, Minnesota, and rose until she became professor of journalism and literature at Augustana College in Sioux Falls, South Dakota. She taught there for thirteen years, lecturing before women's clubs and giving radio talks about books and authors. "In the back of my mind," she writes, "there had always lurked a fear of total blindness. In order to overcome this, I had adopted a cheerful, almost hilarious, attitude toward life."

Then in 1943, when she was fifty-two years old, a miracle happened: an operation at the famous Mayo Clinic. She could now see forty times as well as she had ever been able to see before.

A new and exciting world of loveliness opened before her. She now found it thrilling even to wash dishes in the kitchen sink. "I begin to play with the white fluffy suds in the dishpan," she writes. "I dip my hands into them and I pick up a ball of tiny soap bubbles. I hold them up against the light, and in each of them I can see the brilliant colors of a miniature rainbow."

As she looked through the window above the kitchen sink, she saw "the flapping gray-black wings of the sparrows flying through the thick, falling snow."

She found such ecstasy looking at the soap bubbles and sparrows that she closed her book with these words: "'Dear Lord,' I whisper. Our Father in Heaven, I thank Thee. I thank Thee.'"

Imagine thanking God because you can wash dishes and see rainbows in bubbles and sparrows flying through the snow!

You and I ought to be ashamed of ourselves. All the days of our years we have been living in a fairyland of beauty, but we have been too blind to see, too satiated to enjoy.

Tell the audience what you're going to say, say it; then tell them what you've said.

—Dale Carnegie

The essence of all art is to have pleasure in giving pleasure.

—Dale Carnegie